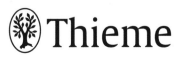

Management of Smell and Taste Disorders

A Practical Guide for Clinicians

Antje Welge-Luessen, MD
Department of Otorhinolaryngology
University Hospital Basel
Basel, Switzerland

Thomas Hummel, MD
Smell and Taste Clinic
Department of Otorhinolaryngology
Technical University of Dresden
Dresden, Germany

With contributions by

Nasreddin Abolmaali, Victor Ching, Michael Damm, Terence M. Davidson, Ron DeVere, John E. Duda, Joel Epstein, Johannes Frasnelli, Jessica Freiherr, Miriam Grushka, Antje Haehner, Josef G. Heckmann, David E. Hornung, Cornelia Hummel, Tino Just, Robert C. Kern, Tatsu Kobayakawa, David G. Laing, Basile N. Landis, Donald A. Leopold, Randy M. Leung, Michael Meredith, Takaki Miwa, Axel Muttray, Steven Nordin, Hisashi Ogawa, Carl Philpott, Nancy E. Rawson, Philippe Rombaux, Masafumi Sakagami, Benoist Schaal, Dennis Shusterman, Dana M. Small, Boris A. Stuck, Hely Tuorila, Martin Wiesmann, Martin Witt

140 illustrations

Thieme
Stuttgart · New York

Library of Congress Cataloging-in-Publication Data is available from the publisher.

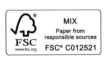

© 2014 Georg Thieme Verlag KG,
Rüdigerstrasse 14, 70469 Stuttgart, Germany
http://www.thieme.de
Thieme Medical Publishers, Inc.,
333 Seventh Avenue, New York, NY 10001, USA
http://www.thieme.com

Illustrator:
Cover design: Thieme Publishing Group
Typesetting by Prepress Projects, Perth, UK
Printed in China by Asia Pacific Offset,
Hong Kong

ISBN 978-3-13-154521-3

Also available as an e-book:
eISBN 978-3-13-164531-9

Contributors

Nasreddin Abolmaali, MD
Institute and Polyclinic for Diagnostic Radiology
Biological and Molecular Imaging, OncoRay
  – National Center for Radiation Research in
  Oncology;
Medical Faculty and University Clinics Carl Gustav
  Carus, Technical University of Dresden
Dresden, Germany

Victor Ching, BScN
Manitoulin Health Center
Little Current, Ontario, Canada

Michael Damm, MD
Department of Otorhinolaryngology, Head and
  Neck Surgery
University of Cologne Medical Center
Cologne, Germany

Terence M. Davidson, MD, FACS
Department of Otolaryngology – Head and Neck
  Surgery
UC San Diego School of Medicine
San Diego, California, USA

Ron DeVere, MD, FAAN, FAADEP
Taste and Smell Disorders Clinic
Austin, Texas, USA

John E. Duda, MD
Parkinson's Disease Research, Education and
  Clinical Center
Philadelphia Veterans Affairs Medical Center;
University of Pennsylvania School of Medicine
Philadelphia, Pennsylvania, USA

**Joel Epstein, DMD, MSD, FRCD(C), FDS,
  RCS(Edin)**
Division of Otolaryngology and Head and Neck
  Surgery
City of Hope
Duarte, California, USA

Johannes Frasnelli, MD
Centre for Research in Neuropsychology and
  Cognition
Department of Psychology
University of Montreal
Montreal, Quebec, Canada

Jessica Freiherr, PhD
RWTH Aachen University
Clinic of Diagnostic and Interventional
  Neuroradiology
Aachen, Germany

Miriam Grushka, DDS
Department of Surgery
William Osler Health Center
Toronto, Ontario, Canada

Antje Haehner MD, PhD
Department of Otorhinolaryngology
and Department of Neurology
Technical University of Dresden
Dresden, Germany

Josef G. Heckmann, MD
Department of Neurology
Municipal Hospital Landshut
Landshut, Germany

David E. Hornung, BS, MS, PhD
Biology Department
St. Lawrence University
Canton, New York, USA

Cornelia Hummel, MD
Smell and Taste Clinic
Department of Otorhinolaryngology
Technical University of Dresden
Dresden, Germany

Thomas Hummel, MD
Smell and Taste Clinic
Department of Otorhinolaryngology
Technical University of Dresden
Dresden, Germany

Tino Just, MD
Department of Otorhinolaryngology – Head and
  Neck Surgery
Rostock University Medical Center
Rostock, Germany

Robert C. Kern, MD, MS, FACS
Department of Otolaryngology – Head and Neck
  Surgery
Northwestern University Feinberg School of
  Medicine
Chicago, Illinois, USA

Tatsu Kobayakawa, PhD
Multimodal Integration Research Group
Human Technology Research Institute
National Institute of Advanced Industrial Science
  and Technology (AIST)
Tsukuba, Ibaraki, Japan

David G. Laing, PhD
School of Women's and Children's Health
University of New South Wales;
Faculty of Medicine
Sydney Children's Hospital
Randwick, New South Wales, Australia

Basile N. Landis, MD
Smell and Taste Outpatient Clinic
Department of Otorhinolaryngology – Head and
  Neck Surgery
University Hospital of Geneva
Geneva, Switzerland

Donald A. Leopold, MD
University of Vermont
Burlington, Vermont, USA

Randy M. Leung, MD, FRCSC
Department of Otolaryngology – Head and Neck
  Surgery
University of Toronto
Toronto, Ontario, Canada

Michael Meredith, PhD
Florida State University
Department of Biological Science
Tallahasse, Florida, USA

Takaki Miwa, MD, PhD
Department of Otorhinolaryngology
Kanazawa Medical University
Kahoku, Ishikawa, Japan

Axel Muttray, MD
Johannes Gutenberg University Mainz
Institute of Occupational, Social and
  Environmental Medicine
Mainz, Germany

Steven Nordin, PhD
Department of Psychology
Umeå University
Umeå, Sweden

Hisashi Ogawa, MD, DMSc
Taste Disorders Outpatient Clinic
Kumamoto Kinoh Hospital
Kumamoto, Japan

**Carl Philpott, MB ChB, FRCS (ORL-HNS), DLO,
  MD, PGCME**
Norwich Medical School
University of East Anglia
Norwich, UK;
The Smell and Taste Clinic
James Paget University Hospital NHS Foundation
  Trust
Gorleston
Norfolk, UK

Nancy E. Rawson, PhD
Monell Chemical Senses Center
Philadelphia, Pennsylvania, USA

Philippe Rombaux, MD, PhD
Catholic University of Louvain
Institute of Neurosciences
Department of Otorhinolaryngology and Head
  and Neck Surgery
University Clinic St Luc
Brussels, Belgium

Masafumi Sakagami, MD, PhD
Department of Otolaryngology
Hyogo College of Medicine
Nishinomiya City, Hyogo, Japan

Benoist Schaal, PhD
Center for Taste, Smell and Food Science
University of Burgundy
Dijon, France;
Dijon–Dresden European Laboratory for Taste and
  Smell Studies
Technical University of Dresden
Dresden, Germany

Dennis Shusterman, MD, MPH
Division of Occupational & Environmental
  Medicine
University of California
San Francisco, California, USA

Dana M. Small, PhD, MSc
Department of Psychiatry
Yale University School of Medicine
New Haven, Connecticut, USA

Boris A. Stuck, MD
Department of Otorhinolaryngology – Head and
  Neck Surgery
University Hospital Mannheim
Mannheim, Germany

Hely Tuorila, PhD
Department of Food and Environmental Sciences
University of Helsinki
Helsinki, Finland

Antje Welge-Luessen, MD
Department of Otorhinolaryngology
University Hospital Basel
Basel, Switzerland

Martin Wiesmann, MD
RWTH Aachen University
Clinic of Diagnostic and Interventional
  Neuroradiology
Aachen, Germany

Martin Witt, MD
Department of Anatomy
Rostock University Medical Center
Rostock, Germany

Preface

We are very happy to present this book focusing on the chemical senses of smell and taste, their pathophysiology, their disorders, and their treatment. The chemical senses contribute significantly to the quality of our lives: they warn us of dangers, they play a role in social communication, and they help us to enjoy foods and drinks. However, olfactory loss and its consequences appear to be underestimated by many clinicians. Just consider that approximately 5% of the general population is functionally anosmic—the highest frequency being in elderly people. In addition, research into the chemical senses is not prominent. It was not until 2004, when two North American researchers (Buck and Axel) received the Nobel Prize for their discoveries of "odorant receptors and the organization of the olfactory system," that the sense of smell received major attention. It is perhaps not surprising, then, that many patients suffering from olfactory disorders feel that clinicians often fail to provide profound advice.

This book, written by an international faculty, mainly medical doctors, is aimed at clinicians who care about patients with chemosensory problems. We hope that it will not only help to increase knowledge of these "forgotten" senses in the clinical population, but also help to improve treatment and advice for suffering patients and help to increase awareness in the general population of the significance of the chemical senses in our daily lives.

Finally, we would like to thank all our colleagues and friends who have contributed to this project, and our partners at Thieme for their help, patience, and advice!

We hope that you enjoy reading and using this book!

Antje Welge-Luessen and Thomas Hummel

Abbreviations

2D	two dimensional
3D	three dimensional
ABRS	acute bacterial rhinosinusitis
AED	antiepileptic drug
ALE	activation likelihood estimation
AOB	accessory olfactory bulb
AON	anterior olfactory nucleus
APS	anterior perforated substance
AR	allergic rhinitis
ARS	acute rhinosinusitis
ASCIC	acid-sensing ion channel
AST	alcohol sniff test
ATP	adenosine triphosphate
BNST	bed nucleus of stria terminalis
CBD	corticobasal degeneration
CISS	constructive interference in steady-state precession
CK	cytokeratin
CNG	cyclic nucleotide-gated channel
CNV	contingent negative variation
CRS	chronic rhinosinusitis
CRSsNP	chronic rhinosinusitis without nasal polyps
CRSwNP	chronic rhinosinusitis with nasal polyps
CSERP	chemosensory event-related potential
CSF	cerebrospinal fluid
CSL VII	Code of Social Law VII
CT	computed tomography
CTN	chorda tympani nerve
DaTSCAN	dopamine transporter scan
ECD	equivalent current dipole
EEG	electroencephalography
EGM	electrogustometry
EnaC	epithelial sodium channel
EPOS	European position paper on rhino-sinusitis and nasal polyps
ERP	event-related potential
ESS	endoscopic sinus surgery
FDG	[18F]-fluorodeoxyglucose
FDG-PET/CT	[18F]-fluorodeoxyglucose positron emission tomography–computed tomography
FLAIR	fluid-attenuated inversion recovery
fMRI	functional magnetic resonance imaging
FPD	filter paper disc
FPR	formyl-peptide receptors
GA	gestational age
GBC	globose basal cells
GCRP	G protein–coupled receptor protein
GERD	gastroesophageal reflux disease
GLN	lossopharyngeal nerve
GnRH	gonadotrophin releasing hormone
HLA	human lymphocyte antigens
IA	isolated anosmia
ICA	independent component analysis
ICAM	intercellular adhesion molecule
IL-8	interleukin 8
IMN	intermediate nerve of Wrisberg
IR	idiopathic rhinitis
LBD	Lewy body disease
LN	lingual branch of the trigeminal nerve
LOT	lateral olfactory tract
MEG	magnetoencephalography
MRI	magnetic resonance imaging
MRT	magnetic resonance tomography
MS	multiple sclerosis
MSA	multiple system atrophy
MSG	monosodium glutamate
MTST	match-to-sample odor identification test
N1	first major negative peak (in event-related potential testing)
NMP	negative mucosal potential
NPD	persistent nasopalatine duct
NTS	solitary tract nucleus
NV/I	branch I of the trigeminal nerve
NV/II	branch II of the trigeminal nerve
NV/III	branch III of the trigeminal nerve
OB	olfactory bulb
OE	olfactory epithelium
OERP	olfactory event-related potential
OFC	orbitofrontal cortex
OFO	orbitofrontal operculum
OMP	olfactory marker protein
OMP-ir	OMP-immunoreactive
ON	olfactory nerve
OR	olfactory receptor
ORN	olfactory receptor neuron
OS	olfactory sulcus
OSN	olfactory sensory neuron
OT	olfactory tract
P1	first positive peak (in event-related potential testing)
PEA	phenylethylalcohol
PET	positron emission tomography
PGA	primary gustatory cortex

pirC	piriform cortex	**SMT**	sniff magnitude test
PKD1L3	polycystic kidney disease protein 1L3	**SNOD**	sensorineural olfactory disorders
		T1R	taste receptor type 1
PKD2L1	polycystic kidney disease protein 2L1	**T2R**	taste receptor type 2
		TDI	Threshold, discrimination, and identification
PrCO	precentral operculum		
PROP	6-n-propylthiouracil	**TIRM**	turbo inversion recovery magnitude
PSP	progressive supranuclear palsy	**TLE**	temporal lobe epilepsy
PTA	post-traumatic anosmia	**TN**	trigeminal nerve
PTC	phenylthiocarbamide	**TRC**	taste receptor cell
RARS	recurrent acute rhinosinusitis	**TRP**	transient receptor potential
rCBF	regional cerebral blood flow	**TRPM5**	transient receptor potential protein M5
RF	receptive field		
RSV	respiratory syncytial virus	**TSE**	turbo spin echo
RTF	rhinosinusitis task force	**UPSIT**	University of Pennsylvania Smell Identification Test
RUDS	reactive upper airways dysfunction syndrome		
		URTI	upper respiratory tract infection
SA	short axon	**UTE**	ultra-short echo time
SCA	spinocerebellar ataxia	**VCD**	vocal cord dysfunction
SCC	solitary chemoreceptor cells	**VN**	vagal nerve
SCHGT	Sydney Children's Hospital gustatory test	**VND**	vomeronasal duct
		VNO	vomeronasal organ
SDOIT	San Diego odor identification test	**VNS**	vagal nerve stimulator
SGP	superficial greater petrosal nerve	**VPMpc**	parvocellular part of the ventromedial posterior nucleus
SIT	specific immunotherapy		

Table of Contents

1   Loss of Smell and Taste: Epidemiology and Impact on Quality of Life   1

Introduction 1
Epidemiology of Smell and Taste Loss 2
Age-related Loss in Smell and Taste 3
Impact of Smell and Taste Loss on Quality of Life 5
Impact of Ambient Odorants on Behavior and Health 6
Acknowledgments 7
References 7

I   Sense of Smell   9

2   Functional Anatomy of the Olfactory System I: From the Nasal Cavity to the Olfactory Bulb   10

Structural Considerations 10
Neurophysiological Considerations 17
Acknowledgments 23
References 23

3   Functional Anatomy of the Olfactory System II: Central Relays, Pathways, and their Function   27

Introduction 27
Outline of Olfactory Pathways 27
Cortical Olfactory Areas and their Function 29
Functional Characteristics of Olfactory Processing 35
References 37

4   The Human Vomeronasal System   39

The Vomeronasal Organ is Functional in Many Nonhuman Vertebrates and has Defined Components 39
Anatomy of the Vomeronasal System in Humans 39
Evidence For and Against a Functioning Human Vomeronasal Organ 42
Outlook and Practical Advice for Physicians 46
References 46

5   Smell and Taste Disorders—Diagnostic and Clinical Work-Up   49

Introduction 49
Examination of the Patient 50
Quantification of Smell Disorder 53
Additional Work-up 54
References 56

6   Assessment of Olfaction and Gustation   58

Why Assess the Chemical Senses? 58
Tests of Olfaction 59
Assessment of Taste Function 68
Investigation of the Intranasal Trigeminal System 71
Summary and Outlook 72
References 72

7 Sinonasal Olfactory Disorders 76

Introduction and Epidemiolgy 76
Acute Viral Rhinitis—Acute Bacterial
Rhinosinusitis 78
Allergic Rhinitis 81

Atrophic Rhinitis 83
Chronic Rhinosinusitis 84
Case Study 88
References 88

8 Postinfectious and Post-traumatic Olfactory Disorders 91

Etiology, Prevalence, and
Pathophysiology 91
Typical Clinical Findings 95

Treatment, Prognosis and Case Reports 97
Conclusion 102
References 102

9 Miscellaneous Causes of Olfactory Dysfunction 106

Introduction 106
Toxicants and Industrial Agents 106
Therapeutic Agents 108
Idiopathic Olfactory Disorder 108
Endocrine Disorders 109
Congenital Olfactory Disorder 109

Tumoral Causes of Olfactory Disorder 110
Complications of Surgery and Olfactory
Dysfunction 112
The Olfactory Cleft Syndrome 113
Conclusions 114
References 114

10 Chemosensory Function in Infants and Children 116

Development of Chemosensory
Functionality 116
Importance of Chemoreception in Infancy
and Childhood 118

Evaluation of Chemosensory Functions in
Newborns and Infants 119
Measurement of Chemosensory Functions
in School-age Children 120
References 124

11 Neurological Diseases and Olfactory Disorders 126

Olfactory Loss in Neurodegenerative
Disorders 126

Non-neurodegenerative Disorders 134
References 135

12 Clinical Disorders of the Trigeminal System 138

Introduction 138
Functional Neuroanatomy of the
Trigeminal System 138
Responsiveness to Physical and Chemical
Stimuli 141

Clinical Disorders of the Trigeminal
System 144
Conclusion 146
Acknowledgments 146
References 146

II Sense of Taste   149

13 Functional Anatomy of the Gustatory System: From the Taste Papilla to the Gustatory Cortex   150

General Aspects of Taste Sensation 150
Taste Reception 150
Peripheral Taste Nerves 153
Central Pathways: Taste Relay Nucleus and Related Structures 155
Gustatory Cortices in Subhuman Primates 158
Gustatory Cortices in Humans 161
References 165

14 Taste Testing   168

General Remarks on Gustatory Testing 168
Patient History 168
Psychophysical Taste Testing 169
Objective Measurements 173
Case Reports 174
References 176

15 Taste Disorders   179

Introduction 179
Typical Clinical Findings 179
Classification of Taste Disorders 180
Pathophysiology 182
Etiology of Taste Disorders 182
Diagnosis 185
Therapy of Taste Disorders 185
Acknowledgments 186
References 186

16 Burning Mouth Syndrome and Qualitative Taste and Smell Disorders   189

Burning Mouth Syndrome 189
Qualitative Taste Disorder: Dysgeusia 191
Qualitative Smell Disorder: Parosmia and Phantosmia 192
References 193

17 Structural Imaging in Chemosensory Dysfunction   195

Imaging Technique 195
Olfactory Imaging 199
Trigeminal Imaging 202
Gustatory Imaging 204
Conclusion 205
Acknowledgments 205
References 205

18 Providing Expert Opinion on Olfactory and Gustatory Disorders   207

Introduction 207
Providing Expert Opinion 207
Expert Opinion in Olfactory Disorders 208
Expert Opinion in Gustatory Disorders 214
Case Studies 216
References 217

19 Flavor: Interaction Between the Chemical Senses   219

Introduction 219
Flavor Perception 219
Conclusions 226
References 226

1 Loss of Smell and Taste: Epidemiology and Impact on Quality of Life

Steven Nordin, Hely Tuorila

Introduction

From an evolutionary perspective, the chemical senses are the oldest of our senses, and therefore differ considerably with regards to role and function from the younger senses, such as vision and hearing. The life-preserving role of the chemical senses requires smell and taste loss to be taken seriously by the clinician.

The most important role of the human sense of smell is to guide our attention toward hazards (e.g., poisonous fumes and spoiled food) and toward items that in a general sense have positive connotations (e.g., nutritious food). This guidance is primarily driven by the hedonic value (i.e., pleasantness or unpleasantness of an odorous item [e.g., food]), which, to a large extent, is determined by the individual's personal history with that item. The relatively strong positive or negative emotions often evoked by smells are also shaped by prior experience, and believed to enhance the appropriate behavioral response. Apart from being an important chemical warning system for safety issues and for regulating food intake, the sense of smell is involved in social communication.[1] An infinite number of volatile chemical compounds can evoke a smell sensation, and a smell is, in many cases, an integrated sensation caused by a combination of such compounds.

The sense of taste functions as a gatekeeper of the internal milieu, acting to guide ingestive and avoidance behaviors.[2] As with smell, hedonic value is an important perceptual dimension of taste, with close ties to motivational behavior. Taste qualities provide information about the presence of useful substances or dangers: carbohydrate energy sources in sweetness, sodium in saltiness, and proteins in umami ("meaty," "brothy") perception; and possible danger from acids and toxins in sour and bitter perceptions, respectively.

The most common cause of a loss in smell or taste is aging, a natural condition applying to an increasing number of people in the developed world. Typically, *age-associated* loss in the chemical senses appears progressively after the age of 60 years, and shows large individual variation, greatly afflicting some and leaving others intact. *Pathological losses* in smell and taste are caused by disease, trauma, working conditions, and lifestyle, and can appear either abruptly or progressively. *Congenital losses* in smell and taste are rare.

A complete smell or taste loss is called *anosmia* or *ageusia*, respectively, whereas diminished smell and taste sensitivity is called *hyposmia* and *hypogeusia*, respectively. The terms functional anosmia and functional ageusia are commonly used in clinical work, referring to some sensations being evoked, but not sufficiently for smell and taste to be useful in daily life (see also Chapter 5 Diagnostic and Clinical Work-Up). The smell loss can be temporary (e.g., during viral disease), causing some discomfort or loss of appetite, but with no major disturbance. In contrast, long-term or permanent smell or taste loss is a clinically challenging condition.

Persons may also seek medical attention for hypersensitivity to ambient odorants, with a symptom profile that can vary considerably between individuals. Those who consider themselves to be sensitive to odors report higher annoyance from odors than those who perceive themselves to be less sensitive.[3] However, this hypersensitivity appears to be predominantly cognitive in origin, as persons with these complaints typically have normal smell detection sensitivity. It has been documented that practitioners request more knowledge and clinical guidelines for the management of this groups of patients.[4]

The objective of this chapter is to provide a review of what we know today about the epidemiology of loss in smell and taste, and its impact on quality of life (QoL). As aging accounts for much of these sensory losses, and as ear, nose, and throat (ENT) and related clinicians also meet patients with hypersensitivity to ambient odorants, these issues will also be reviewed briefly.

Epidemiology of Smell and Taste Loss

Smell Loss

The olfactory epithelium is directly exposed to potentially neurotoxic compounds in surrounding air, making this sensory system vulnerable to pathology. Furthermore, the system depends on only one cranial nerve to mediate information from the epithelium to the brain.

Smell loss is a common condition. Large-scale population-based studies with clinical examination show a prevalence of smell loss of 19% in Swedish adults (≥ 20 years),[5] 22% in German adults (25 to 75 years),[6] and 24% in US adults (≥ 53 years).[7] These prevalence rates per se may lead one astray if not specified by age factor. The typical increase in prevalence with aging, and the slightly higher prevalence in men than in women is illustrated in **Fig. 1.1**. The prevalence of smell loss in the general adult population, when based on self-reports, has been reported to vary between 9.5 and 15.3%.[7,8] Although self-reports of smell loss underestimate prevalence rates obtained by smell testing,[7,9] it can be assumed that it is predominantly the individual's self-evaluation of his or her sense of smell that will determine whether he or she will seek medical attention. The under-reporting of smell loss is likely to be related to unawareness of smell loss, which is common in old age.

Regarding clinical populations, a review[10] of studies focusing on consecutive cases at smell and taste clinics in the United States, Europe and Japan suggests that the most common etiologies of smell loss are postviral upper respiratory tract infection (URTI) (18 to 45% of the clinical population) and nasal or sinus disease (7 to 56%), followed by head trauma (8 to 20%), exposure to toxins or drugs (2 to 6%), and congenital loss (0 to 4%). Another study of ENT patients in Germany, Austria and Switzerland shows similar results.[11] Conversely, the percentage of patients with these conditions who have clinically proven smell loss is rather high: 76 to 95% in postviral URTI, 72 to 98% in nasal/sinus disease, 86 to 94% in head trauma, 67% in exposure to toxins/drugs, and 100% in congenital cases.[10] Loss due to postviral URTI, head trauma, and exposure to toxins or drugs are, in some cases, spontaneously reversible, whereas many cases of nasal or sinus disease can be treated with medication or with a combination of medical and surgical treatment.

Certain volatile compounds are perceived by some individuals, but not by others. An example of such a compound is androstenone, a hormone-based substance to which 20 to 40% of the population are anosmic.[12] Such *specific anosmia* emphasizes the individuality of the perceptual world, but this type of loss is not likely to have a major consequence for QoL.

Taste Loss

Taste sensitivity is for several reasons robust compared with smell sensitivity. Not only are there three types of papilla and three cranial nerves on each side involved in mediating taste, but there is also so-called taste constancy that contributes to the robustness. This constancy is believed to be based on inhibitory feedback loops among the cranial nerves, so that damage to one taste nerve releases inhibition on others, resulting in intensification of sensations from other regions of the oral cavity. Despite this robustness, taste loss can result from damage to any location of the neural gustatory pathway, from the taste buds via the peripheral (facial, glossopharyngeal, and vagal nerve) and central nervous system (brainstem and thalamus) to the cerebral cortex.[13]

The inability to taste the bitter compounds phenylthiocarbamide and n-propylthiouracil is genetically determined and extensively studied,[14] but, in general, there is a lack of population-based studies on taste loss with clinical examination. However, in a German population aged 25 to 75 years, 20% recognized three or fewer of the four tastants (sucrose, sodium chloride, citric acid, and quinine hydrochloride) when presented at supra-threshold concentrations.[6] In contrast, only 0.14% of the US adult population indicated a loss in taste function.[15] The large discrepancy in prevalence between these two studies (20 vs. 0.14%) may be attributable to a rather loose criterion for taste loss in the former study, and perhaps to unawareness of loss in the latter. A recent, large study examining over 700 individuals in Switzerland using psychophysical testing with two types of stimulus administration (taste spray and taste strips) revealed a 5% prevalence of taste disorder. However, none of the participants showed complete ageusia.[16] Naming a taste, even in a cued task (multiple choice options provided), easily leads to confusion either between sour and bitter in both adults and children[17,18] or between sour, bitter, and salty,[16] because persons seldom receive training in chemosensory tasks. In any case, it is apparent that further epidemiological studies of taste loss and its consequences in the general population are needed.

Taste and chemesthetic perception, together with retronasal odor perception, constitute what we call the flavor of food. Owing to this integrated perception whereby retronasal odors are localized in the oral cavity, a considerable proportion of patients at ENT clinics who seek medical attention for taste loss do instead show smell loss. This is illustrated by data from the University of Pennsylvania Smell and Taste Center, showing that 66% of the patients complained of taste loss, but only 5% of these had a measured taste loss. The most common etiology was head trauma (30%), followed by postviral URTI, toxic exposure, medication induced, and idiopathic (13% for each etiology).[19] The literature suggests a very large variability in the proportion of patients with measured taste loss (between 1 and 30%),[19-22] probably because of the lack of consensus on appropriate clinical measures. Sparse documentation of recovery from taste loss indicates complete or incomplete recovery in 5 out of 10 cases.[22]

Summary

Smell loss is common in the general adult population (19 to 24%), but with a rather low self-awareness. Importantly, both prevalence and awareness are associated with increasing age. Common etiologies of smell loss among patients at smell and taste clinics include postviral URTI, nasal/sinus disease, and head trauma. A combination of too few population-based studies and large differences in the criteria used to diagnose taste loss makes it difficult to provide a good estimate of the prevalence of taste loss in the general population, although it has been reported at 5% in a non population-based study.[16] Common etiologies of taste loss among patients at smell and taste clinics are head trauma, postviral URTI, toxic exposure, and use of medication.

Age-related Loss in Smell and Taste

Smell Loss

Apart from gross anatomical changes in the nasal cavity, aging is typically accompanied by structural neurological abnormalities in the olfactory epithelium, olfactory bulb, and central olfactory cortices.[23] As a result, a vast number of studies have demonstrated age-related decline in detection sensitivity, intensity and quality discrimination, identification, and perceived intensity.[24] Data shown in **Fig. 1.1** indicate only a slight increase in prevalence of smell loss from the 20-to-29-year strata (9% across gender) to the 50-to-59-year strata (14%), but a rapid increase above that age (80+ year strata, 83%).[5] In another such study, the prevalence increased from 8% at 25 to 34 years to 33% at 65 to 74 years.[6] In yet another study, the prevalence of smell loss increased from 6% at 53 to 59 years to 62% at 80+ years.[7] The impact of age on smell function has further been shown by a large-scale population-based study in which performance on a relatively difficult task of odor identification fell from ~64% correct identifications for the age strata 45 to 50 years to 43% for the 85-to-90-year strata.[25] The strong influence of aging on smell sensitivity has also been demonstrated among patients at ENT clinics.[26,27]

There is a clear trend of increasing heterogeneity of the population in the course of aging, as illustrated in **Fig. 1.2**.[28] The figure shows that some elderly people perform just as well as the best-performing young adults. Why do some elderly people perform well whereas others do not? Mackay-Sim and associates[29] studied healthy, nonmedicated nonsmokers with no history of nasal problems, as well as participants who were medicated, smokers, or had a history of nasal problems. Based on a composite score of detection, discrimination, and identification, they found that the age-related decline in smell function was considerably less in the nonmedicated and nonsmoking participants with no history of nasal problems. Taking this reasoning a step further, a recent study compared odor-detection sensitivity between elderly people (77 to 87 years), considered to be "successfully aged" in terms of medical health and cognitive ability, and young adults (20 to 24 years).[30] The two age groups had very similar

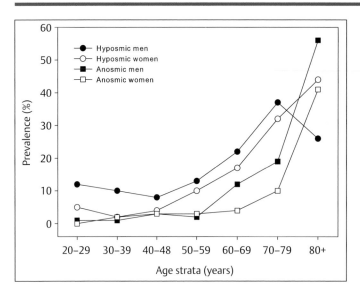

Fig. 1.1 Prevalence of hyposmia and anosmia in men (*n* = 668) and women (*n* = 719) across age strata assessed with the Scandinavian Odor Identification Test. (Adapted from Brämerson et al.[5])

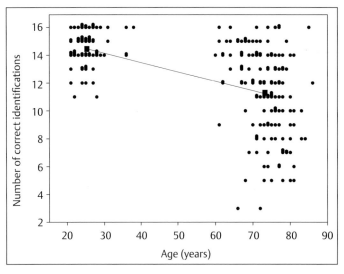

Fig. 1.2 Distribution of number of correct odor identifications on the Scandinavian Odor Identification Test (max = 16) in young (*n* = 72) and elderly (*n* = 147) adults. Mean numbers of correct odor identifications for the two age groups are shown. (Adapted from Mustonen et al.[28])

detection thresholds and psychometric detection functions (**Fig. 1.3**), implying that deficits in smell sensitivity in the course of aging may not be inevitable, and that factors secondary to aging, such as poor medical health status and cognitive decline, may contribute to deficits in odor detectability in normal aging.

Taste Loss

Age-related taste loss is less prominent than age-related smell loss, presumably because of the robustness of this sensory system described on pp. 168–178. Nevertheless, poor detection sensitivity, intensity and quality discrimination, and identification of tastes have been documented, as well as attenuated perceived intensity. Importantly, there seem to be quality-specific age-related changes in taste perception. Although the results are not fully consistent across studies, bitter sensitivity seems to be most affected by age and sweet sensitivity least affected, whereas salty and sour sensitivities fall in between.[24,31] The prevalence of self-reported taste problems has been reported to increase gradually across age groups from 0.3% at 18 to 24 years to 3.8% at 85+ years.[15] However, these prevalence rates include unspecified taste problems other than taste loss.

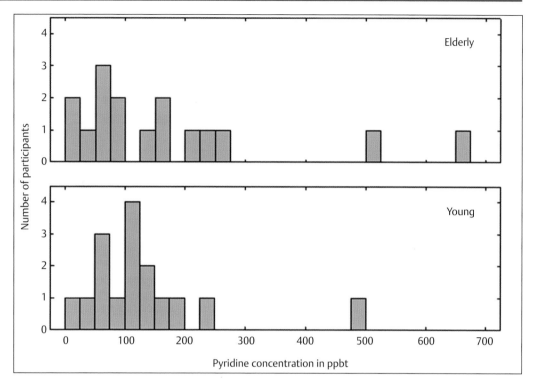

Fig. 1.3 Frequency distributions of individual odor detection thresholds for pyridine for "successfully aged" elderly (mean = 105 ppb; *n* = 16) and young adults (mean = 100 ppb; *n* = 16). (Reproduced with kind permission of Springer Science from Nordins, Almkvist O, Berglund B. Is loss in odor sensitivity inevitable to the aging individual? A study of "successfully-aged" elderly. Chemosens Percept 2012;5:188–196.)

Summary

Age-related anatomical and neurological changes in the nasal cavity and olfactory nervous system result in the decline of various smell functions in normal aging. However, smell loss may not be inevitable in aging individuals. Age-related taste loss is less prominent than age-related smell loss, probably because of the general robustness of the taste system. There does seem to be a quality-specific age-related loss in taste perception.

Impact of Smell and Taste Loss on Quality of Life

Smell Loss

Olfaction is important as a chemical warning system with emotional impact, in the regulation of food intake, and in interpersonal relations, and studies of patients with smell loss show conse-

quences for all these aspects of life.[32,33] Clinical investigations have demonstrated poor general QoL, depression and mood changes, feelings of vulnerability, and difficulties in daily life. Vulnerability is related to worries and actual experience of safety issues (e.g., fire and gas leaks), as well as worries of poor personal hygiene. A negative consequence of smell loss from a nutritional perspective is its impact on food intake: loss of appetite, changed food preferences, change in body weight, cooking difficulties, and poor detection of spoiled food are frequent complaints of these patients. Change in body weight may be either loss or gain, the gain presumably due to compensation for diminished flavor by means of larger food intake. A more detailed description of the influence of smell loss on dietary behavior has been provided by Aschenbrenner and associates.[34] Smell loss has also been associated with decreased social interaction with friends and colleagues, and decreased intimacy with a partner. It has been suggested that olfactory loss may not have a direct impact on sexual appetite, but that depression caused by olfactory loss causes a decrease in sexual appetite.[35] A limitation in these studies of QoL is that they have investigated heterogeneous groups with respect to either the type of smell disorder (sensitivity loss, smell distortion, or phantom smell) or the primary etiology underlying the disorder, making it difficult to conclude to what extent the impact on QoL can be referred to a specific type of disorder or etiology. However, a recent study[36] shows a very similar impact on QoL in a patient group with smell disorder (smell loss only) and etiology (nasal polyposis) to that of an earlier studied heterogeneous group.

Taste Loss

Taste is the core sensory property of foods, a fact underscored in Western cultures by a division of foods into "sweet" versus "salty" (or "savory") categories. Almost all foods and beverages have either a sweet or a salty taste, and, depending on the food, these are accompanied by sour, bitter, or umami tastes. With eating and food being a prominent source of enjoyment, decreased sensitivity to tastes could potentially change the perceived quality and pleasure derived from food. Clinically diagnosed ageusia or hypogeusia lead to decreased appetite and food enjoyment,[37] but they are rare in the general population. Research addressing the relationship between taste sensitivity (determined by threshold concentrations or suprathreshold intensity perception of taste compounds) and pleasantness of foods has mainly involved unselected populations with individual variations in perception, or elderly populations. In general, no particular relationship between lower-than-average sensitivity and preference for a taste has been demonstrated. Thus, for example, optimal perceived saltiness does not vary with individual detection thresholds for sodium chloride. It seems that culturally learned preferences override individual variations in taste perception.

Consistent with this, elderly people whose perception of tastes has been impaired do not show altered preferences for taste intensities.[38,39] A long history of repeated exposure to culturally typical foods supports the adjustment to progressively fading taste perceptions. Current knowledge does not support the notion that impairment of taste would be a primary cause of loss of appetite or body weight changes in the elderly population.

Summary

Smell loss may have adverse effects on general QoL and can lead to depression, feelings of vulnerability, practical issues in daily life, altered food intake, reduced social interaction, and decreased intimacy with a partner. Although taste loss may contribute to decreased appetite and food enjoyment, it may only be a partial explanation for loss of appetite or body weight changes in elderly people.

Impact of Ambient Odorants on Behavior and Health

A smell elicits psychological and physiological responses to guide the individual toward appropriate behavior. Whether the response will be positive or negative in character depends predominantly on the hedonics of the smell. An odorous compound will not have a direct impact on behavior or health. Instead, the positive or negative hedonic evaluation of the compound will moderate emotions evoked from this evaluation and will have positive or negative consequences on mood, behavior, and health (e.g., calm state, good cognitive performance and no symptoms versus anxiety, poor cognitive performance and headache). An example of a powerful negative impact of odors on QoL is industrial wastewater management or animal production facilities emitting strong smells in surrounding residential areas (for a review, see ref. 40).

The negative impact of smells on behavior and health has vast public health consequences. About one-third of the general population report annoyance and symptoms from strong smells; in about one-fifth of the population, everyday smells have strong affective and behavioral consequences; and about 1 in 20 meet criteria for a clinical diagnosis of hypersensitivity to smells.[41,42] Symptoms may vary considerably among afflicted individuals, but airway (e.g., cough and nasal congestion) and general symptoms (e.g., headache and nausea) seem to dominate.[43] Results from a controlled experimental study suggest that mold smell per se may act as a warning signal and significantly strengthen symptoms, and thus contribute to building-related illness.[44]

Acknowledgments

This work was supported by grants to Steven Nordin from the European territorial cooperation program Botnia-Atlantica, Region Västerbotten (Sweden), and the Regional Council of Ostrobothnia (Finland).

References

1. Stevenson RJ. An initial evaluation of the functions of human olfaction. Chem Senses 2010;35(1):3–20
2. Smith DV, Scott TR. Gustatory neural coding. In: Doty RL, ed. Handbook of Olfaction and Gustation. New York, NY: Marcel Dekker; 2003:731–758.
3. Knaapila A, Tuorila H, Kyvik KO, et al. Self-ratings of olfactory function reflect odor annoyance rather than olfactory acuity. Laryngoscope 2008;118(12): 2212–2217
4. Skovbjerg S, Johansen JD, Rasmussen A, Thorsen H, Elberling J. General practitioners' experiences with provision of healthcare to patients with self-reported multiple chemical sensitivity. Scand J Prim Health Care 2009;27(3):148–152
5. Brämerson A, Johansson L, Ek L, Nordin S, Bende M. Prevalence of olfactory dysfunction: the Skövde population-based study. Laryngoscope 2004;114(4): 733–737
6. Vennemann MM, Hummel T, Berger K. The association between smoking and smell and taste impairment in the general population. J Neurol 2008;255(8):1121–1126
7. Murphy C, Schubert CR, Cruickshanks KJ, Klein BE, Klein R, Nondahl DM. Prevalence of olfactory impairment in older adults. JAMA 2002;288(18): 2307–2312
8. Nordin S, Brämerson A, Bende M. Prevalence of self-reported poor odor detection sensitivity: the Skövde population-based study. Acta Otolaryngol 2004; 124(10):1171–1173
9. Shu CH, Hummel T, Lee PL, Chiu CH, Lin SH, Yuan BC. The proportion of self-rated olfactory dysfunction does not change across the life span. Am J Rhinol Allergy 2009;23(4):413–416
10. Nordin S, Brämerson A. Complaints of olfactory disorders: epidemiology, assessment and clinical implications. Curr Opin Allergy Clin Immunol 2008; 8(1):10–15
11. Damm M, Temmel A, Welge-Lüssen A, et al. Olfactory dysfunctions. Epidemiology and therapy in Germany, Austria and Switzerland. [Article in German] HNO 2004;52(2):112–120
12. Bremner EA, Mainland JD, Khan RM, Sobel N. The prevalence of androstenone anosmia. Chem Senses 2003;28(5):423–432
13. Heckmann JG, Lang CJ. Neurological causes of taste disorders. Adv Otorhinolaryngol 2006;63:255–264
14. Tepper BJ. Nutritional implications of genetic taste variation: the role of PROP sensitivity and other taste phenotypes. Annu Rev Nutr 2008;28:367–388
15. Hoffman HJ, Cruickshanks KJ, Davis B. Perspectives on population-based epidemiological studies of olfactory and taste impairment. Ann N Y Acad Sci 2009;1170:514–530
16. Welge-Lüssen A, Dörig P, Wolfensberger M, Krone F, Hummel T. A study about the frequency of taste disorders. J Neurol 2011;258(3):386–392
17. O'Mahony M, Goldenberg M, Stedmon J, Alford J. Confusion in the use of taste adjectives 'sour' and 'bitter'. Chem Senses 1979;4:301–318
18. Oerlemans P, Mustonen S, Esselström H, Tuorila H. Sensory and food related perceptions of 8-, 9-, 10- and 11-year-old school children: baseline measurements. EKT series 1362. Department of Food Technology, University of Helsinki; 2006.
19. Deems DA, Doty RL, Settle RG, et al. Smell and taste disorders, a study of 750 patients from the University of Pennsylvania Smell and Taste Center. Arch Otolaryngol Head Neck Surg 1991;117(5):519–528
20. Goodspeed RB, Gent JF, Catalanotto FA. Chemosensory dysfunction. Clinical evaluation results from a taste and smell clinic. Postgrad Med 1987; 81(1):251–257, 260
21. Cowart BJ, Young IM, Feldman RS, Lowry LD. Clinical disorders of smell and taste. Occup Med 1997;12(3):465–483
22. Pribitkin E, Rosenthal MD, Cowart BJ. Prevalence and causes of severe taste loss in a chemosensory clinic population. Ann Otol Rhinol Laryngol 2003; 112(11):971–978
23. Kovács T. Mechanisms of olfactory dysfunction in aging and neurodegenerative disorders. Ageing Res Rev 2004;3(2):215–232
24. Nordin S. Sensory perception of food and ageing. In: Raats MM, van Staveren W, de Groot L, eds. Food for the Ageing Population. Cambridge: Woodhead Publishing; 2009:73–94.
25. Larsson M, Nilsson L-G, Olofsson JK, Nordin S. Demographic and cognitive predictors of cued odor identification: evidence from a population-based study. Chem Senses 2004;29(6):547–554
26. Harris R, Davidson TM, Murphy C, Gilbert PE, Chen M. Clinical evaluation and symptoms of chemosensory impairment: one thousand consecutive cases from the Nasal Dysfunction Clinic in San Diego. Am J Rhinol 2006;20(1):101–108
27. Hummel T, Kobal G, Gudziol H, Mackay-Sim A. Normative data for the "Sniffin' Sticks" including tests of odor identification, odor discrimination, and olfactory thresholds: an upgrade based on a group of more than 3,000 subjects. Eur Arch Otorhinolaryngol 2007;264(3):237–243
28. Mustonen S, Vento S, Tuorila H. Hajuaistin toiminnan mittaaminen. [Measurement of olfactory function, abstract in English] Finn Med J 2007; 62:3177–3183
29. Mackay-Sim A, Johnston AN, Owen C, Burne TH. Olfactory ability in the healthy population: reassessing presbyosmia. Chem Senses 2006;31(8): 763–771
30. Nordin S, Almkvist O, Berglund B. Is loss in odor sensitivity inevitable to the aging individual? A study of "successfully-aged" elderly. Chemosens Percept 2012;5:188–196

31. Koskinen S, Kälviäinen N, Tuorila H. Perception of chemosensory stimuli and related responses to flavored yoghurts in the young and elderly. Food Qual Prefer 2003;14:623–635

32. Hummel T, Nordin S. Olfactory disorders and their consequences for quality of life. Acta Otolaryngol 2005;125(2):116–121

33. Smeets MAM, Veldhuizen MG, Galle S, et al. Sense of smell disorder and health-related quality of life. Rehabil Psychol 2009;54(4):404–412

34. Aschenbrenner K, Hummel C, Teszmer K, et al. The influence of olfactory loss on dietary behaviors. Laryngoscope 2008;118(1):135–144

35. Gudziol V, Wolff-Stephan S, Aschenbrenner K, Joraschky P, Hummel T. Depression resulting from olfactory dysfunction is associated with reduced sexual appetite—a cross-sectional cohort study. J Sex Med 2009;6(7):1924–1929

36. Nordin S, Blomqvist EH, Olsson P, Stjärne P, Ehnhage A; NAF2S2 Study Group. Effects of smell loss on daily life and adopted coping strategies in patients with nasal polyposis with asthma. Acta Otolaryngol 2011;131(8):826–832

37. Mattes RD. Nutritional implications of taste and smell. In: Doty RL, ed. Handbook of Olfaction and Gustation. New York, NY: Marcel Dekker; 2003: 881–903.

38. Koskinen S, Nenonen A, Tuorila H. Intakes of cold cuts in the elderly are predicted by olfaction and mood, but not by flavor type or intensity of the products. Physiol Behav 2005;85(3):314–323

39. Kremer S, Bult JH, Mojet J, Kroeze JH. Compensation for age-associated chemosensory losses and its effect on the pleasantness of a custard dessert and a tomato drink. Appetite 2007;48(1):96–103

40. Schiffman SS, Williams CM. Science of odor as a potential health issue. J Environ Qual 2005;34(1): 129–138

41. Johansson Å, Brämerson A, Millqvist E, Nordin S, Bende M. Prevalence and risk factors for self-reported odour intolerance: the Skövde population-based study. Int Arch Occup Environ Health 2005;78(7):559–564

42. Johansson Å, Millqvist E, Nordin S, Bende M. Relationship between self-reported odor intolerance and sensitivity to inhaled capsaicin: proposed definition of airway sensory hyperreactivity and estimation of its prevalence. Chest 2006;129(6): 1623–1628

43. Andersson MJ, Andersson L, Bende M, Millqvist E, Nordin S. The idiopathic environmental intolerance symptom inventory: development, evaluation, and application. J Occup Environ Med 2009; 51(7):838–847

44. Claeson A-S, Nordin S, Sunesson A-L. Effects on perceived air quality and symptoms of exposure to microbially produced metabolites and compounds emitted from damp building materials. Indoor Air 2009;19(2):102–112

I Sense of Smell

2   Functional Anatomy of the Olfactory System I:
    From the Nasal Cavity to the Olfactory Bulb   10

3   Functional Anatomy of the Olfactory System II:
    Central Relays, Pathways, and their Function   27

4   The Human Vomeronasal System   39

5   Smell and Taste Disorders—Diagnostic and Clinical Work-Up   49

6   Assessment of Olfaction and Gustation   58

7   Sinonasal Olfactory Disorders   76

8   Postinfectious and Post-traumatic Olfactory Disorders   91

9   Miscellaneous Causes of Olfactory Dysfunction   106

10 Chemosensory Function in Infants and Children   116

11 Neurological Diseases and Olfactory Disorders   126

12 Clinical Disorders of the Trigeminal System   138

2 Functional Anatomy of the Olfactory System I: From the Nasal Cavity to the Olfactory Bulb

Structural Considerations

David E. Hornung

The nasal air passageways are delineated in the anterior plane by the nasal valve, in the lateral plane by the superior, middle, and inferior conchae (turbinates), and in the medial plane by the nasal septum. As seen in **Figs. 2.1 and 2.2**, these structures define the organizational borders for the nasal air passages, which provide the conduit through which air and odorant molecules are delivered to the airspace above the olfactory receptors.[1]

The olfactory receptors are located high in the nose along the septum and on the superior concha. Because of their location, and because the airspaces defined by the middle and inferior conchae are much larger than those leading up to the olfactory receptor region, during a sniff only ~10% of the inspired air is directed toward the airspace in contact with the olfactory receptors.[2,3]

The septum and conchae produce multiple and convoluted (sometimes turbulent) flow paths for the inspired air (**Fig. 2.3**). By affecting the rate at which odorant molecules are delivered to the olfactory receptor sheet, the structure of the nose itself may be one of the mechanisms involved with odor detection and discrimination. In addition, some investigators have suggested that the relatively low air volume, coupled with the convoluted air flow path leading to the receptors, may help protect the olfactory processing system from particulate pollutants.[4]

> The nasal air passageways, which can have a dramatic effect on olfactory ability, are delineated by the superior, middle, and inferior turbinates. Alterations in these nasal air passageways often have an effect on odorant perception.

Nasal Air Conditioning, Conduction Problems and the Nasal Cycle

The nose serves important functions beyond odorant identification. These nonolfactory nasal functions together will be referred to as "nasal air conditioning." During the process of air conditioning, the inspired air is brought to the temperature and humidity of the lungs. In addition, a filtration process occurs in which particles in the inspired air, ranging from combustion products to airborne bacteria, are trapped in the mucus and removed. Some aspects of nasal air conditioning are briefly discussed below because these nonolfactory physiological processes can have a profound effect on the ability to detect odorants.[5]

> The major function of the nose is to provide the lower airways with clean, humidified, and warm air.

The epithelial cells lining the structures of the internal nose have a very rich blood supply and are covered by watery mucus that is continually flowing into the back of the throat. By regulating the amount of blood in the dense capillary beds servicing the structures of the internal nose, the size of the airspace defined by these organizational structures can be changed quickly and dramatically. Because of the speed and the amount of change that can occur around the inferior concha, these areas of the nose are called "swell spaces."[1]

If olfactory complaints are due to the problem of odorant molecules not getting to the head space above the olfactory receptors (a conduction problem), breathing warm, humidified air can sometimes temporarily restore some lost olfactory ability by increasing the size of the nasal air passageways. Given the impact the swell spaces can have on nasal patency, questions about how olfactory ability changes as the ambient temperature or humidity change should be included as part of a routine history for patients with olfactory complaints.

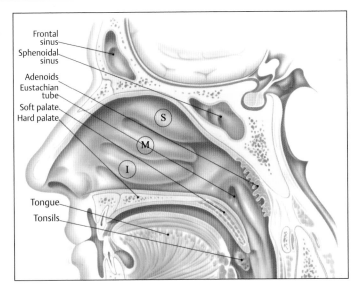

Fig. 2.1 A cross-sectional view of the human head. The inferior (I), middle (M), and superior (S) conchae are located above the hard palate. The location of the olfactory receptor cell area is around the superior turbinate. (Modified from Hornung 2006.[1])

Frontal sinus
Sphenoidal sinus
Adenoids
Eustachian tube
Soft palate
Hard palate
Tongue
Tonsils
S
M
I

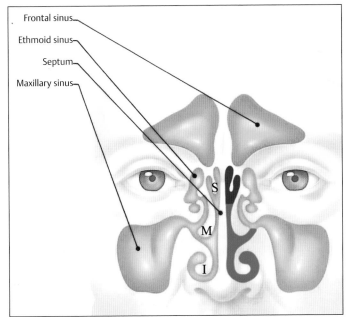

Fig. 2.2 A cross-sectional view of the airspaces on the human nose. The airspace for the left nostril (the right-hand side of the drawing) is filled in. The blue color indicates the airspace adjacent to the olfactory receptor region and the rest of the airspace is delineated by the green. S, superior concha; M, middle concha; I, inferior concha. (Modified from Hornung 2006.[1])

Frontal sinus
Ethmoid sinus
Septum
Maxillary sinus
S
M
I

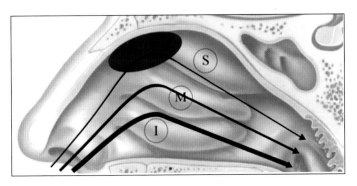

Fig. 2.3 Cartoon showing the general direction of nasal airflow in the airspaces defined by the inferior (I), middle (M), and superior (S) turbinates. The thicker the line, the larger the percentage of airflow that moves along that particular flow path. The olfactory receptor is the shaded area located around the anterior portion of the superior turbinate.

S
M
I

Conduction problems can happen as a result of structural blockages or as a result of temporary changes in the nasal air passageways due to conditions such as allergic rhinitis.[6] Structural blockages can occur as a result of conditions such as polyposis or as a result of an alteration in the nasal passageways, such as a severely deviated nasal system or facial trauma. With conduction problems, restoring the patency of the nasal passageways often restores olfactory function.[1]

> Inflammatory processes may produce conduction problems. However, inflammatory processes may also produce olfactory loss in the presence of open nasal passages.

When the cause of a complaint is an access problem, olfactory ability can sometimes be restored even after a considerable period of time. For example, when, after many years, patients who had under gone laryngectomy were able to move air through their noses by connecting a tube from the stoma to the mouth, olfactory ability was restored to normal levels for most patients.[7]

As a word of caution, in rats with conduction problems like those accompanying allergic rhinitis, an increase in the size and number of Bowman glands and the infiltration of several kinds of white blood cell have been observed in addition to the blocked nasal passages. If observations from ani-mal models can be applied to humans, restoring nasal airflow may not immediately resolve the olfactory complaint as the increase in gland activity could contribute to olfactory problems.[8]

The degree of openness of the nasal cavity at some level contributes to the feeling of "comfortable breathing." In addition, the stimulation of cold receptors and other trigeminal receptors and the presence of a dry mucosa can all contribute to the sensation of stuffiness. Total nasal resistance may also contribute, although there are some data to support the hypothesis that the obstruction on the more open side of the nose is primarily responsible for the presence or absence of nasal complaints.[9,10]

To add to the complexity of the relationship between nasal anatomy and olfactory ability, a pattern has been observed in most human noses in which congestion on one side of the nose is accompanied by decongestion on the other (**Fig. 2.4**). This pattern is called the nasal cycle. The periodicity of the cycle is between 50 minutes and 7 hours. There has even been a correlation reported between handedness and the nostril which is open for a larger percent of a 24-hour period, such that left-handed individuals are more likely to have a more open left nostril and vice versa for right handers. The relationship among single-nostril olfactory ability, binasal olfactory ability, and the nasal cycle has not yet been well described.[11]

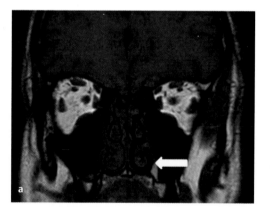 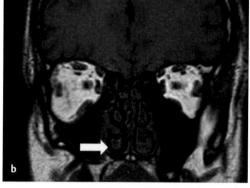

Fig. 2.4 Magnetic resonance images showing the effect of the nasal cycle on nasal patency.

a The white arrow is pointing to the airspace in the left nostril defined by the inferior turbinate.

b The nasal cavity of the same patient 75 minutes later. The white arrow is pointing to the airspace in the right nostril defined by the inferior turbinate. In 75 minutes the dominant nostril has changed from the left nostril to the right nostril.

Humidification and the Partitioning of Odorant Molecules in the Nasal Mucus

The humidification of incoming air is possible as the respiratory and olfactory mucus layers are mostly composed of water. Thus, when the inspired air is dry, water evaporates from the mucus into the inspired air. The watery mucus can also sorb odorants as they make their way through the nose toward the olfactory receptors. As described in detail below, this sorption is especially noteworthy for water-soluble odorants and it can significantly reduce the number of odorant molecules delivered to the headspace adjacent to the olfactory receptors.[12]

Using a combination of experimental and modeling techniques, odorant solubility in human nasal and olfactory mucosa has been determined for some odorants. Mucosal odorant solubility is odorant specific and usually follows the trend that odorants with lower water solubility are more soluble in the mucosa than would be predicted from their water solubility alone. Additionally there is a odorant-independent increase in the effective diffusive resistance of the olfactory mucosa compared with that of water alone.[13]

In addition to supplying water for humidification purposes, the nasal mucus serves as a trap for particulate matter, including smoke and dust particles, and even airborne bacteria. The respiratory and olfactory cells lining the nasal passageways contain cilia, which beat in a slow wavelike action and so move the mucus through the nose to the back of the throat. The flow of mucus toward the back of the throat is one of the mechanisms by which water-soluble odorant molecules sorbed to the mucus bathing the olfactory receptors are cleared. Molecules sorbed in the mucus can also be cleared from the olfactory mucosa through odorant uptake by the circulatory system.[1]

Ciliopathies, diseases in which the structure and function of cilia are significantly altered, are often accompanied by olfactory problems. This observation underscores the important role cilia play in olfactory transduction.[14]

Inherent and Imposed Patterns

When odorant molecules are delivered to the headspace above the mucus-coated olfactory receptors, they bind to receptor sites on the cilia of olfactory receptor neurons (ORNs). This produces a change in the membrane potential at the tip of the olfactory receptor cell that, in turn, creates an electronic signal that flows along the axon of the olfactory neuron to the olfactory bulb. The olfactory bulb is composed of several different types of cell, although the axons of the olfactory receptor cells first make contact with glomerular cells.[1]

Like-tuned receptor cells (there are ~400 different functioning receptor cell types in the human olfactory mucosa) send their signals to specific glomerular cells. With a few exceptions, like-tuned olfactory sensory neurons are segregated to a limited part of the olfactory epithelium (OE) and are thought to be confined to one of the four nonoverlapping zones (**Fig. 2.5**).[15-17]

> The physiochemical properties of incoming odorants and the distribution of like-tuned olfactory receptors are apparently both important in the peripheral coding of olfactory information.

Most odorants stimulate more than one type of receptor cell and all produce a response pattern across the olfactory mucosa that is unique for that particular odorant. The axons for like-tuned olfactory neurons innervate a limited number of glomeruli which are usually found in a specific locus in the medial glomerular layer and another specific locus in the lateral glomerular layer. As a result, the mucosal activity pattern is maintained, and perhaps even sharpened, in the glomerular cell layer of the olfactory bulb.[15-17] There is also recent evidence from OE recordings that is consistent with the hypothesis that there is a zonal expression of ORNs in humans.[18]

> ORNs are expressed in certain zones of the olfactory epithelium.

There is an increasing body of evidence to suggest that the mucosa and bulb patterns play a key role in odorant detection and discrimination.[19,20] For example, using voltage-sensitive dyes, Youngentob and his coworkers demonstrated that odorant-induced activity patterns in the mucosa were sharpened as animals learned an odorant identification task (**Figs. 2.5 and 2.6**).[21]

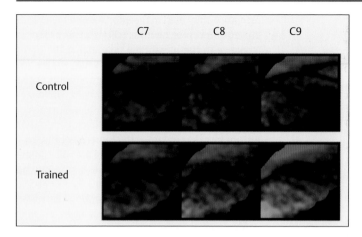

Fig. 2.5 Mouse septal olfactory mucosal activity patterns recorded using optical techniques and the voltage-sensitive dye di-4-ANEPPS. The panels show the composite average response of a set of trained and untrained (control) mice to C7–C9 aldehydes. The pink areas show when the response for the odorant of interest is larger than the response averaged across all animals and all pixels. Black represents equal responsiveness. For the control animals, the response patterns for each of the aldehydes is different from the patterns for the other two, indicating that each odorant produces a different mucosal activity pattern. Comparing the control and trained responses for each odorant, the area of responsiveness seen after training is larger than the response seen before training, indicating that training increases the size of the activity patterns. (Figure courtesy of Dr. Steven Youngentob, SUNY, Upstate Medical University, Syracuse, NY.)

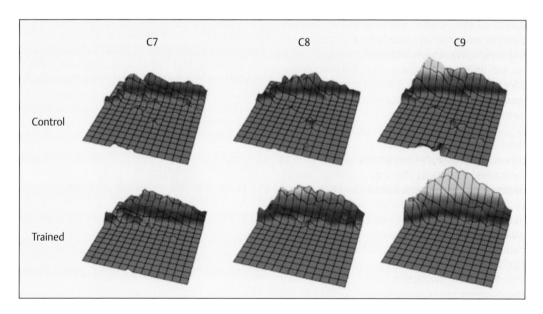

Fig. 2.6 Composite color scale-enhanced surface plots for the septal olfactory mucosa of the data shown in **Fig. 2.5**. The height of the z-axis corresponds to a change in response for a given odorant at a particular pixel compared with the average of all odorants for that pixel. Only the region of maximal activity or "hot spot" for the odorants is shown. The remaining areas are set to zero (green pixels). Again, for the control animals, the response patterns for each aldehyde are different from the patterns for the other two, and comparing the control and trained responses for each odorant, the area of responsiveness seen after training is larger than the response seen before training. (Figure courtesy of Dr. Steven Youngentob, SUNY, Upstate Medical University, Syracuse, NY.)

In summary, as receptor cells of similar sensitivity are grouped in particular locations along the olfactory receptor sheet, different smells produce different patterns of electrical activity in both the mucosa and the olfactory bulb. These patterns are thought to be one of the ways in which the brain can identify a particular smell. The electrical pattern of activity created by the specific tuning and location of olfactory receptor cells is called the "inherent" mucosal activity pattern. Again, this pattern is maintained at the level of the olfactory bulb.[22]

In rats, odorant receptor (OR) expression patterns in the olfactory mucosa are restored even after a high exposure to methyl bromide gas. These reconstituted neurons have been shown to have olfactory function. This observation suggests that olfactory problems observed after severe peripheral injuries are not likely to be caused by a lack of regrown olfactory neurons, but rather by a more central problem.[22]

Because the olfactory receptors are located at some distance from the tip of the nose, incoming odorant molecules interact with the mucous surface of the respiratory epithelium as they are directed toward the airspace adjacent to the superior concha. The nature of this interaction depends on the physical and chemical properties of the odorant molecules themselves. For example, one would expect there to be considerable sorption of mucosa-soluble odorant molecules to the surface of the respiratory mucosa. As a result, fewer of these molecules would reach the olfactory receptor area, and those that did would take longer than molecules of odorants that were not very soluble in the mucosa. In addition, there would be a spatial distribution pattern across the receptor sheet itself, with most of the mucosa-soluble odorant molecules being concentrated early in the flow path compared with a more even mucosal distribution pattern for less mucosa-soluble odorants. The different arrival times and mucosal distribution patterns resulting from an odorant's solubility may be another of the mechanisms by which the central nervous system identifies smells. These distribution patterns are called "imposed" patterns,[23,24] and are likely to be the basis for the differences between nasal and retronasal perception of odors.[25,26]

There is considerable evidence supporting the existence of imposed patterns in animals. Electrophysiological, gas chromatographic, and radioisotopic studies in frogs and rats have provided strong evidence that the degree of mucosal solubility can affect spatial and temporal distribution patterns along the respiratory and olfactory mucosas.[1]

Stimulus Parameters

Regardless of the odorant, within physiological limits, there is thought to be a direct relationship between the olfactory response and the number of odorant molecules delivered to the olfactory receptors. That is, more odorant molecules means a more intense smell. However, the olfactory stimulus is actually defined by three "primary" variables: the number of molecules (N); the duration of the sniff (T); and the volume of the sniff (V). These primary variables in turn define the three "derived" variables of concentration: ($C = N/V$); delivery rate ($D = N/T$); and flow rate ($F = V/T$).[1,27]

From an analysis of variance, Mozell and his coworkers[27] generated a model using the three primary variables (NVT) to account for the variability (R) in the olfactory receptor neural activity in bullfrogs. The model was:

$$R \sim N^{0.35}V^{-0.28}T^{0.22}$$

The model proposes that the magnitude of the response **increases** as the sniff volume **decreases**, whereas the magnitude of the olfactory nerve response **increases** as the number of molecules and sniff time **increase**. This model provides a good explanation of the variability in the response of the bullfrog olfactory nerve to subthreshold concentrations of octane.

The relationship among the sniff variables, which influences the interaction of odorants and the olfactory mucosa, is complex, and changing a variable such as flow rate, either experimentally or clinically, also changes other variables that can affect the olfactory response.

Because the primary variables can be represented as derived variables, Mozell was able to test other possible models that included combinations of the primary and derived variables. From this analysis, a model emerged that was even better than the NVT model in explaining the variability in the olfactory nerve response. This model was:

$$R \sim F^{-0.25}N^{0.35}$$

In the *FN* model, the effects of volume and time are equal and opposite, whereas the number of molecules is independent of the other two. Of all 11 models tested, the *FN* model was the best at explaining the variability in the olfactory nerve response.[1,27]

The *FN* model was generated from bullfrog neural activity. As, in the bullfrog, there is no splitting of the inspired air into different flow channels, all of the inspired air flows over the olfactory sheet. Therefore, if applicable to humans at all, perhaps the *FN* model best describes the results of the airflow delivered to the olfactory sheet, not what comes into the tip of the nose.

The results from human psychophysical studies looking at the relationship between the olfactory response and changes in the primary and secondary variables have been equivocal. As changing the primary variables also obviously changes the derived variables, determining the appropriateness of any of the above models to human olfactory response has been difficult.

Techniques using Nasal Dilators and Computational Fluid Dynamics

As a research tool, nasal dilators provide a way to temporarily alter nasal anatomy and thus, when combined with computational fluid dynamics, provide a way of beginning to evaluate the *FN* model.

Nasal dilators are elastic strips with plastic springs running along their long axis. When applied externally to the skin covering the nose, the springs increase the diameter of the nasal cavity in the region of the nasal valve. Psychophysical recordings have shown that nasal dilators increase perceived odorant intensity, reduce odorant detection thresholds, and increase odorant identification. In addition, pneumotachograph recordings have demonstrated that the mean flow rate, maximum flow rate, and volume and duration of the sniff at the tip of the nose are all increased when nasal dilators are worn.[28,29]

At first glance, there appears to be a contradiction between the results of the *FN* model and the observation that when wearing nasal dilators the olfactory perception is increased because of higher flows, larger sniff volumes, and longer sniffs. However, the increases in the flow characteris-

tics reported from the nasal dilator studies were recorded at the tip of the nose. Any estimates of the actual flow to the olfactory receptor region and the subsequent odorant deposition patterns in this part of the nose have been a matter of only speculation.

Computational fluid dynamics techniques have been used in the past to predict the impact of regional airway changes on airflow and odorant distribution patterns, especially to the olfactory region.[23] Three-dimensional numerical nasal models for numerical simulation of nasal airflow were constructed in dilated and nondilated conditions.

The data from these modeling studies may provide a glimpse into the appropriateness of the *FN* model in humans. The dilator-induced increase in size of the lower part of the nose directs more of the inspired air along the floor of the nose and therefore reduces the flow to the olfactory area.[30] Obviously, there is some limit to the applicability of the *FN* model in explaining the olfactory response. At its extreme, a really low flow would not be expected to generate any olfactory response. Therefore, the model needs to be considered as describing events within certain physiological limits. The description of these limits awaits further studies.

Because of the location of the olfactory receptors in humans, changes along the flow conduit leading up to the receptors may have surprising effects on olfactory ability. Widening the nasal air passageways or increasing the air flow at the tip of the nose may not necessarily improve olfactory ability.

Clearly there is not yet a full understanding of the relationship between olfactory ability and the primary and secondary stimulus variables. The *FN* model (and similar attempts to quantify the olfactory response in terms of stimulus characteristics) at best provides a stepping stone for future work. The possibility of nasal cycle changes either complementing or reducing the effect of any experimental nasal manipulation adds another level of complexity to the analysis of any data generated.

The relationship between nasal anatomy and olfactory ability is complex. Patients should be warned about the complex nature of this relationship, so that they will not have unrealistic expectations following nasal surgery.

Neurophysiological Considerations

Nancy E. Rawson

The OE is uniquely suited to its function and position as the chemosensory sentinel informing the owner about the nature of a host of volatile compounds present in our environment. The anatomy and neurophysiological capacity of the OE is specialized for sensitivity, scope of response, and robustness in the face of a harsh and changing environment. This sensory neuroepithelium occupies the olfactory cleft and projects onto the dorsal portion of the superior turbinate. By 5 months of gestation, the OE is well ordered and contiguous, extending from the roof of the nasal cavity to the mid-portion of the nasal septum and onto the superior turbinate.[31,32] It has been estimated that the human OE occupies an area of 1–4 cm^2 containing ~6 million olfactory neurons.[31–33] While comprehensive studies have not been reported, in our studies of several hundred biopsy specimens from generally healthy patients, we did not observe marked gender- or ethnicity-related differences in the likelihood of obtaining functional neurons from biopsies obtained from the superior turbinate (refs. 34 and 35 and unpublished observations), suggesting that the overall number may

be relatively consistent. In adult humans, sensory epithelium is often intermingled with nonsensory tissue along the superior turbinate and septum, in contrast to the rodent, in which there is a clear delineation between epithelial types.[36] Functionally, human ORNs exhibit general characteristics similar to those of most mammals, with a large diversity of receptor proteins and a signaling cascade designed to amplify and specifically transmit odorant-binding events to the olfactory bulb using electrical action potentials (**Fig. 2.7**). However, specific aspects of ORN function diverge across species, including the diversity and number of receptor protein types and certain aspects of the signaling cascades. Such similarities and differences should be considered in evaluating the clinical relevance of research on rodent models.

> The olfactory sensory epithelium is designed for detection of and protection from volatile stimuli, and is composed of multiple cell types in a pseudostratified arrangement.

The olfactory neuroepithelium is a pseudostratified epithelium consisting of multiple cell types sitting on a basal lamina that separates the epithelium from the submucosal lamina propria (**Fig. 2.8**). The lamina propria includes fibrous and glandular tissue, along with axonal fibers, blood

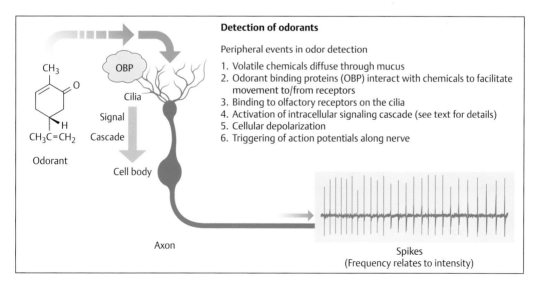

Detection of odorants

Peripheral events in odor detection

1. Volatile chemicals diffuse through mucus
2. Odorant binding proteins (OBP) interact with chemicals to facilitate movement to/from receptors
3. Binding to olfactory receptors on the cilia
4. Activation of intracellular signaling cascade (see text for details)
5. Cellular depolarization
6. Triggering of action potentials along nerve

CH$_3$

OBP

O

Cilia

Signal

CH$_3$C=CH$_2$ Cascade

Odorant

Cell body

Axon

Spikes
(Frequency relates to intensity)

Fig. 2.7 When an odorous substance (e.g., L-carvone, which smells like mint) makes contact with olfactory receptors on the cilia of a receptor cell, it sets off a chain of events leading to activation of electrical currents. This makes the cell fire a sequence of action potentials—voltage signals or spikes—the frequency of which relates to the intensity of the odor. The spikes are sent out along the nerve fiber to the glomeruli in the olfactory bulb (see Chapter 3).

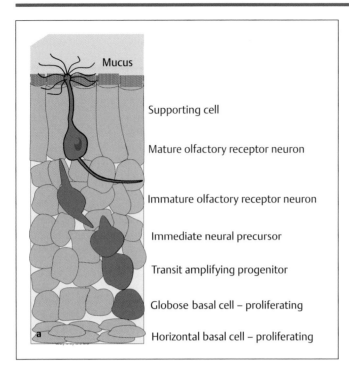

Mucus

Supporting cell

Mature olfactory receptor neuron

Immature olfactory receptor neuron

Immediate neural precursor

Transit amplifying progenitor

Globose basal cell – proliferating

Horizontal basal cell – proliferating

Fig. 2.8a, b Cell types of the olfactory epithelium.

a Diagram depicting cell types within the olfactory epithelium.

b Human olfactory epithelium immunostained with an antibody to olfactory marker protein to show mature odorant receptor neurons (brown cell bodies).

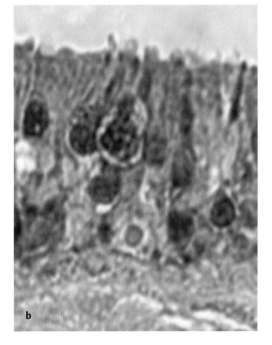

bind distinct classes of volatile compounds and are thought to facilitate odorant transport.[37,38] A population of resident macrophages and other immune cell types is also typical within both healthy and pathological OE.[39,40] In addition to axons of the ORNs, fibers of the trigeminal nerve project to the surface of the OE, and both cholinergic and adrenergic fibers are also present within the epithelium and lamina propria.[41] Adrenergic fibers within the lamina propria act on glands to control nasal mucus secretion, and on vascular elements to regulate blood flow. Dispersal of odorants via the mucus and through the lamina propria into the blood constitutes an important mechanism for odorant removal.[42] Accordingly, age-related decline in the density of adrenergic fibers, or medications that influence adrenergic pathways, can impair olfactory performance in part via reduced odorant clearance rates.[43]

> Olfactory sensory neurons are bipolar receptor cells that are replaced throughout life.

vessels and immune cells. Bowman glands secrete watery mucus, which forms a protective layer coating the OE surface. Odorant-binding proteins, related to lipocalins, are a family of proteins that

ORNs are bipolar cells with an apical dendritic knob bearing cilia and a basal cell body with a single axonal process that projects through the submucosa. The axonal processes assemble into a bundle within nonmyelinating ensheathing glial cells and extend through the cribriform plate to synapse within the olfactory bulb (see Chapter 3). Mature ORNs are classically identified by their expression of olfactory marker protein (OMP), and also express characteristic signaling, structural, and receptor proteins.[44] Mature ORNs are derived from a population of slowly dividing basal cells that replicate asynchronously to produce more rapidly dividing progenitors, and are the only primary sensory neuron type to undergo replacement throughout life. This feature helps ensure the maintenance of this vital sensory system, and the lifespan of mature ORNs depends in part on exposure to toxic or infectious xenobiotics. While ORNs are susceptible to destruction by neurovirulent influenza A, preventing its transmission to the brain, they are resistant to other viruses and can serve as an avenue for infection of the central nervous system by several viruses (e.g., herpes simplex, parainfluenza).[45] While neuronal cell replacement is part of the normal OE, activation by odorants appears to promote survival of ORNs.[46] Thus, the population of ORNs is plastic and responsive to the environment in a way that helps to ensure the ability to sense both novel and diverse compounds, while also being tuned to the most salient and prevalent volatile signals in the individual's environment.

Nonolfactory sensory and supporting cell types also occur within the OE.

Several other types of sensory or cell types have been reported in the OE of rodents, but have yet to be described in human OE. Among these are solitary chemoreceptor cells (SCCs), which express bitter taste receptors and signaling components common to taste receptor cells.[47] These cells appear to synapse with nerve endings from the trigeminal system, and have apical processes positioned to detect a variety of noxious stimuli too lipophilic to penetrate the mucosa to reach the trigeminal nerve endings.[48,49] Like taste cells and olfactory neurons, they are replaced throughout life, although the local progenitor is unclear.[50] In rodent OE, SCCs are present in both the nasopharyngeal region and the anterior nasal cavity within the respiratory epithelium, and have recently been reported in the nasal epithelium and vomeronasal glands of humans.[51] Two populations of microvillous cells express-

ing the thermally sensitive, nonselective cation channel transient receptor potential M5 (TRPM5) have also been identified in rodent OE.[52] One type is morphologically and immunocytochemically similar to the bipolar ORNs, is sparsely distributed, and is restricted to the lateral and ventral OE. The other is scattered throughout the OE, and has a pear- or flasklike cell body smaller than an ORN, residing in the apical third of the OE. The microvilli may be short and brushlike or have a more tuftlike arrangement.[52] These microvillous cells do not express the neuronal marker protein gene product 9.5 or proteins characteristic of ORNs (e.g., OMP and the cyclic nucleotide-gated channel), nor do they express markers seen in SCCs (e.g., phospholipase C β2 or α-gustducin). Neither do they express markers of neuroendocrine cells (e.g. chromogranin), but most do express cytokeratin 18, a marker of brush cells. While not yet established in human OE, brush cells are present in other parts of the human respiratory tract, and cells with this morphology are observed in human OE specimens (personal observation). It is possible that the microvillar cells expressing the retinoic acid receptor reported by Yee and Rawson[53] are a subset of these TRPM5-expressing cells, based on morphology. However, further studies are needed to establish the distribution, molecular identity, and role of these cells in the human OE.

Supporting cells serve trophic and detoxification roles.

Supporting or sustentacular cells are large, columnar cells that extend nearly the full width of the OE. They are identified in rodents by the sustentacular cell antibody (SUS antibody), and express cytokeratin 8.[54] In contrast, cytokeratin 5 labels this cell population in human OE, and the SUS antibody is ineffective (Borgmann-Winter K, personal communication). Supporting cells provide trophic and protective support, expressing detoxification enzymes such as cytochrome P450[55] and glutathione-S-peroxidase.[56]

Horizontal basal cells are less defined in human than rodent OE.

Horizontal basal cells may serve a function comparable to a blood–brain barrier, and provide structural and trophic support for proliferating cells, although little is known about their physiological properties. They are molecularly defined by the expression of specific cytokeratins and the epidermal growth factor receptor and in adult human, but not rodent, OE, express p75-nerve growth factor receptor.[57,58] While this cell class is easily recognized morphologically within the rodent OE, it appears more sparse, or perhaps more heterogeneous morphologically, in the human OE (Borgmann-Winter K, personal communication, and ref. 36).

> The development and lifespan of olfactory receptor neurons are dependent on the cellular context and the external environment.

In the rodent, globose basal cells (GBCs) can be selected on the basis of expression of the GBC-2 protein, and represent multipotent precursors capable of giving rise to ORNs, supporting cells and additional GBCs.[59-61] This marker fails to identify any cells in human OE, and it has been difficult to identify a specific population of slowly dividing precursors with characteristics of stem cells or early fate-specified progenitors within the OE.[62] However, the presence of such cells is supported both by the regenerative capacity of the tissue, demonstrated even into advanced age, and by studies showing that biopsied human OE can be used to generate long-term primary cultures containing cells with multipotent capabilities.[63,64] ORN precursors differentiate into immature neurons expressing Gap-43 and neuron-specific tubulin,[65] and ultimately to mature ORNs expressing OMP along with receptors and their associated signaling molecules.[61,66,67] ORNs whose axons fail to synapse with their respective mitral cells within the olfactory bulb, because of injury, inflammation, or surgical intrusion, undergo apoptosis.[68] Cells expressing markers of most stages of this lineage have been characterized and localized within human OE,[36,62] but questions remain regarding the molecular characteristics and localization of the earliest progenitor. Cells expressing markers of proliferation and cell death are more numerous under conditions of inflammation, reflecting the capacity of the tissue to respond to the need for neuronal replacement under these conditions (**Fig. 2.9**).[58]

> Human OE tends to be less organized and less robust in the face of age and disease than rodent OE.

The structure of the OE in adult humans tends to be far less organized than that in rodents, with respect to both apical to basal stratification and to homogeneity of sensory versus respiratory regions across the epithelial sheet. Whether this is due to a true species difference, or to differences in environmental exposure, incidence of allergy, and sinus infections and inflammation, is unclear. Unlike the very orderly layers of OMP-immunoreactive (OMP-ir)–ORNs observed in the rodent OE, the frequency of OMP-ir–ORNs in the human middle turbinate tends to be sparse and scattered. This accounts for the comparatively smaller likelihood of obtaining sensory epithelium from biopsies obtained from this region than from the olfactory cleft.[69,70] It is clear that, with age and disease, the human OE becomes increasingly patchy and interspersed with respiratory or fibrotic tissue.[71] Under these conditions, olfactory neurons may persist as a population within the tissue, but exhibit abnormal morphology, may be displaced below a keratinized epithelium, or may be entirely absent (**Fig. 2.9**).[39,58,72]

It is possible that the comparative OE disorder often observed in human biopsy specimens reflects a less robust regenerative capacity than rodent OE. In rodents, the regenerative capacity of the OE is such that even following total ablation with chemical irritant, complete recovery can be accomplished within a few months.[73] In human patients, OE recovery following damage due to infection, trauma, or chemical irritants may be prolonged and accompanied by long-term or permanent olfactory impairment.[72,74,75] Unfortunately, OE integrity based on tissue biopsies typically does not correlate well with olfactory function,[58,76] and it is likely that substantial damage can occur without overt consequences on performance depending on the location and nature of the damage. With age, in both humans and animal models, this neuroepithelial sheet becomes increasingly disordered and patchy, with a higher proportion of respiratory epithelium infiltrating the sensory regions.[31,76] However, the extent and degree of degeneration is highly variable among individuals, and is probably influenced by exposures, infections, and other factors that impair the ability of the tissue to regenerate.

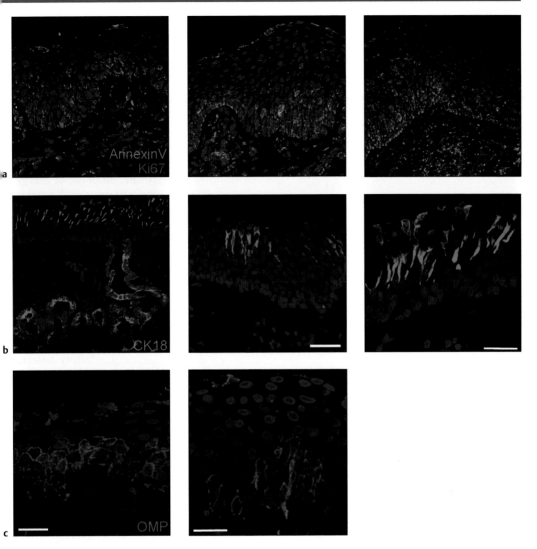

Fig. 2.9 Immunofluorescent staining of human olfactory epithelial biopsies. Nuclei are stained blue with DAPI. Scale bars are 20 μm. (Methods as in Kern 2000.[10] Images courtesy of Karen K Yee, Monell Chemical Senses Center, Philadelphia, PA.)

a Tissue exhibiting altered morphology due to chronic inflammation, with horizontally aligned squamous cells along the surface. Annexin V, a marker of apoptotic cell death is shown in green. Ki67, a marker of cell division, is labeled in red.

b Supporting cell localization of cytokeratin 18 (CK18).

c Olfactory marker protein (OMP) immunostaining in cells that are dysmorphic and abnormally situated in inflamed tissue.

> Odorants are detected via a large family of G-protein-coupled receptors that use a signaling cascade that amplifies each binding event to enable detection of extremely low concentrations of volatile stimuli.

Odorants are bound to receptors of the G-protein-coupled receptor (GPCR) class, which, in humans, is estimated to have 300 to 400 functional members with perhaps twice as many pseudogenes.[77,78] The majority of these putative ORs remain orphans, although data suggest that each OR binds to a small number of odorant ligands, and that each odorant ligand is recognized by a small number of ORs.[79] Each mature ORN appears to express only a single type of OR, although expression of multiple ORs may occur transiently.[80,81] This structural configuration provides the basis for odor recognition via activation of a unique pattern of ORNs projecting to distinct glomeruli in the olfactory bulb (see Chapter 3). Binding to these receptors is transduced to an action potential in the majority of ORNs via a cascade involving activation of adenylate cyclase, opening of a cyclic nucleotide-gated, nonselective cation channel, and cellular depolarization (**Fig. 2.10**). This pathway is relatively inefficient as a result of the low affinity of odorant binding and relatively inefficient synthesis of cyclic adenosine monophosphate. To accommodate this, ORNs accumulate chloride, particularly within the cilia, and rapid chloride efflux via Na^+/K^+/2Cl^- co-transport[82] and a calcium-gated chloride channel[83] enable a depolarization of significant rate and magnitude to trigger an action potential along the axon. This signal detection and amplification process, together with the convergence of signals in the olfactory bulb, supports detection of volatile stimuli as low as parts per trillion for certain odorants, even by the often underappreciated human nose![84] Termination of the signal occurs as calcium is removed via Ca^{2+}/ATPase and, to a lesser degree, through Na^+/Ca^{2+} exchange (**Fig. 2.10**).[85] Calcium also results in adaptation via calcium-dependent kinases and subsequent phosphorylation of proteins within the signaling cascade.[86] In addition to ORs, ORNs express over 30 other types of GPCRs, including noradrenergic, cholinergic,[87] dopaminergic,[88,89] and purinergic[90] receptors. Thus, modulation of ORN function is complex, even at the initial steps in odor perception, and it is easy to envision why many pharmaceuticals, xenobiotics, and health conditions affecting these pathways may also have a disruptive impact on our sense of smell.

> Olfactory epithelial biopsies can be obtained from living subjects for primary culture and as a source of stem cell–like cells with multipotent differentiation capacity.

In humans, the olfactory neuroepithelium is accessible via biopsy using relatively simple procedures, and olfactory epithelial biopsies have been established as a viable approach to obtain fresh sensory epithelial tissue for physiological and molecular studies.[34,69,91] Such tissue represents a uniquely accessible neuroepithelium available from living

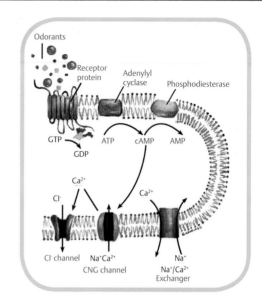

Fig. 2.10 Signaling cascade of events occurring within the olfactory cilia involved in translating the odorant binding event into an electrical signal carried along the axon to the olfactory bulb and termination of the odorant binding signal. (Artwork by Courtney Loveless.)

AMP, adenosine monophosphate; ATP, adenosine triphosphate; Ca^{2+}, calcium ions; cAMP, cyclic AMP; Cl^-, chloride ions; GDP, guanosine diphosphate; GTP, guanosine triphosphate; Na^+, sodium ions.

subjects, and studies using this tissue have provided novel insights into the neuropathology of psychiatric disorders such as bipolar depression,[92] schizophrenia[93,94] and Rett syndrome.[95] While ex vivo preparations provide the ability to examine the native cells, they are subject to the effects of dissociation and tissue extraction trauma, which may compromise and alter their cellular physiology. Accordingly, methods have been developed to use biopsied epithelium as the source of precursor cells, which may be grown under conditions conducive to the generation of neuronal[63,64] or non-neuronal[96,97] cells. In these cultures, cells may be generated that express both molecular and functional properties of the desired cell type. The OE-derived precursor cells express markers and multipotent capacity indicative of mesenchymal stem cells.[97–101] Rapid advances are being made in our understanding of the growth factors and conditions under which these cells function in vivo, and may be differentiated in vitro to express functional characteristics of osteogenic, adipogenic, audiogenic, or neurogenic cells. The ability to obtain such cells from a living patient for their own use, avoiding concerns of rejection, make it likely that these cells will serve a prominent role in regenerative medicine in the future.

While remarkable in its ability to overcome the daily onslaught of environmental exposure, the human OE is also sensitive to damage from infection, irritation, aging, and the direct and indirect consequences of many diseases and their treatments. Being aware of these consequences will help the clinician understand the potential causes for their patient's olfactory dysfunction and the factors that may contribute to improvement.

Acknowledgments

The author acknowledges the fine technical assistance of Grant J. Currie and Lucas D. Wright of St. Lawrence University in the preparation of **Figs. 2.1, 2.2 and 2.3** and the generosity of Dr. Steven Youngentob of SUNY, Upstate Medical University, Syracuse, NY, for providing **Figs. 2.5 and 2.6**.

References

1. Hornung D. Nasal anatomy and the sense of smell. In Hummel T and Welge-Lüssen A, eds. Advances in Oto-Rhino-Laryngology, Taste and Smell: An Update. Basel: Karger Press; 2006:1–22.
2. Simmen D, Scherrer JL, Moe K, Heinz B. A dynamic and direct visualization model for the study of nasal airflow. Arch Otolaryngol Head Neck Surg 1999;125(9):1015–1021
3. Schroeter JD, Garcia GJ, Kimbell JS. A computational fluid dynamics approach to assess interhuman variability in hydrogen sulfide nasal dosimetry. Inhal Toxicol 2010;22(4):277–286
4. Kelly JT, Prasad AK, Wexler AS. Detailed flow patterns in the nasal cavity. J Appl Physiol 2000; 89(1):323–337
5. Zhao K, Dalton P. The way the wind blows: implications of modeling nasal airflow. Curr Allergy Asthma Rep 2007;7(2):117–125
6. Doty RL, Mishra A. Olfaction and its alteration by nasal obstruction, rhinitis, and rhinosinusitis. Laryngoscope 2001;111(3):409–423
7. Mozell M, Schwartz D, Youngentob S, Leopold D, Hornung D, Sheehe P. Reversal of hyposmia in laryngectomized patients. Chem Senses 1986;11: 397–410
8. Ozaki S, Toida K, Suzuki M, et al. Impaired olfactory function in mice with allergic rhinitis. Auris Nasus Larynx 2010;37(5):575–583
9. Damm M, Eckel HE, Jungehülsing M, Hummel T. Olfactory changes at threshold and suprathreshold

levels following septoplasty with partial inferior turbinectomy. Ann Otol Rhinol Laryngol 2003; 112(1):91–97
10. Kern RC. Chronic sinusitis and anosmia: pathologic changes in the olfactory mucosa. Laryngoscope 2000;110(7):1071–1077
11. Searleman A, Hornung D, Stein E, Brzuszkiewicz L. Nostril dominance: differences in nasal airflow and preferred handedness. Laterality 2005;10(2): 111–120
12. Keyhani K, Scherer PW, Mozell MM. A numerical model of nasal odorant transport for the analysis of human olfaction. J Theor Biol 1997;186(3):279–301
13. Kurtz DB, Zhao K, Hornung DE, Scherer P. Experimental and numerical determination of odorant solubility in nasal and olfactory mucosa. Chem Senses 2004;29(9):763–773
14. Jenkins PM, McEwen DP, Martens JR. Olfactory cilia: linking sensory cilia function and human disease. Chem Senses 2009;34(5):451–464
15. Schwob JE, Gottlieb DI. The primary olfactory projection has two chemically distinct zones. J Neurosci 1986;6(11):3393–3404
16. Buck L, Axel R. A novel multigene family may encode odorant receptors: a molecular basis for odor recognition. Cell 1991;65(1):175–187
17. Ressler KJ, Sullivan SL, Buck LB. A zonal organization of odorant receptor gene expression in the olfactory epithelium. Cell 1993;73(3):597–609
18. Lapid H, Shushan S, Plotkin A, et al. Neural activity at the human olfactory epithelium reflects olfactory perception. Nat Neurosci 2011;14(11):1455–1461
19. Youngentob SL, Margolis FL, Youngentob LM. OMP gene deletion results in an alteration in odorant quality perception. Behav Neurosci 2001;115(3): 626–631
20. Kent PF, Mozell MM, Youngentob SL, Yurco P. Mucosal activity patterns as a basis for olfactory discrimination: comparing behavior and optical recordings. Brain Res 2003;981(1–2):1–11
21. Youngentob SL, Kent PF. Enhancement of odorant-induced mucosal activity patterns in rats trained on an odorant identification task. Brain Res 1995; 670(1):82–88
22. Iwema CL, Fang H, Kurtz DB, Youngentob SL, Schwob JE. Odorant receptor expression patterns are restored in lesion-recovered rat olfactory epithelium. J Neurosci 2004;24(2):356–369
23. Kent PF, Mozell MM, Murphy SJ, Hornung DE. The interaction of imposed and inherent olfactory mucosal activity patterns and their composite representation in a mammalian species using voltage-sensitive dyes. J Neurosci 1996;16(1):345–353
24. Zhao K, Scherer PW, Hajiloo SA, Dalton P. Effect of anatomy on human nasal air flow and odorant transport patterns: implications for olfaction. Chem Senses 2004;29(5):365–379
25. Small DM, Gerber JC, Mak YE, Hummel T. Differential neural responses evoked by orthonasal versus retronasal odorant perception in humans. Neuron 2005;47(4):593–605
26. Scott JW, Acevedo HP, Sherrill L, Phan M. Responses of the rat olfactory epithelium to retronasal air flow. J Neurophysiol 2007;97(3):1941–1950

27. Mozell MM, Sheehe PR, Swieck SW Jr, Kurtz DB, Hornung DE. A parametric study of the stimulation variables affecting the magnitude of the olfactory nerve response. J Gen Physiol 1984;83(2):233–267

28. Hornung DE, Chin C, Kurtz DB, Kent PF, Mozell MM. Effect of nasal dilators on perceived odor intensity. Chem Senses 1997;22(2):177–180

29. Hornung DE, Smith DJ, Kurtz DB, White T, Leopold DA. Effect of nasal dilators on nasal structures, sniffing strategies, and olfactory ability. Rhinology 2001;39(2):84–87

30. Zhao K, Hornung D, Leopold D. The relationship between nasal airflow and olfactory perception. Abstracts of the AchemS Annual Meeting April 13–17, 2011; Florida; 2011;P129:69–70

31. Nakashima T, Kimmelman CP, Snow JB Jr. Structure of human fetal and adult olfactory neuroepithelium. Arch Otolaryngol 1984;110(10):641–646

32. Leopold DA, Hummel T, Schwob JE, Hong SC, Knecht M, Kobal G. Anterior distribution of human olfactory epithelium. Laryngoscope 2000;110(3 Pt 1):417–421

33. Moran DT, Jafek BW. III JCR. The ultrastructure of the human olfactory mucosa. In: Laing DG, Doty RL, Breipohl W, eds. The Human Sense of Smell. Berlin: Springer-Verlag; 1991:395.

34. Rawson NE, Gomez G, Cowart B, et al. Selectivity and response characteristics of human olfactory neurons. J Neurophysiol 1997;77(3):1606–1613

35. Rawson NE, Gomez G, Cowart BJ, Kriete A, Pribitkin E, Restrepo D. Age-associated loss of selectivity in human olfactory sensory neurons. Neurobiol Aging 2012;33(9):1913–1919

36. Holbrook EH, Wu E, Curry WT, Lin DT, Schwob JE. Immunohistochemical characterization of human olfactory tissue. Laryngoscope 2011;121(8):1687–1701

37. Briand L, Eloit C, Nespoulous C, et al. Evidence of an odorant-binding protein in the human olfactory mucus: location, structural characterization, and odorant-binding properties. Biochemistry 2002;41(23):7241–7252

38. Pelosi P. The role of perireceptor events in vertebrate olfaction. Cell Mol Life Sci 2001;58(4):503–509

39. Yee KK, Pribitkin EA, Cowart BJ, Rosen D, Feng P, Rawson NE. Analysis of the olfactory mucosa in chronic rhinosinusitis. Ann N Y Acad Sci 2009;1170:590–595

40. Mellert TK, Getchell ML, Sparks L, Getchell TV. Characterization of the immune barrier in human olfactory mucosa. Otolaryngol Head Neck Surg 1992;106(2):181–188

41. Hall RA. Autonomic modulation of olfactory signaling. Sci Signal 2011;4(155):pe1

42. Getchell TV, Margolis FL, Getchell ML. Perireceptor and receptor events in vertebrate olfaction. Prog Neurobiol 1984;23(4):317–345

43. Chen Y, Getchell TV, Sparks DL, Getchell ML. Patterns of adrenergic and peptidergic innervation in human olfactory mucosa: age-related trends. J Comp Neurol 1993;334(1):104–116

44. Baker H, Grillo M, Margolis FL. Biochemical and immunocytochemical characterization of olfactory marker protein in the rodent central nervous system. J Comp Neurol 1989;285(2):246–261

45. Mori I, Goshima F, Imai Y, et al. Olfactory receptor neurons prevent dissemination of neurovirulent influenza A virus into the brain by undergoing virus-induced apoptosis. J Gen Virol 2002;83(Pt 9):2109–2116

46. Zhao H, Reed RR. X inactivation of the OCNC1 channel gene reveals a role for activity-dependent competition in the olfactory system. Cell 2001;104(5):651–660

47. Tizzano M, Cristofoletti M, Sbarbati A, Finger TE. Expression of taste receptors in solitary chemosensory cells of rodent airways. BMC Pulm Med 2011;11:3

48. Finger TE, Böttger B, Hansen A, Anderson KT, Alimohammadi H, Silver WL. Solitary chemoreceptor cells in the nasal cavity serve as sentinels of respiration. Proc Natl Acad Sci U S A 2003;100(15):8981–8986

49. Lin W, Ogura T, Margolskee RF, Finger TE, Restrepo D. TRPM5-expressing solitary chemosensory cells respond to odorous irritants. J Neurophysiol 2008;99(3):1451–1460

50. Gulbransen BD, Finger TE. Solitary chemoreceptor cell proliferation in adult nasal epithelium. J Neurocytol 2005;34(1–2):117–122

51. Braun T, Mack B, Kramer MF. Solitary chemosensory cells in the respiratory and vomeronasal epithelium of the human nose: a pilot study. Rhinology 2011;49(5):507–512

52. Lin W, Ezekwe EA Jr, Zhao Z, Liman ER, Restrepo D. TRPM5-expressing microvillous cells in the main olfactory epithelium. BMC Neurosci 2008;9:114

53. Yee KK, Rawson NE. Immunolocalization of retinoic acid receptors in the mammalian olfactory system and the effects of olfactory denervation on receptor distribution. Neuroscience 2005;131(3):733–743

54. Schwob JE. Neural regeneration and the peripheral olfactory system. Anat Rec 2002;269(1):33–49

55. Getchell ML, Chen Y, Ding X, Sparks DL, Getchell TV. Immunohistochemical localization of a cytochrome P-450 isozyme in human nasal mucosa: age-related trends. Ann Otol Rhinol Laryngol 1993;102(5):368–374

56. Krishna NS, Getchell TV, Dhooper N, Awasthi YC, Getchell ML. Age- and gender-related trends in the expression of glutathione S-transferases in human nasal mucosa. Ann Otol Rhinol Laryngol 1995;104(10 Pt 1):812–822

57. Holbrook EH, Szumowski KE, Schwob JE. An immunochemical, ultrastructural, and developmental characterization of the horizontal basal cells of rat olfactory epithelium. J Comp Neurol 1995;363(1):129–146

58. Yee KK, Pribitkin EA, Cowart BJ, et al. Neuropathology of the olfactory mucosa in chronic rhinosinusitis. Am J Rhinol Allergy 2010;24(2):110–120

59. Goldstein BJ, Schwob JE. Analysis of the globose basal cell compartment in rat olfactory epithelium using GBC-1, a new monoclonal antibody against globose basal cells. J Neurosci 1996;16(12):4005–4016

60. Jang W, Youngentob SL, Schwob JE. Globose basal cells are required for reconstitution of olfactory epithelium after methyl bromide lesion. J Comp Neurol 2003;460(1):123–140

61. Schwob JE, Huard JM, Luskin MB, Youngentob SL. Retroviral lineage studies of the rat olfactory epithelium. Chem Senses 1994;19(6):671–682

62. Hahn CG, Han LY, Rawson NE, et al. In vivo and in vitro neurogenesis in human olfactory epithelium. J Comp Neurol 2005;483(2):154–163

63. Borgmann-Winter KE, Rawson NE, Wang HY, et al. Human olfactory epithelial cells generated in vitro express diverse neuronal characteristics. Neuroscience 2009;158(2):642–653

64. Gomez G, Rawson NE, Hahn CG, Michaels R, Restrepo D. Characteristics of odorant elicited calcium changes in cultured human olfactory neurons. J Neurosci Res 2000;62(5):737–749

65. Verhaagen J, Oestreicher AB, Gispen WH, Margolis FL. The expression of the growth associated protein B50/GAP43 in the olfactory system of neonatal and adult rats. J Neurosci 1989;9(2):683–691

66. Huard JM, Youngentob SL, Goldstein BJ, Luskin MB, Schwob JE. Adult olfactory epithelium contains multipotent progenitors that give rise to neurons and non-neural cells. J Comp Neurol 1998;400(4):469–486

67. Packard A, Giel-Moloney M, Leiter A, Schwob JE. Progenitor cell capacity of NeuroD1-expressing globose basal cells in the mouse olfactory epithelium. J Comp Neurol 2011;519(17):3580–3596

68. Schwob JE, Szumowski KE, Stasky AA. Olfactory sensory neurons are trophically dependent on the olfactory bulb for their prolonged survival. J Neurosci 1992;12(10):3896–3919

69. Féron F, Perry C, McGrath JJ, Mackay-Sim A. New techniques for biopsy and culture of human olfactory epithelial neurons. Arch Otolaryngol Head Neck Surg 1998;124(8):861–866

70. Lane AP, Gomez G, Dankulich T, Wang H, Bolger WE, Rawson NE. The superior turbinate as a source of functional human olfactory receptor neurons. Laryngoscope 2002;112(7 Pt 1):1183–1189

71. Paik SI, Lehman MN, Seiden AM, Duncan HJ, Smith DV. Human olfactory biopsy. The influence of age and receptor distribution. Arch Otolaryngol Head Neck Surg 1992;118(7):731–738

72. Upadhyay UD, Holbrook EH. Olfactory loss as a result of toxic exposure. Otolaryngol Clin North Am 2004;37(6):1185–1207

73. Schwob JE, Youngentob SL, Mezza RC. Reconstitution of the rat olfactory epithelium after methyl bromide-induced lesion. J Comp Neurol 1995;359(1):15–37

74. Collet S, Grulois V, Bertrand B, Rombaux P. Posttraumatic olfactory dysfunction: a cohort study and update. B-ENT 2009;5(Suppl. 13):97–107

75. Rombaux P, Martinage S, Huart C, Collet S. Post-infectious olfactory loss: a cohort study and update. B-ENT 2009;5(Suppl. 13):89–95

76. Holbrook EH, Leopold DA, Schwob JE. Abnormalities of axon growth in human olfactory mucosa. Laryngoscope 2005;115(12):2144–2154

77. Malnic B, Godfrey PA, Buck LB. The human olfactory receptor gene family. Proc Natl Acad Sci U S A 2004;101(8):2584–2589

78. Mombaerts P. The human repertoire of odorant receptor genes and pseudogenes. Annu Rev Genomics Hum Genet 2001;2:493–510

79. Buck LB. Olfactory receptors and odor coding in mammals. Nutr Rev 2004;62(11 Pt 2):S184–188; discussion S224–S241

80. Mombaerts P. Odorant receptor gene choice in olfactory sensory neurons: the one receptor–one neuron hypothesis revisited. Curr Opin Neurobiol 2004;14(1):31–36

81. Rawson NE, Eberwine J, Dotson R, Jackson J, Ulrich P, Restrepo D. Expression of mRNAs encoding for two different olfactory receptors in a subset of olfactory receptor neurons. J Neurochem 2000; 75(1):185–195

82. Hengl T, Kaneko H, Dauner K, Vocke K, Frings S, Möhrlen F. Molecular components of signal amplification in olfactory sensory cilia. Proc Natl Acad Sci U S A 2010;107(13):6052–6057

83. Reisert J, Lai J, Yau KW, Bradley J. Mechanism of the excitatory Cl⁻ response in mouse olfactory receptor neurons. Neuron 2005;45(4):553–561

84. Cometto-Muñiz JE, Abraham MH. Odor detection by humans of lineal aliphatic aldehydes and helional as gauged by dose-response functions. Chem Senses 2010;35(4):289–299

85. Antolin S, Reisert J, Matthews HR. Olfactory response termination involves Ca^{2+}-ATPase in vertebrate olfactory receptor neuron cilia. J Gen Physiol 2010;135(4):367–378

86. Matthews HR, Reisert J. Calcium, the two-faced messenger of olfactory transduction and adaptation. Curr Opin Neurobiol 2003;13(4):469–475

87. Li YR, Matsunami H. Activation state of the M3 muscarinic acetylcholine receptor modulates mammalian odorant receptor signaling. Sci Signal 2011;4(155):ra1

88. Hegg CC, Lucero MT. Dopamine reduces odor- and elevated-K(+)-induced calcium responses in mouse olfactory receptor neurons in situ. J Neurophysiol 2004;91(4):1492–1499

89. Koster NL, Norman AB, Richtand NM, et al. Olfactory receptor neurons express D2 dopamine receptors. J Comp Neurol 1999;411(4):666–673

90. Hegg CC, Greenwood D, Huang W, Han P, Lucero MT. Activation of purinergic receptor subtypes modulates odor sensitivity. J Neurosci 2003;23(23): 8291–8301

91. Rawson NE, Gomez G, Cowart B, Restrepo D. The use of olfactory receptor neurons (ORNs) from biopsies to study changes in aging and neurodegenerative diseases. Ann N Y Acad Sci 1998;855:701–707

92. Hahn CG, Gomez G, Restrepo D, et al. Aberrant intracellular calcium signaling in olfactory neurons from patients with bipolar disorder. Am J Psychiatry 2005;162(3):616–618

93. McCurdy RD, Féron F, Perry C, et al. Cell cycle alterations in biopsied olfactory neuroepithelium in schizophrenia and bipolar I disorder using cell culture and gene expression analyses. Schizophr Res 2006;82(2–3):163–173

94. Féron F, Perry C, Hirning MH, McGrath J, Mackay-Sim A. Altered adhesion, proliferation and death in neural cultures from adults with schizophrenia. Schizophr Res 1999;40(3):211–218

95. Ronnett GV, Leopold D, Cai X, et al. Olfactory biopsies demonstrate a defect in neuronal

development in Rett's syndrome. Ann Neurol 2003; 54(2):206–218

96. Féron F, Mackay-Sim A, Andrieu JL, Matthaei KI, Holley A, Sicard G. Stress induces neurogenesis in non-neuronal cell cultures of adult olfactory epithelium. Neuroscience 1999;88(2):571–583

97. Murrell W, Féron F, Wetzig A, et al. Multipotent stem cells from adult olfactory mucosa. Dev Dyn 2005;233(2):496–515

98. Mackay-Sim A. Stem cells and their niche in the adult olfactory mucosa. Arch Ital Biol 2010;148(2): 47–58

99. Sicard G, Féron F, Andrieu JL, Holley A, Mackay-Sim A. Generation of neurons from a nonneuronal precursor in adult olfactory epithelium in vitro. Ann N Y Acad Sci 1998;855:223–225

100. Tomé M, Lindsay SL, Riddell JS, Barnett SC. Identification of nonepithelial multipotent cells in the embryonic olfactory mucosa. Stem Cells 2009; 27(9):2196–2208

101. Delorme B, Nivet E, Gaillard J, et al. The human nose harbors a niche of olfactory ectomesenchymal stem cells displaying neurogenic and osteogenic properties. Stem Cells Dev 2010;19(6):853–866

3 Functional Anatomy of the Olfactory System II: Central Relays, Pathways, and their Function

Jessica Freiherr, Martin Wiesmann, Martin Witt

Introduction

The first steps of central olfactory processing are accomplished in phylogenetically old brain structures located in the basal forebrain and medial temporal lobe, which are activated simultaneously or consecutively. Higher order olfactory processes, including conscious olfactory perception, convergence, lateral inhibition, adaptation/habituation, and central integration of olfactory inputs with other sensory stimuli (e.g., gustatory, trigeminal, mechanosensory, auditory, and visual afferents), are mediated in the mentioned brain structures as well as in neocortical areas that are not specific for olfactory processing. Collectively, these processes enable an individual to create adequate reaction patterns to a changing external environment.

This chapter aims to provide insights into the anatomical brain structures involved in olfactory processing. Most canonical features of the central olfactory anatomy were studied in animals in a laboratory setting; data derived from observations in humans are mentioned when necessary. Moreover, the authors intend to link the respective functionality of a brain area to its anatomical features.

> **Key Hypotheses of Central Olfactory Processing**
> - In contrast to other ascending sensory systems, olfactory fibers project directly to the telencephalon, mainly without a thalamic relay. Thus, incoming olfactory information is not filtered and monitored in the thalamus before entering neocortical areas.
> - The main central gate for olfactory inputs is the olfactory bulb, in which the first topical map for odor representation is generated.
> - The olfactory system is organized in an anatomically unilateral manner. Very few, if any, canonical olfactory fibers use commissural tracts to enter contralateral brain areas.

> - Evidence of olfactory lateralization (i.e., representation of specific olfactory tasks within one hemisphere) is provided.

Outline of Olfactory Pathways

Olfactory pathways subdivide into bulbofugal fibers originating in the olfactory bulb (OB) and terminating in cortical areas and corticofugal fibers in reversed orientation (arising in the cortex and projecting to the OB). The latter probably mediate top-down modulation of olfactory perception at an early processing level.

Bulbofugal Fibers

Axons of olfactory receptor neurons (ORNs) collect into ~20 bundles, the *olfactory fila*, which pass through 1- to 2-mm-wide holes in the cribriform plate and connect to *mitral/tufted cells* in the OB. Collectively, these projections make up the *olfactory nerve (cranial nerve I)*. Axons of mitral/tufted cells form the *olfactory tract*. The fact that the olfactory tract divides into a medial, an intermedial, and a lateral portion, or stria, has been derived from animal observation and cannot be found in humans.[1] Therefore, in humans, the *lateral olfactory tract (LOT)* is considered the only projection from the OB terminating in a set of structures. The commonly used terminology, *primary/secondary/tertiary olfactory cortex*, for projection areas from the OB is somewhat misleading, as the OB already comprises typical cortical layers and accomplishes functional processes comparable to those of primary cortices in other modalities.[2] Therefore, in our opinion, the OB should be considered a *primary olfactory structure*. The target areas of the bulbar mitral/tufted cells as *secondary olfactory structures* are the *anterior olfactory nucleus (AON)*, *piriform cortex (pirC)*, *medial nuclei of the amygdala*, *periamygdaloid cortex*, and the *entorhinal cortex* (**Figs. 3.1 and 3.2**). The entorhinal cortex

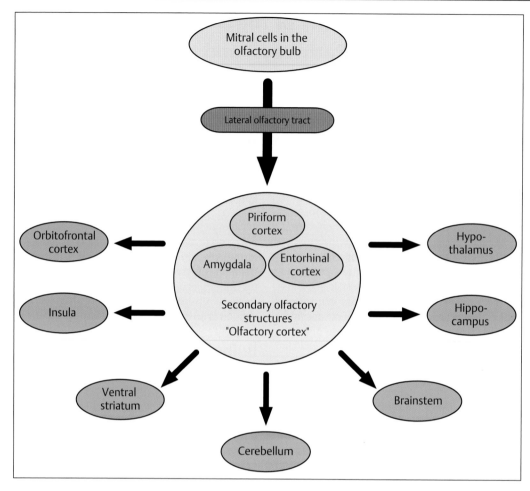

Fig. 3.1 Simplified schematic drawing of the essential bulbofugal olfactory pathways, deriving from mitral cells of the olfactory bulb. The lateral olfactory tract carries direct connections to secondary olfactory structures ("olfactory cortex"), before tertiary olfactory structures are reached. Contralateral projections and other afferents to the olfactory bulb are not indicated.

occupies the anterior part of the parahippocampal gyrus (Brodmann area 28), and probably targets an area underlying the anterior perforated substance, namely the *ventral striatum,* especially its major structure, *the nucleus accumbens.*[3] The entities of those areas are commonly named "olfactory cortex."

Fiber connections from the above-mentioned structures project to associated neocortical areas, *tertiary olfactory structures,* which are not exclusively specific olfactory areas: the *orbitofrontal gyri* and, in close proximity, the *anterior insula,* which is reached either directly or through a relay in the *dorsomedial thalamic nucleus.*[4] A series of either diencephalic or telencephalic structures is reached from the amygdala or entorhinal cortices, for example, *septal nuclei, bed nucleus of stria terminalis (BNST) in the hypothalamus, and hippocampal formation.*

Furthermore, a subset of mitral cell collaterals project from the anterior olfactory nucleus to the contralateral olfactory bulb using the anterior commissure.

> The entity of the olfactory fila in the olfactory epithelium in the upper nose is termed the *nervus olfactorius* or *first cranial nerve.*

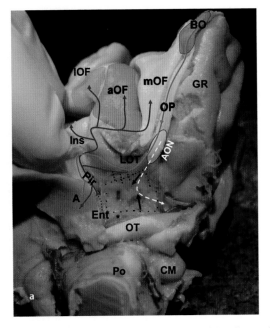

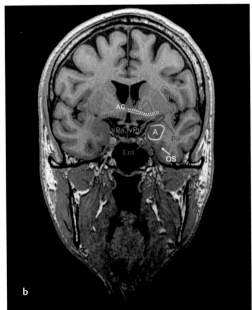

Fig. 3.2a, b Projections from the mitral cells of the olfactory bulb to central olfactory areas.

a Olfactory projections at the right human basal forebrain (top, anterior; right, medial). Most olfactory structures are visible on the surface of the brain without further dissection. The left hemisphere is removed. Red line indicates projections from the olfactory bulb (OB) via the lateral olfactory tract (LOT) to the piriform (Pir) and entorhinal (Ent) cortex and to the medial amygdala and periamygdalar cortex (A). From there, the blue line indicates projections into neocortical targets: insula (Ins) and orbitofrontal gyri (aOF, anterior; lOF, lateral; mOF, medial orbitofrontal gyrus), and probably to the ventral striatum (dotted blue lines dorsal to the anterior perforated substance, which is indicated by the dotted rectangle). The white dotted line indicates projections to the contralateral olfactory bulb via the anterior commissure. The anterior olfactory nucleus (AON) is situated diffusely within the oval of the olfactory peduncle (OP). CM, corpus mamillare; GR, rectal gyrus; OT, optical tract; Po, Pons. The asterisk anterior to the OT marks the diagonal band of Broca, carrying fibers from the amygdala to septal nuclei. The right temporal pole is somewhat repositioned to show the sharp bend of the olfactory tract into the piriform cortex and projections to the insula.

b Central olfactory projections and cortical areas overlaid on a structural T1-weighted magnetic resonance image (coronal plane at the anterior commissure [AC]). The lateral olfactory tract projects into the piriform cortex (Pir, red) and in medial amygdalar regions (A, yellow) ending in the entorhinal cortex (Ent, red). Underneath the striatum (CN, caudate nucleus; Pu, putamen) and pallidum (Pa), one can find the ventral pallidum (vPa) situated more medially and the ventral striatum (vPu) situated more laterally. OS, olfactory sulcus; Ins, insula.

Corticofugal Fibers

Though not entirely established in humans, animal data provide evidence for several glutamatergic, adrenergic, cholinergic, and serotonergic projections terminating in the AON and OB. They are believed to partly take the same route as the "medial olfactory tract (stria)" in animals, although its existence in humans has been questioned (see above). The functional significance of corticofugal fibers has not been investigated yet; however, they are assumed to mediate top-down modulation of olfactory information, such as olfactory learning or memory.[5]

Cortical Olfactory Areas and their Function

The First Olfactory Processing Relay: Olfactory Bulb

The OB is the first relay for incoming ORNs and is responsible for a condensation and amplification of olfactory information. It is located bilaterally upon the cribriform plate and is surrounded by the subarachnoid space filled with cerebrospinal fluid. In humans, its size varies considerably (ranging from 0.5 to 1.5 mm; **Fig. 3.3**) depending on indi-

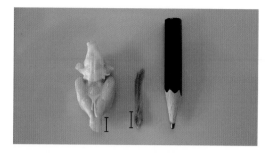

vidual olfactory performance.[6,7] As an extension of the prosencephalon, the OB presents a laminar structure that is similar to the laminar structure of cortical areas (**Fig. 3.4**). Occasionally, a vesicle may be preserved as a developmental relict.[8,9]

Fig. 3.3 Olfactory bulb (OB) of a rat (left) and a human brain (right). The absolute size of the human OB is very similar to that of the rat, but, in relation to the total brain mass (1500 g versus 2 g), rather small. (OBs delineated in brackets.)

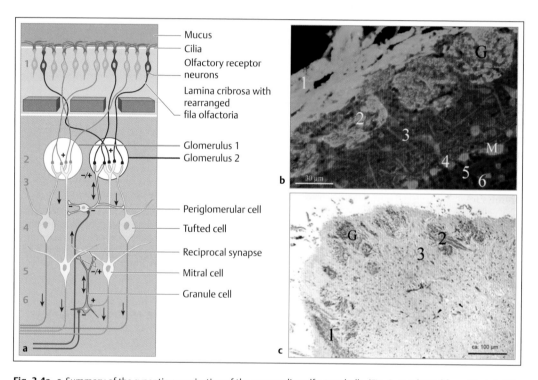

Fig. 3.4a–c Summary of the synaptic organization of the mammalian olfactory bulb. (Fig. 3.4a adapted from Mori et al.[2])

a Schematic organization of the olfactory bulb. Arabic numbers indicate the cortical structure: 1, nerve fiber layer; 2, glomerular layer; 3, external plexiform layer; 4, mitral/tufted cell layer; 5, internal plexiform layer; 6, granule cell layer. Glomerular coding: Axons of receptor cell expressing the same olfactory receptor project to only a few analogous glomeruli (e.g., "blue" olfactory receptor neurons converge with "blue" glomeruli). Efferent (bulbofugal, blue) fibers project from mitral/tufted cells to secondary olfactory structures; afferent (centrofugal, gray) fibers project either from contralateral mitral cells or ipsilateral central nuclei and synapse to glomerular or granule cells, respectively.

b,c Immunohistochemical features of the mouse (**b**) and human (**c**) olfactory bulb (OB). Arabic numbers again indicate the cortical structure (see (**a**)). Double immunofluorescence of the mouse OB (**b**) using antibodies against OMP (green) and the pan-neuronal marker PGP 9.5 (red) shows a more distinct lamination than in an 80-year-old human. OMP, reactive neurons or glomeruli; G, glomerulus; M, mitral cell.

Cell Layers

As mentioned above, the OB shows a cortical lamination. It mainly consists of the olfactory nerve layer, the glomerular layer, the internal plexiform layer, the mitral/tufted cell layer, the external plexiform layer, and the granule cell layer (**Fig. 3.4**). ORNs assemble on the OB´s surface and immerse in easily detectable spherical structures, *glomeruli*, in which they connect with dendrites of *mitral cells*. Glomeruli are surrounded by two major groups of inhibitory interneurons, *periglomerular cells* and short axon (SA) cells, which are responsible for fine tuning olfactory information mediated through mitral cells. The deepest cortex layer consists of columnar arrangements of another cell type—*granular cells*—derived from precursor neurons that migrate from the rostral migratory stream and the subventricular zone. The regenerative capacity of those interneurons is extraordinarily high. Genetic tracer studies suggest the arrival of ~30,000 new neurons per day in the OB.[10] However, only a subset of these neurons climbs up to convert to the interneurons mentioned above.[11] Both kinds of OB interneurons are also target neurons for inhibitory projections from the contralateral anterior olfactory nucleus through the anterior portion of the anterior commissure.

Convergence

From rodent studies it is known that several olfactory neurons expressing the same receptor converge onto two glomeruli. In consequence, a given odorant elicits a characteristic spatial pattern of glomerular activities,[12,13] initiating an odor-specific activation pattern already at the OB level. Odor-related spatial positions are conserved across different individuals of the same species. However, this topographic organization has not yet been demonstrated in neocortical brain areas.

Processes of GABAergic periglomerular cells project to a single glomerulus for intraglomerular processing, whereas GABA- and dopaminergic SA cells extend to multiple glomeruli, thus providing interglomerular crosstalk.[14] Local circuits among large projection neurons (mitral/tufted cells) and small OB interneurons mediate lateral inhibition among glomerular units to enhance contrast related to odor information that is forwarded to higher order olfactory structures.[2]

> The olfactory bulb is the first relay for incoming olfactory information. Lateral inhibition and convergence at the level of the olfactory bulb seem to be important for contrasting different olfactory perceptions against each other.

What is Special about the Human Olfactory Bulb?

Compared with laboratory animals, the volume of the human OB is much smaller relative to total brain size (**Figs. 3.3 and 3.5**). Furthermore, data obtained from 42 human autopsies (mean age 77 years) revealed a remarkable interindividual variability in OB size (mean: 83 μL; range: 50 to 142 μL).[8] As mentioned above, magnetic resonance imaging (MRI) studies revealed a strong correlation between OB size and olfactory performance.[6] However, precise information on wiring, presorting of individual ORNs in the periphery, and receptor-specific glomerular unit organization has not yet been determined in humans.

Besides this, the number of glomeruli in the human OB is considerably higher than animal models would predict. Animal studies provide evidence that ORNs expressing one particular receptor project to only two receptor-specific glomeruli. This 2:1 model (two glomeruli per receptor) assumes that if 1,000 functional receptor genes exist (as in mice), there are 2,000 glomeruli per OB.[15] In humans, however, who have only ~340 to 400 functional receptor genes,[16,17] one might predict 680 to 800 glomeruli, which is clearly contradicted by histomorphological estimations ranging from 2,975 to 9,325 glomeruli per human OB.[18,19] Thus the 2:1 ratio originating from other mammals is greater by a factor of eight (16:1) in humans. These results suggest that the convergence described for rodents or other mammals might be distinct from that in humans, pointing to a fundamental difference in human OB organization.[19]

> **Projection Targets of Mitral Cells in the Olfactory Bulb ("Secondary Olfactory Structures")**
> - Anterior olfactory nucleus
> - Anterior perforated substance and underlying ventral striatum (nucleus accumbens)
> - Piriform cortex
> - Periamygdalar cortex/medial amygdala
> - Entorhinal cortex

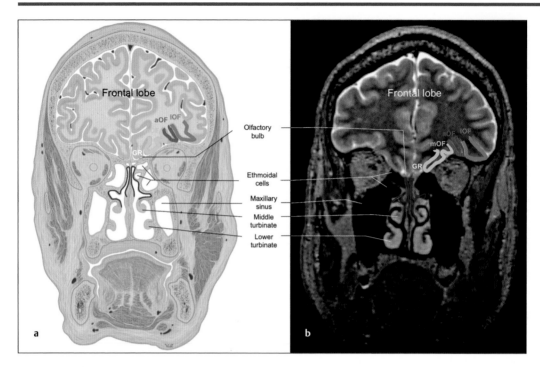

Fig. 3.5a, b Olfactory brain regions in the orbitofrontal area in a schematic drawing (**a**) and overlaid onto a structural, T2-weighted magnetic resonance image (**b**). The blue line delineates the olfactory epithelium in the upper turbinate of the human nose (aOF, anterior; lOF, lateral; mOF, medial orbitofrontal gyrus; GR, rectal gyrus). (Fig. 3.5a adapted from Schünke et al. 2007.[66])

Anterior Olfactory Nucleus as Inhibitor of Contralateral Information

The olfactory peduncle contains mitral cell axons bundled in the LOT and is situated laterally to the rectal gyrus and adjacent to the olfactory sulcus of the basal forebrain (**Fig. 3.2**). The term *olfactory peduncle* is usually used for describing the AON and the anterior part of the LOT as a whole.

The AON is a predominantly two-layered structure composed of neurons scattered across the course of the olfactory peduncle. It is the major relay for fibers to and from the contralateral OB. In contrast to ipsilateral connections, contralateral neuropeptide Y projections through the anterior commissure seem to decrease rapidly after birth in cats.[20] The significance of the AON for processing of olfactory stimuli is unclear. It is known that the AON mainly contains inhibitory fibers to enhance the contrast of ipsilateral olfactory information. Notably, the AON is one of the first nuclei affected in patients with Parkinson disease or multiple system atrophy.[21–23]

Anterior Perforated Substance and Underlying Ventral Striatum Mediate the Induction of Sexual Arousal via Olfactory Cues

The olfactory tubercle, a prominent structure in animals, is rarely distinguishable in humans. Instead, the anterior perforated substance (APS) might be considered as its human homologue (**Fig. 3.2a**). The APS is a three-layered cortex with characteristic cell clusters, the islands of Calleja. The function of the APS in humans is largely unknown. The ventral parts of the caudate nucleus, putamen, pallidum, and nucleus accumbens (brain areas that are situated adjacent to the APS) are conjointly referred to as the ventral striatum (**Fig. 3.2b**). As recently reviewed by Heimer's group,[3,24] animal studies point to a direct projection pathway from the olfactory cortex toward the basal ganglia (ventral striatum) rather than to the hypothalamus. The functional significance of this projection probably involves the mediation of sexual arousal elicited by learned olfactory cues.[5]

Different Levels of Cortical Processing Take Place in the Piriform Cortex

The piriform cortex (pirC) is a three-layered, pear-shaped allocortical structure spanning the junction of the medial frontal and temporal lobes. It is the main and most important projection area of mitral/tufted cell axons in the OB (**Fig. 3.2**). From here, projections terminate in subsequent subcortical areas via allocorticostriatal pathways into the ventral striatum and hypothalamus. Further neocortical olfactory areas include the insula and orbitofrontal gyri (see below).

Early olfactory neuroimaging experiments revealed that the pirC is involved in basic processing of passive olfactory stimulation.[25-28] However, the recent development of modern olfactometry, as well as functional neuroimaging methods and study designs, has enabled researchers to provide further insights, leading to a change of concept regarding the function of the pirC. It has been shown that the pirC can be subdivided into an anterior, or frontal, and a posterior, or temporal, portion, and, although histologically similar, these portions show a functional heterogeneity.[29] They are involved in different olfactory processing steps. While the anterior portion is considered primarily to be involved in basic or low level olfactory processing such as passive smelling and encoding of the chemical or molecular structure of an odorant, the posterior portion is rather responsible for higher order olfactory processing such as hedonic quality evaluation or discrimination and encoding of the perceptual character of an odorant.[30-33] The pirC, as a prominent target structure of OB afferents, is also critically involved in olfactory memory and learning as well as multisensory integration processes. The results of a recent meta-analysis[34] imply that the piriform cortex is consistently activated across a set of olfactory functional imaging experiments (**Fig. 3.6**).

The Amygdala Encodes Behavioral Salience of an Odor

Olfactory projections pass either directly or via pirC to a superficially located subdivision of the amygdala, the periamygdalar complex, and to the anterior cortical nucleus of the amygdala (**Fig. 3.2a**). Deeper subnuclei are not directly linked to LOT projections. In animals, amygdalar structures not only coordinate the mediation of aggressive and predator behavior, but also are linked to sexual development and olfactory recognition of offspring.[35] Amygdalar nuclei are also canonical targets of vomeronasal input in most animal species.[36] As the existence of a vomeronasal system in humans is questionable (see Chapter 4), stimuli processed via the olfactory system may contribute to gender-specific reactions to odorants or pheromone-like substances.[37] It is known that the anterior cortical nucleus and the periamygdaloid complex are highly responsive to odorants.[36] Some authors have connected the function of the centromedial amygdalar nuclei with that of the BNST,[38] a hypothalamic nucleus involved in a neuronal circuit also involving the OB, anterior piriform cortex, and preoptic area.

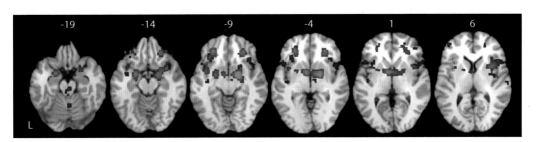

Fig. 3.6 The results of a meta-analysis of functional imaging studies using the technique of activation likelihood estimation.[34] Depicted are brain areas that are commonly recruited owing to trigeminal stimulation (red) and pure olfactory stimulation (blue). Typical olfactory brain areas are the piriform cortex (bilaterally in slice −14), orbitofrontal cortex (bilaterally in slice −9), and insula (bilaterally in slice 6). (Adapted from Albrecht 2010.[34])

Several research teams used functional imaging techniques to answer the important question of whether the amygdala is involved in coding odor intensity or valence.[39–42] The results of their studies suggest that the amygdala encodes the behavioral salience of an olfactory stimulus, and thus a combination of intensity and valence is important.[43] There is also evidence that the amygdala is involved in associative learning along with olfactory memory.[29]

Entorhinal Cortex: A Gate for Olfactory Memory

The entorhinal cortex is the most distant target area of LOT axons (**Fig. 3.2**) and constitutes a transition zone from three-layered allocortex into six-layered neocortex. Its strongest projection turns into the hippocampal formation. Therefore, it is assumed that the entorhinal cortex is involved in olfactory memory processes. Results of a functional MRI (fMRI) study reveal that activation of the entorhinal cortex correlates with perceived intensity of olfactory stimuli and thus is considered to be involved in a gating process of intense olfactory stimuli to the hippocampus.[44] The entorhinal cortex shows specific neuropathologies in Alzheimer disease.[45]

Projection Targets of Secondary Olfactory Structures

- Insula
- Orbitofrontal cortex
- Ventral striatum (e.g., nucleus accumbens)
- Hippocampus
- Septal nuclei
- Hypothalamus (bed nucleus of stria terminalis, preoptic area)

The Insula is Responsible for Integration of Different Chemosensory Stimuli

The insula is an agranular cortical area buried in the depths of the lateral sulcus and overlaid by opercula ("lids") from the frontal, parietal, and temporal lobes (**Fig. 3.2**). The anterior part of the insula in particular is considered to be the primary taste cortex. Nevertheless, in rats, the insula receives olfactory projections either directly from the pirC or indirectly through a thalamic relay.[46] In humans, fMRI and positron emission tomography (PET) studies show activation of the anterior insula in relation to odorant stimulation.[47] The precise role of the insula in odor processing remains somewhat unclear. Results of a recent meta-analysis support the view that the insula plays an important role during the integration of olfaction with other chemosensory modalities.[33] The authors reviewed scientific literature and submitted the results of all functional neuroimaging experiments utilizing (1) olfactory, (2) trigeminal, and (3) gustatory stimulation to an activation likelihood estimation (ALE) meta-analysis. A conjunction of the three ALE maps representing the brain areas that are recruited across all studies in the three modalities reveals that a part of the anterior insula is recruited during all three conditions (**Fig. 3.7**). Thus it seems highly likely that the anterior portion of the insula is responsible for integration of different chemosensory experiences.

The Orbitofrontal Cortex is the Integration Site with Other Sensory Modalities

The orbitofrontal gyri interposed between the rectal gyrus medially and the insula laterally are considered to compose the orbitofrontal cortex (OFC; **Figs. 3.2a** and **3.5**). It consists of an agranular (five-layered) cortex and receives direct input mainly from the pirC and indirect input via the thalamus. Although data from tracer studies in humans are not available, reports from monkey studies suggest a very early stage of olfactory information processing, in conjunction with adjacent gustatory and visual processing areas in frontal portions of the OFC.[29,48] Projections from and to other brain regions are extensive, especially for integration of several sensory modalities. The integrative function of the OFC is probably involved in generating the sensation of flavor associated with different foods.[48,49] The OFC is considered to be involved in olfactory working memory and discrimination processes.[50] In addition, recognition and reward value of an odor is represented in the OFC.[51,52]

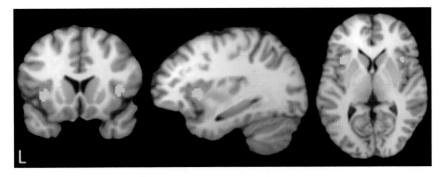

Fig. 3.7 Results of a recent activation likelihood estimation (ALE) meta-analysis[33] investigating common brain activation across all olfactory, trigeminal, and gustatory functional imaging studies. The conjunction of all three ALE maps reveals that the anterior portion of the insula is important for processing of stimuli in all three modalities (yellow). Thus it is suggested that the anterior insula is involved in multisensory integration processes. (Adapted from Lundström et al. 2011.[33])

> For illustration of cortical processes during smell perception in humans, imaging techniques such as fMRI, electroencephalography, or PET, in combination with constant flow olfactometry, are used. The development of sophisticated statistical analysis tools such as voxel-based morphometry, independent component analysis, dynamical causal modeling, and ALE warrants further insights.

Non-Specific Olfactory Brain Regions

Functional imaging records reveal that many other brain areas are activated by olfactory stimuli, without a direct anatomical link to primary olfactory structures.[53] The pathways appear diffuse and include neocortical areas as well as, for example, the cerebellum, which seems to play a role in motor control of olfaction. One hypothesis suggests that sniffing activity is regulated by a feedback mechanism using data on odor concentration.[53]

Functional Characteristics of Olfactory Processing

The Role of the Thalamus in Olfaction—More Important than Previously Thought

Common anatomical work in animals and humans implies no direct thalamic activity during central olfactory processing. Canonical pathways include only two relays from ORNs via mitral/tufted cells into the piriform cortex, and from there directly into mainly medial and lateral OFC projection areas without further synapse.

However, several animal models suggest at least one indirect connection between the piriform cortex and neocortical areas (OFC) via the medioposterior thalamic nucleus, but this route seems less important than direct pathways, as it contains considerably fewer fibers.[54] The first evidence of a more important thalamic interaction with odor processing was found during an fMRI study[55] and recently during an investigation utilizing multisensory stimulation.[4] Both studies suggest that attention to smells enhances the participation of the thalamocortical pathway, which appears to be a modulatory target of olfactory attentional processing.

As to the necessity of a thalamic interneuron in olfaction, one might assign computational issues such as convergence and sorting out olfactory information ("bottleneck functions") as key tasks of the OB and thus compare its activity to that of the thalamus in other sensory systems.[56]

Task-specific Odor Processing

The number and size of secondary olfactory structures is tremendous, including the olfactory nucleus, cortical nuclei of amygdala, periamygdalar complex, anterior and posterior pirC, entorhinal area, and the anterior perforated substance with adjacent ventral striatum (or the olfactory tubercle as its homologue in animals), not to mention all tertiary neocortical, diencephalic, and brainstem areas targeted by projections of the former regions. One should wonder if, after sniffing a simple odor, the entire brain might be involved and occupied with processing this particular sensation. Certainly, it is not. An approach to determine the specialization of diverse olfactory-related brain areas was introduced by measuring the effects of task-specific stimulation. There are, for example, hemispheric differences in perception of familiar/unfamiliar or pleasant/unpleasant stimuli. The left hemisphere is more engaged in processing familiar odors, and the right hemisphere in that of unpleasant odors.[57] Further, olfactory detection, discrimination, and memory recovery from experience implies the hierarchical recruitment of different structural and functional relays within the olfactory system.[58]

Lateralization

As previously introduced, there is some evidence for olfactory lateralization (i.e., specific olfactory tasks are represented in one hemisphere). Olfactory nerve fibers project ipsilaterally up to the level of the pirC (see above). The anatomical substrate for lateralized cortical odorant processing seems to be the anterior part of the anterior commissure, but proof of this possibility is still lacking. A recently published, event-related source imaging study provides evidence that olfactory information is processed in different steps, starting with ipsilateral activation of the amygdala, parahippocampal gyrus, superior temporal gyrus, and insula. Subsequently, the corresponding contralateral structures are activated and, finally, frontal areas of both hemispheres are involved.[59] Accordingly, monorhinally presented odorants activate bilateral higher order brain areas independent of the side of presentation.[57,59] In patients with Parkinson disease, neuronal activity in the right amygdala and hippocampus seems to be diminished, and it is assumed that the selective impairment within these brain areas causes the olfactory dysfunction.[60] In our opinion, olfactory lateralization effects should be carefully considered in the context of the interconnectivity of the nasal, oral, and pharyngeal cavities, which renders a pure unilateral olfactory stimulation almost impossible.

Adaptation – Habituation

Adaptation

In the periphery, a long-lasting olfactory stimulus leads to a decreased response of ORNs. Intracellular calcium ions (Ca^{2+}) interact with calmodulin and calmodulin kinase II. As soon as the Ca^{2+}/calmodulin complex has bound to cyclic nucleotide-gated channels, the latter decrease their sensitivity to cyclic adenosine monophosphate (cAMP) and close again. This results in a diminished number of action potentials despite a successful ligand–receptor interaction, which is equal to adaptation. The contribution of the enzyme phosphodiesterase-1c2, which catalyzes cAMP, has been recently questioned.[61] Short-term adaptation is defined as a decrease in excitability during a short odor presentation within a few seconds. Also, a longer adaptation (over minutes) has been observed.[62] The duration of adaptation depends on the activity of the Na^+/Ca^{2+} exchanger complex, which transports Ca^{2+} out of the cell. Adaptation occurs in peripheral ORNs, but it has been shown that desensitization is smaller than the decrease of intensity estimates.[63] The pirC might therefore play a more important role in adaptation than the OB or the olfactory receptors. The pirC processes information from mitral cells of the OB and might react with a temporary synaptic depression (cortical adaptation).[64]

Habituation

In contrast to peripheral or central adaptation, the term *habituation* implies a more complex, central, multineuronal learning process, which protects the organism against persistent, "non-important" signals from its environment. It is dependent on the input of olfactory signals, but also employs a series of non-olfactory circuits, such as brainstem nuclei involved in cardiovascular regulation.[65] This phenomenon ("sensory gating") may be triggered by various stimuli or by cortical desensitization.

> The piriform cortex seems to play a more important role in adaptation processes than olfactory receptor cells or the olfactory bulb.

References

1. Sakamoto N, Pearson J, Shinoda K, Alheid GF, de Olmos JS, Heimer L. The human basal forebrain. Part I. An overview. In: Bloom FE, Björklund A, Hökfelt T, eds. Handbook of Chemical Neuroanatomy, Vol. 15: The Primate Nervous System, Part III: Elsevier Science BV; 1999:1–13.

2. Mori K, Nagao N, Yoshihara Y. The olfactory bulb: coding and processing of odor molecule information. Science 1999;286(5440):711–715

3. Heimer L. Basal forebrain in the context of schizophrenia. Brain Res Brain Res Rev 2000;31(2–3): 205–235

4. Plailly J, Howard JD, Gitelman DR, Gottfried JA. Attention to odor modulates thalamocortical connectivity in the human brain. J Neurosci 2008; 28(20):5257–5267

5. Talbot K, Woolf NJ, Butcher LL. Feline islands of Calleja complex: II. Cholinergic and cholinesterasic features. J Comp Neurol 1988;275(4):580–603

6. Buschhüter D, Smitka M, Puschmann S, et al. Correlation between olfactory bulb volume and olfactory function. Neuroimage 2008;42(2):498–502

7. Gudziol V, Buschhüter D, Abolmaali N, Gerber J, Rombaux P, Hummel T. Increasing olfactory bulb volume due to treatment of chronic rhinosinusitis—a longitudinal study. Brain 2009; 132(Pt 11):3096–3101

8. Smitka M, Abolmaali N, Witt M, et al. Olfactory bulb ventricles as a frequent finding in magnetic resonance imaging studies of the olfactory system. Neuroscience 2009;162(2):482–485

9. Curtis MA, Kam M, Nannmark U, et al. Human neuroblasts migrate to the olfactory bulb via a lateral ventricular extension. Science 2007;315(5816): 1243–1249

10. Lledo PM, Alonso M, Grubb MS. Adult neurogenesis and functional plasticity in neuronal circuits. Nat Rev Neurosci 2006;7(3):179–193

11. Winner B, Cooper-Kuhn CM, Aigner R, Winkler J, Kuhn HG. Long-term survival and cell death of newly generated neurons in the adult rat olfactory bulb. Eur J Neurosci 2002;16(9):1681–1689

12. Mori K, Takahashi YK, Igarashi KM, Yamaguchi M. Maps of odorant molecular features in the Mammalian olfactory bulb. Physiol Rev 2006;86(2): 409–433

13. Stewart WB, Kauer JS, Shepherd GM. Functional organization of rat olfactory bulb analysed by the 2-deoxyglucose method. J Comp Neurol 1979; 185(4):715–734

14. Parrish-Aungst S, Kiyokage E, Szabo G, Yanagawa Y, Shipley MT, Puche AC. Sensory experience selectively regulates transmitter synthesis enzymes in interglomerular circuits. Brain Res 2011;1382:70–76

15. Mombaerts P. Odorant receptor gene choice in olfactory sensory neurons: the one receptor–one neuron hypothesis revisited. Curr Opin Neurobiol 2004;14(1):31–36

16. Malnic B, Godfrey PA, Buck LB. The human olfactory receptor gene family. Proc Natl Acad Sci U S A 2004;101(8):2584–2589

17. Olender T, Lancet D, Nebert DW. Update on the olfactory receptor (OR) gene superfamily. Hum Genomics 2008;3(1):87–97

18. Meisami E. A new morphometric method to estimate the total number of glomeruli in the olfactory bulb. Chem Senses 1990;15:407–418

19. Maresh A, Rodriguez Gil D, Whitman MC, Greer CA. Principles of glomerular organization in the human olfactory bulb—implications for odor processing. PLoS ONE 2008;3(7):e2640

20. Sanides-Kohlrausch C, Wahle P. Morphology of neuropeptide Y–immunoreactive neurons in the cat olfactory bulb and olfactory peduncle: postnatal development and species comparison. J Comp Neurol 1990;291(3):468–489

21. Pearce RK, Hawkes CH, Daniel SE. The anterior olfactory nucleus in Parkinson's disease. Mov Disord 1995;10(3):283–287

22. Kovács T, Papp MI, Cairns NJ, Khan MN, Lantos PL. Olfactory bulb in multiple system atrophy. Mov Disord 2003;18(8):938–942

23. Witt M, Bormann K, Gudziol V, et al. Biopsies of olfactory epithelium in patients with Parkinson's disease. Mov Disord 2009;24(6):906–914

24. de Olmos JS, Heimer L. The concepts of the ventral striatopallidal system and extended amygdala. Ann N Y Acad Sci 1999;877:1–32

25. Zatorre RJ, Jones-Gotman M, Evans AC, Meyer E. Functional localization and lateralization of human olfactory cortex. Nature 1992;360(6402):339–340

26. Savic I, Berglund H. Passive perception of odors and semantic circuits. Hum Brain Mapp 2004; 21(4):271–278

27. Bengtsson S, Berglund H, Gulyas B, Cohen E, Savic I. Brain activation during odor perception in males and females. Neuroreport 2001;12(9):2027–2033

28. Weismann M, Yousry I, Heuberger E, et al. Functional magnetic resonance imaging of human olfaction. Neuroimaging Clin N Am 2001;11(2):237–250, viii

29. Gottfried JA. Smell: central nervous processing. Adv Otorhinolaryngol 2006;63:44–69

30. Gottfried JA, Winston JS, Dolan RJ. Dissociable codes of odor quality and odorant structure in human piriform cortex. Neuron 2006;49(3):467–479

31. Howard JD, Plailly J, Grueschow M, Haynes JD, Gottfried JA. Odor quality coding and categorization in human posterior piriform cortex. Nat Neurosci 2009;12(7):932–938

32. Gottfried JA. Central mechanisms of odour object perception. Nat Rev Neurosci 2010;11(9):628–641

33. Lundström JN, Boesveldt S, Albrecht J. Central processing of the chemical senses: an overview. ACS Chem Neurosci 2011;2(1):5–16

34. Albrecht J, Kopietz R, Frasnelli J, Wiesmann M, Hummel T, Lundström JN. The neuronal correlates of intranasal trigeminal function—an ALE meta-analysis of human functional brain imaging data. Brain Res Brain Res Rev 2010;62(2):183–196

35. Heimer L. A new anatomical framework for neuropsychiatric disorders and drug abuse. Am J Psychiatry 2003;160(10):1726–1739

36. Aggleton JP, Saunders RC. The amygdala—what's happened in the last decade? 1.4 The amygdala

and olfactory processing. In: Aggleton JP, ed. The Amygdala. 2nd ed. New York: Oxford University Press; 2000:8–15.

37. Wysocki CJ, Preti G, Larry RS. Pheromones in mammals. In: Encyclopedia of Neuroscience. Oxford: Academic Press; 2009:625–632.

38. Swaab DF. Chapter 7 Bed nucleus of the stria terminalis (BST) and the septum. In: Handbook of Clinical Neurology: Elsevier; 2003:149–162.

39. Zald DH. The human amygdala and the emotional evaluation of sensory stimuli. Brain Res Brain Res Rev 2003;41(1):88–123

40. Hudry J, Perrin F, Ryvlin P, Mauguière F, Royet JP. Olfactory short-term memory and related amygdala recordings in patients with temporal lobe epilepsy. Brain 2003;126(Pt 8):1851–1863

41. Gottfried JA, Deichmann R, Winston JS, Dolan RJ. Functional heterogeneity in human olfactory cortex: an event-related functional magnetic resonance imaging study. J Neurosci 2002;22(24):10819–10828

42. Anderson AK, Christoff K, Stappen I, et al. Dissociated neural representations of intensity and valence in human olfaction. Nat Neurosci 2003;6(2):196–202

43. Winston JS, Gottfried JA, Kilner JM, Dolan RJ. Integrated neural representations of odor intensity and affective valence in human amygdala. J Neurosci 2005;25(39):8903–8907

44. Zald DH, Pardo JV. Functional neuroimaging of the olfactory system in humans. Int J Psychophysiol 2000;36(2):165–181

45. Thompson MD, Knee K, Golden CJ. Olfaction in persons with Alzheimer's disease. Neuropsychol Rev 1998;8(1):11–23

46. Price JL. Olfactory system. In: Paxinos G, ed. The Human Nervous System. San Diego: Academic Press; 1990:979–1001.

47. Yousem DM, Maldjian JA, Hummel T, et al. The effect of age on odor-stimulated functional MR imaging. AJNR Am J Neuroradiol 1999;20(4):600–608

48. Ongür D, Price JL. The organization of networks within the orbital and medial prefrontal cortex of rats, monkeys and humans. Cereb Cortex 2000;10(3):206–219

49. Small DM, Gerber JC, Mak YE, Hummel T. Differential neural responses evoked by orthonasal versus retronasal odorant perception in humans. Neuron 2005;47(4):593–605

50. Plailly J, Radnovich AJ, Sabri M, Royet JP, Kareken DA. Involvement of the left anterior insula and frontopolar gyrus in odor discrimination. Hum Brain Mapp 2007;28(5):363–372

51. Rolls ET. Convergence of sensory systems in the orbitofrontal cortex in primates and brain design for emotion. Anat Rec A Discov Mol Cell Evol Biol 2004;281(1):1212–1225

52. Rolls ET. The functions of the orbitofrontal cortex. Brain Cogn 2004;55(1):11–29

53. Sobel N, Johnson BN, Mainland JD. Functional neuroimaging of human olfaction. In: Doty RL, ed. Handbook of Olfaction and Gustation. New York, Basel: Marcel Dekker, Inc; 2003:251–273.

54. Price JL. Beyond the primary olfactory cortex: olfactory-related areas in the neocortex, thalamus and hypothalamus. Chem Senses 1985;10:239–258

55. Sobel N, Prabhakaran V, Zhao Z, et al. Time course of odorant-induced activation in the human primary olfactory cortex. J Neurophysiol 2000;83(1):537–551

56. Kay LM, Sherman SM. An argument for an olfactory thalamus. Trends Neurosci 2007;30(2):47–53

57. Savic I. Brain imaging studies of the functional organization of human olfaction. Neuroscientist 2002;8(3):204–211

58. Savic I, Gulyas B, Larsson M, Roland P. Olfactory functions are mediated by parallel and hierarchical processing. Neuron 2000;26(3):735–745

59. Lascano AM, Hummel T, Lacroix J-S, Landis BN, Michel CM. Spatio-temporal dynamics of olfactory processing in the human brain: an event-related source imaging study. Neuroscience 2010;167(3):700–708

60. Westermann B, Wattendorf E, Schwerdtfeger U, et al. Functional imaging of the cerebral olfactory system in patients with Parkinson's disease. J Neurol Neurosurg Psychiatry 2008;79(1):19–24

61. Dougherty DP, Wright GA, Yew AC. Computational model of the cAMP-mediated sensory response and calcium-dependent adaptation in vertebrate olfactory receptor neurons. Proc Natl Acad Sci U S A 2005;102(30):10415–10420

62. Hummel T, Knecht M, Kobal G. Peripherally obtained electrophysiological responses to olfactory stimulation in man: electro-olfactograms exhibit a smaller degree of desensitization compared with subjective intensity estimates. Brain Res 1996;717(1–2):160–164

63. Linster C, Henry L, Kadohisa M, Wilson DA. Synaptic adaptation and odor-background segmentation. Neurobiol Learn Mem 2007;87(3):352–360

64. Yadon CA, Wilson DA. The role of metabotropic glutamate receptors and cortical adaptation in habituation of odor-guided behavior. Learn Mem 2005;12(6):601–605

65. Schünke E, Schulte E, Schumacher U. Prometheus—Kopf und Neuroanatomie. Stuttgart: Thieme; 2007.

4 The Human Vomeronasal System

Martin Witt, Michael Meredith

One of the most intriguing chemosensory subsystems in humans is the "vomeronasal organ" (VNO). Since its discovery in man by Frederic Ruysch in 1703[1] and more systematic observations in domesticated animals by Ludwig Lewin Jacobson in 1811, few organs have undergone more illustrious functional interpretations than the VNO. One of the most common misunderstandings concerning its functionality reflects inappropriate analogies with nonhuman vertebrates with respect to influences on social and sexual behavior.

In many nonhuman mammals, the VNO is a complex of different component structures that detects specific chemical communication signals (commonly referred to as pheromones) and conveys the information to the central nervous system.

The Vomeronasal Organ is Functional in Many Nonhuman Vertebrates and has Defined Components

The VNO is present in most amphibians, reptiles, and mammals, but is lacking in some successful phylogenetic groups, such as crocodiles, birds, or marine mammals. The anatomy of the VNO varies considerably among the different classes. Except in amphibians, the VNO is anatomically separated from the main olfactory epithelium. It is composed of different tissues and entities, such as the vomeronasal duct (VND), seromucous glands, the vomeronasal nerve, a vomeronasal capsule, and a venous pumping system (**Fig. 4.1**).[2] The VND in rodents is a blind-ending channel running in the lower nasal septum parallel to the floor of the nasal cavity. On its medial side it is lined with a pseudostratified sensory epithelium that contains sensory neurons, supporting cells, and basal cells, a cellular organization similar to that of the main olfactory epithelium. The vomeronasal epithelium (VNE) is much thicker and contains two main types of vomeronasal sensory neurons, which express two families of vomeronasal receptor genes: guanosine triphosphate–binding proteins

(G-proteins); and TRPC2 transduction-channel proteins. These, and olfactory marker protein (OMP, **Fig. 4.1b**), are components of the accepted (canonical) vomeronasal transduction pathway, but they are missing in humans. The axons of vomeronasal sensory neurons project to the accessory olfactory bulb (AOB),[3] which is also missing in humans. AOB output passes principally to the medial nucleus of the amygdala, which integrates chemosensory and hormonal information,[4] and is thought to interpret the meaning of chemical signals.[5] Outputs from the medial amygdala, and from other nuclei receiving independent AOB input, are directed to hypothalamic and preoptic nuclei, the control centers for neuroendocrine functions and social behavior.[6–8] Several volatile and nonvolatile compounds in mouse urine and various skin secretions stimulate specific VNO sensory neurons,[9] but data linking particular ligands to specific receptors are still scarce.

Anatomy of the Vomeronasal System in Humans

Prenatal Development and Regression in Humans: "Classical" Vomeronasal Organ Structure Suggests Possibility of Prenatal Function

Development

Initial vomeronasal structures in staged human embryos are observed between weeks 4 and 5 (Carnegie stages 13 to 15[10]; **Fig. 4.1**). The medial epithelium of the olfactory placode gives rise to the vomeronasal neurons, nervus terminalis, cells expressing gonadotrophin releasing hormone (GnRH), and some further neurons.[11,12] Vomeronasal and terminalis ganglia appear around stages 18 and 19 as clusters of protein gene product 9.5 (PGP 9.5)–immunoreactive cells migrating out of the epithelium (**Fig. 4.2a, c**). Vomeronasal and olfactory axons start to grow into the primitive

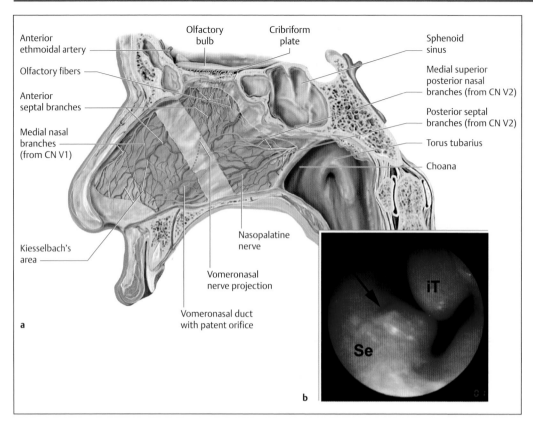

Fig. 4.1a, b The vomeronasal duct in adult humans.

a Location of the vomeronasal duct in adult humans. The dotted line indicates the vomeronasal nerve projection (absent in humans). There is no accessory olfactory bulb. CN V1, cranial nerve V1; CN V2, cranial nerve V2. (Modified from Schünke et al. Thieme Atlas of Anato-

my. Head, Neck and Neuroanatomy. Stuttgart, New York: Thieme; 2007: 116.)

b Endoscopy of the left nasal cavity showing the orifice of the vomeronasal duct (arrow). Se, anterior nasal septum; iT, inferior turbinate.

Fig. 4.2a–d Immunohistochemical features of the human vomeronasal duct (VND). ▷

a Human VND during delevopment, approximately week 8. Immunohistochemical reaction with an antibody against protein gene product 9.5 (black reaction product; PGP 9.5) shows clusters of immunopositive ganglion cells (outwandered epithelial cells; small arrows) and the vomeronasal nerve (or terminal nerve?) close to the vomeronasal duct (large arrows) running in the septal mucosa. Olf, olfactory cleft, lined with PGP 9.5–immunoreactive olfactory epithelium; Se, nasal septum (cartilage). Scale bar: 200 µm.

b In comparison, a frontal section of the nasal septum in a newborn rat reacted with an antibody against olfactory marker protein (brownish reaction product; OMP). The crescent-shaped vomeronasal duct exhibits a lateral nonsensory and a medial sensory epithelium. The latter possesses two levels of OMP-positive cells, superficially and basally located. They project to

different regions in the accessory olfactory bulb. Scale bar: 200 µm.

c Detail of the developing human vomeronasal duct from (**a**). PGP 9.5–immunoreactive cells with dendritic processes (arrowheads) and cluster-like formation of ganglion cells in the lamina propria (arrows) shows structural prerequisites for prenatal function.

d Vomeronasal epithelium in an aged human vomeronasal duct after autopsy. The immunoreactivity against caveolin 1, an integral membrane protein involved in receptor-independent endocytosis, shows slender, bipolar, neuron-like cells (arrowheads), but never reactivity to classical neuron markers. This mirrors the somewhat enigmatic nature of this apparently highly specialized epithelium. Counterstain with haematoxylin. Scale bar: 10 µm.

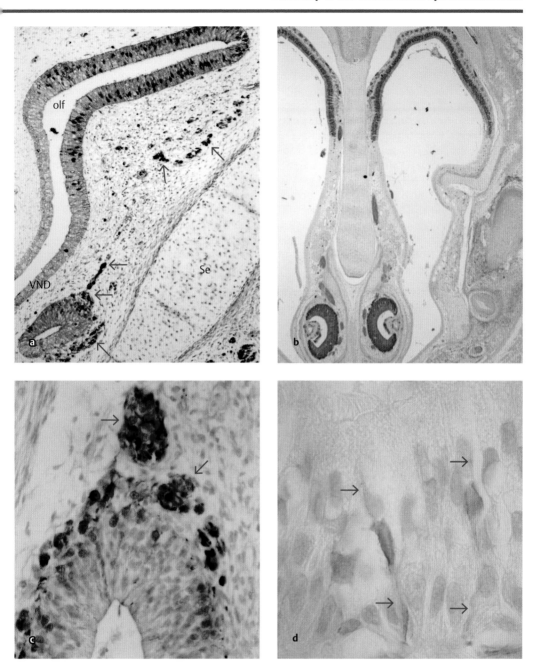

Fig. 4.2a–d

olfactory bulb, and GnRH cells begin to migrate to the hypothalamus, following vomeronasal or nervus terminalis substructures. They normally begin reaching the median eminence by week 8, but some cells may remain along the migration pathway.[13] An intriguing connection between olfaction and sex becomes apparent if GnRH cells fail to reach the hypothalamus, resulting in hypogonadotrophic hypogonadism, often associated with anosmia (Kallmann syndrome).[14,15] Around week 8, a VND similar to that seen in rodents becomes visible (**Fig. 4.1a**). This duct is lined by neuroepithelial cells reactive for neurotubulin, neural cell adhesion molecule, and PGP 9.5, but not for OMP, a reliable marker for functional olfactory and rodent vomeronasal neurons. In contrast to rodents, humans do not form a clearly separate AOB.[16,17]

Regression

Usually the connection of the neuroepithelium with central nervous system structures degenerates before week 28. There are a few reports of the persistence of the vomeronasal nerve and appropriate G_o- and G_i-positive epithelial cells until the late fetal period,[18] but, lacking other important components, these are probably not functional. The vomeronasal nerve has been described as present until the sixth fetal month,[19] and "vestigial remains" were inconsistently observed until week 18.5.[16] The closure of the vomeronasal duct was interpreted as a sign of "degeneration,"[20] but, in most individuals, the duct remains open to different extents (see below). However, the timing of disconnection of the nerve from epithelial cells has not yet been described.

Most Vomeronasal Organ–related Structures have Disappeared in Adult Humans

Most constituents of the VNO are no longer detectable at birth in humans. The only remaining structure is the VND, which exhibits considerable variability in shape, size, and even presence or detectability. The VND is situated superior to the paraseptal cartilage and runs smoothly craniodorsally. The opening of the VND is less than 2 mm in diameter, sometimes pigmented a brownish-yellow (**Fig. 4.2**). Generally described as a blind-ending duct or a mucosal pouch located in the anterior nasal septum, its length varies between 3 and 22 mm.[17] The frequency of detection depends strongly on the technique of investigation: histological studies reveal a higher percentage of VNDs than rhinoscopic or endoscopic investigations (**Table 4.1**).[29] Unlike in rodents, there is no difference between the two sides of the duct with regard to a possible "sensory" and "nonsensory" epithelium. Histologically, the epithelium of the VND contains portions of sensory-like formations, but neuronal markers are no longer expressed, and nor are there any nerve terminals left in the vicinity of the epithelium.[30] Taken together, the vomeronasal epithelium of the adult human VND expresses highly specialized histochemical features; however, it does not provide the essential requirements for classical neuroepithelial information transfer into the brain. Owing to its exposed location in the anterior septum, the VND can easily be damaged during nasoseptal or orthognatic surgery. Despite occasional anecdotal reports and speculation (e.g., Foltán and Sedý 2009[31]), there are no studies that provide measurable functional evidence that VND damage leads to behavioral changes after nasoseptal surgery.

Evidence For and Against a Functioning Human Vomeronasal Organ

Are There Human Pheromones?

Chemical compounds that convey information from one individual to another of the same species are commonly called pheromones. By original definition (notably in insects which lack a morphological VNO), these are, "substances which are secreted to the outside by an individual and received by a second individual of the same species, in which they release a specific reaction, e.g., a definite behaviour or a developmental process."[32] The mediation of chemosensory signals in social and sexual behavior has been widely documented in animals.[33] A similar function seems likely in humans but has been less widely documented (reviewed by Grammer et al 2005[34]):

- Meredith[35] proposes restricting the definition for *pheromone* by including a requirement for mutual benefit to sender and receiver, putting

Table 4.1 Frequency of vomeronasal duct in adult humans varies according to the investigation technique

Reference	N	Frequency
Potiquet 1891[21]	200	25%
Johnson et al 1985[22]	100	Patients 39% (endoscopy) Postmortem specimens 70% (histology)
Stensaas et al 1991[23]	410	93%
Moran et al 1991[24]	200	100% bilateral
Garcia-Velasco and Mondragon 1991[25]	1,000	90%
Trotier et al 2000[26]	1,842	Patients 26% (endoscopy)
Gaafar et al 1998[27]	200	Patients 76% (endoscopy)
Won et al 2000[28]	78	36%
Knecht et al 2001[29]	173	65% (41% bilateral, 24% unilateral; endoscopy)
Witt et al 2002[30]	25	65% (histology)

pheromone communication in an evolutionary context. The communication function, if any, for example of human odor response, is obscure, so these would not necessarily meet the more restrictive definition for pheromone communication. However, this scientific definition is not universally accepted and the term pheromone is used loosely in both scientific and popular publications.

- The chemical nature of proposed pheromone compounds is heterogeneous, but some pheromone candidates in humans and animals may be chemically related.[36] Possible production sites for human pheromone candidates include urine, smegma-producing urogenital glands, lachrymal glands,[37] axillary apocrine glands, and mammary glands,[38] mirroring known pheromone sources in animals.

- There may also be similarities in the relationship between complex "odor prints" and components of the immune system that confer individual identity (e.g., human lymphocyte antigens [HLA], or the rodent major histocompatibility complex).[39] People have been shown to be capable of identifying odors of closely related persons (from samples of axillary volatiles collected from T-shirts) better than would be expected by chance alone.[40] Thus, there could be "signaler pheromones" that help individuals recognize relatives. There is also some evidence for a physiological response that varies with the reproductive cycle of female odor donors, including modulation of the menstrual cycle in other women and an increase in testosterone in

men.[41,42] The unidentified compounds involved may be classified as "primer pheromones," producing an endocrine response and (maybe) a delayed change in behavior. Less convincingly, pheromones representing paternally inherited HLA alleles may influence mate choice.[43,44]

- In humans, activation of the hypothalamus by some odors is sexually dimorphic (and sexual orientation–specific) in brain imaging studies,[45] but evidence suggests that the detection of such odors is via the main olfactory system, not the vomeronasal organ or VND.

Pheromones are not Necessarily Detected by the Vomeronasal Organ

In no case of proposed human pheromone communication has a direct specific ligand–receptor interaction involving vomeronasal or olfactory chemosensory cells and their regular transduction mechanisms been shown. Cases in which the vomeronasal system was thought to be involved have not been supported by subsequent systematic investigation (see below). Chemosensory detection must involve a ligand–receptor interaction of some kind, but there is no compelling evidence that this occurs in the distinct human VND rather than in the olfactory epithelium, or elsewhere.

- Although there is no universally accepted definition of "pheromone," it is clear that some chemosensory communication signals in animals, which would be pheromones by almost any definition, are detected by the main olfactory system and not the vomeronasal system.[46,47] For example, in newborn rabbits, a molecule secreted by lactating females, the "mammary pheromone," triggers orofacial responses in the pups that help them locate the nipples.[48] Interestingly, these chemosensory cues are learned prenatally via the main olfactory system, emphasizing the functionality of chemosensory organs before birth. Thus, the idea that a functional VNO is necessary for pheromone communication is contradicted by available data. Equally erroneous is the idea that a substance stimulating the VNO must be a pheromone.

Evidence Against Human Vomeronasal Organ Function

Pheromone-like communication in humans probably exists, but a vomeronasal system is not necessary.

All well-studied cases of vomeronasal function in other vertebrates require the presence of specific types of sensory neuron expressing certain stimulus-receptor and -transduction proteins, and possessing neural connections capable of transmitting sensory information to the brain. Humans lack many of these requirements:

- Most of the genes encoding the vomeronasal receptors belong to the V1R and V2R families but, in humans, there are no V2R genes[49] and 95% of all V1R genes are pseudogenes (i.e., cannot produce normal functional proteins).[50] (The remaining V1R genes are discussed below.) Evidence from knockout animals suggests that the TRPC2 transduction channel protein (product of the *trpc2* gene) is critical for normal VNO function in animals. The human *trpc2* gene is also a nonprotein-producing pseudogene.[51] Formyl-peptide receptors (FPR) are alternative chemosensory receptors in rodent VNOs[52] but are not expressed in chemosensory epithelia of nonrodent mammals. Human VND tissue has not been tested for the presence of FPRs, but it lacks the vomeronasal bipolar sensory cells in which V1R, V2R, and FPRs are normally expressed.

- In addition to lacking cellular components such as bipolar neurons, humans have no demonstrable vomeronasal nerve to carry sensory information to the brain, and no AOB, the brain region that normally receives vomeronasal sensory input.

- Electrophysiological experiments[53,54] and positron emission tomography (PET) studies[55] showed that subjects with or without a detectable VND, or with their VND covered, did not differ in olfactory sensitivity or odor threshold for androstenone or androstadienone (previously proposed as human pheromones) or other odors.

Chemical communication involving chemosensory transduction via the classical vomeronasal sensory pathway or via other chemosensory pathways in the vicinity of the human vomeronasal duct is unlikely.

Evidence For Possible Human Vomeronasal Organ/Vomeronasal Duct Function

- Although humans lack most structures required for normal vomeronasal function, they do retain five remnant V1R genes with open reading frames,[56] and could potentially produce human V1R-like (hV1R-L) receptor proteins. In a recent study, all five could facilitate activation of the $G\alpha_o$ signal pathway in cultured HeLa/olf cells in vitro.[57]

- The absence of a functional *trpc2* gene in humans does not absolutely rule out some VNO function. Residual function remains in mice with *trpc2* knocked out,[58] so some noncanonical transduction mechanism could allow VR-type receptors to function—but there is no evidence for their expression in the human VND.

- Expression of one human VR gene (*hV1R-L1*) is reported in human *main olfactory epithelium*,[56] but there is no evidence for displaced *vomeronasal-type* sensory neurons there. If expressed in *olfactory* sensory neurons (not demonstrated), with a compatible transduction pathway, then human V1Rs might behave like olfactory receptors. They could contribute to the regular sense of smell or, with appropriate central connections, they could contribute to pheromone communication. But this is all speculation: there is no evidence that *hV1R-L1* has a chemosensory function of any kind, in olfactory epithelium or in the VND.

- Monti Bloch and colleagues[59] reported a sexually dimorphic electrophysiological response to androstadienone (in women) and estratetraenol (in men), recorded from the region of the VND and associated with an unconscious autonomic response. They called these substances and related steroids "vomeropherins," and claimed they were male and female human pheromones, respectively, based on a mistaken belief that substances stimulating a VNO must be pheromones. These findings have not been supported by later electrophysiological and PET studies (see above). There has also been no confirmation of specific electrophysiological responses to "vomeropherins" in cells isolated from the human VND.[60]
- The recent discovery of a previously unknown vomeronasal receptor family (see above), and the existence of some VNO chemosensory function in the absence of TRPC2, leaves open the possibility that there may be other VNO sensory mechanisms. VR receptor genes differ widely across taxonomic groups, perhaps helping to maintain species isolation.[49] Some mammals, including the nonhuman primate marmosets, lack functional versions of all known vomeronasal receptor genes, V1R, V2R, and FPR, but they do have a classical VNO, which, in a related species, appears to be functional.[61] Thus, there may be vomeronasal receptors yet to be discovered, but they are unlikely to be the basis for chemosensory function in the human VND, because other essential components are missing.

Trigeminal receptors may contribute to odor perception.

- There are no classical vomeronasal sensory neurons in or near the VND in adult humans—but there may be other chemosensory cells. The trigeminal nerve innervates solitary chemosensory cells in the nasal mucosa, which express signal transduction components common to both olfactory and taste systems[62] and respond to odors at high concentrations.

Trigeminal chemoreceptors in the nasal cavity primarily serve to detect irritants and trigger protective reflexes (e.g., sneezing), but they can also contribute to odor perception. Solitary chemoreceptor cells cluster in and around the VND in mice,[63] but their presence and distribution around the human VND is unknown.

Chemical Communication via Vomeronasal Organ– or Vomeronasal Duct–independent Pathways

There is a possibility of chemosensory communication via VNO-independent pathways. The most likely pathway, of course, is the main olfactory system. Trigeminal or other potential chemoreceptors of the nose (e.g., Grüneberg ganglion or nervus terminalis)[62] are also possible (but unlikely) contributors. In addition, chemical compounds could diffuse into blood vessels in the nose or airways, or after ingestion, for detection by (undefined) internal chemoreceptors.[64] There are no prominent capillaries close to the VND,[30] so this is not a likely VND-related mechanism.

- There is no reason that the main olfactory system could not mediate all human chemosensory communication even though other mammals depend in part on their vomeronasal systems. Unlearned communication signals require the identification of particular molecules, which the vomeronasal system achieves via receptors with highly selective responses. Most main olfactory receptors are relatively nonspecific, but the mammalian brain should be able to solve the computational problem of identifying molecules via combinations of input, even if there are no specific olfactory pheromone receptors. In the vomeronasal system, information passes directly to the amygdala, part of the brain's limbic system implicated in unlearned responses to pheromones. The main olfactory system also has projections to limbic circuits, including the amygdala, in primates and other mammals.[65]
- Because vomeronasal input was thought to be essential for pheromone response, and because the amygdala has relatively indirect pathways to the neocortex, some have proposed[59] that response without conscious per-

ception would be the hallmark of pheromone communication—but the initial assumption is now known to be incorrect. Conscious detection of the stimulus is not incompatible with pheromone communication, although it may be independent and unnecessary for pheromone communication.

- The most common (canonical) type of olfactory transduction pathway is via olfactory receptor activation of adenylyl cyclase III to produce cyclic adenosine monophosphate, which opens cyclic nucleotide–gated channels. However, several other olfactory transduction pathways that use either conventional or nonconventional (noncanonical) olfactory receptor molecules are now known to be expressed in small subsets of main olfactory sensory neurons. Thus, an odor response in the absence of the canonical olfactory transduction pathway[66] does not necessarily implicate involvement of vomeronasal receptors. Ironically, some of these specialized olfactory receptor neurons (ORNs) use the phospholipid transduction cascade normally activated by vomeronasal receptors, but vomeronasal receptor molecules are not known to be expressed in any of them. One of the small subgroups of ORN that uses a noncanonical transduction pathway and expresses the TRPM5 transduction channel does project its axons to the ventral olfactory bulb, where projections to limbic circuits may originate in mice,[67] and there is evidence for a limbic projection from these particular neurons.[68]
- Recently, an olfactory receptor (OR7D4) has been found to be activated by steroid-derived odors, including androstenone and androstadienone.[69] The associated gene is intact in humans and may be responsible for human behavioral and physiological responses to volatile steroids previously attributed to VNO function (see above).

Summary

There is reasonably convincing evidence for chemosensory communication in humans. Whether it is learned or unlearned is not clear in all cases, but it is more likely to be accomplished by the main olfactory system than any chemosensory system located in or near the VND.

Outlook and Practical Advice for Physicians

- The detectability of the VND by endoscopy varies considerably from one day to another, as it can be obstructed by mucus or periodic swelling of the nasal mucosa. However, even when the presence of VND(s) can be established, this is unlikely to be helpful with diagnosis of chemosensory or behavioral disorders.
- Occasionally, a VND orifice can be misinterpreted as a (rarely) persistent nasopalatine duct (NPD), a communication between the oral and nasal cavities that usually closes at birth or at the latest in childhood.[70] If any NPD is detectable, the opening is located at the nasal floor, whereas the VND orifice is located more posteriorly ~1 to 2 mm above the nasal floor.
- Patients should be reassured that the best scientific evidence indicates that damage or malfunction of the VNO/VND is unlikely to be a contributor to any adverse symptoms they are experiencing.

References

1. Ruysch F. Thesaurus Anatomicus Tertius. Amstelaedami: Johann Wolters; 1703; 39.
2. Meredith M. Sensory processing in the main and accessory olfactory systems: comparisons and contrasts. J Steroid Biochem Mol Biol 1991;39(4B): 601–614
3. Jia C, Halpern M. Subclasses of vomeronasal receptor neurons: differential expression of G proteins (Gi alpha 2 and G(o alpha)) and segregated projections to the accessory olfactory bulb. Brain Res 1996;719(1–2):117–128
4. Samuelsen CL, Meredith M. Oxytocin antagonist disrupts male mouse medial amygdala response to chemical-communication signals. Neuroscience 2011;180:96–104
5. Meredith M, Westberry JM. Distinctive responses in the medial amygdala to same-species and different-species pheromones. J Neurosci 2004;24(25): 5719–5725
6. Choi GB, Dong HW, Murphy AJ, et al. Lhx6 delineates a pathway mediating innate reproductive behaviors from the amygdala to the hypothalamus. Neuron 2005;46(4):647–660
7. Luo M, Katz LC. Encoding pheromonal signals in the mammalian vomeronasal system. Curr Opin Neurobiol 2004;14(4):428–434
8. Mohedano-Moriano A, Pro-Sistiaga P, Ubeda-Bañón I, Crespo C, Insausti R, Martinez-Marcos A. Segregated pathways to the vomeronasal amygdala: differential projections from the anterior and

posterior divisions of the accessory olfactory bulb. Eur J Neurosci 2007;25(7):2065–2080

9. Leinders-Zufall T, Lane AP, Puche AC, et al. Ultrasensitive pheromone detection by mammalian vomeronasal neurons. Nature 2000;405(6788):792–796

10. Müller F, O'Rahilly R. Olfactory structures in staged human embryos. Cells Tissues Organs 2004;178(2):93–116

11. Schwanzel-Fukuda M. Origin and migration of luteinizing hormone-releasing hormone neurons in mammals. Microsc Res Tech 1999;44(1):2–10

12. Wray S. From nose to brain: development of gonadotrophin-releasing hormone-1 neurones. J Neuroendocrinol 2010;22(7):743–753

13. Quinton R, Hasan W, Grant W, et al. Gonadotropin-releasing hormone immunoreactivity in the nasal epithelia of adults with Kallmann's syndrome and isolated hypogonadotropic hypogonadism and in the early midtrimester human fetus. J Clin Endocrinol Metab 1997;82(1):309–314

14. Kjaer I, Hansen BF. Luteinizing hormone-releasing hormone and innervation pathways in human prenatal nasal submucosa: factors of importance in evaluating Kallmann's syndrome. APMIS 1996;104(9):680–688

15. Balasubramanian R, Dwyer A, Seminara SB, Pitteloud N, Kaiser UB, Crowley WF Jr. Human GnRH deficiency: a unique disease model to unravel the ontogeny of GnRH neurons. Neuroendocrinology 2010;92(2):81–99

16. Humphrey T. The development of the olfactory and the accessory olfactory formations in human embryos and fetuses. J Comp Neurol 1940;73:431–468

17. Witt M, Hummel T. Vomeronasal versus olfactory epithelium: is there a cellular basis for human vomeronasal perception? Int Rev Cytol 2006;248:209–259

18. Takami S, Yukimatsu M, Matsumura G, Nishiyama F. Vomeronasal epithelial cells of human fetuses contain immunoreactivity for G proteins, Go(alpha) and Gi(alpha 2). Chem Senses 2001;26(5):517–522

19. McCotter RE. The connection of the vomero-nasal nerves with the accessory olfactory bulb in the opossum and other mammals. Anat Rec 1912;6:299–318

20. Kallius E. Geruchsorgan (organon olfactus). In: Bardeleben's Handbuch der Anatomie des Menschen. Jena: G Fischer; 1905.

21. Potiquet A. Du canal de Jacobson. De la possibilité de le reconnaitre sur le vivant et de son role probable dans la pathogénie de certaines lésions de la cloison nasale. Rev Laryngol Otol Rhinol (Bord) 1891;24:737–753

22. Johnson A, Josephson R, Hawke M. Clinical and histological evidence for the presence of the vomeronasal (Jacobson's) organ in adult humans. J Otolaryngol 1985;14(2):71–79

23. Stensaas LJ, Lavker RM, Monti-Bloch L, Grosser BI, Berliner DL. Ultrastructure of the human vomeronasal organ. J Steroid Biochem Mol Biol 1991;39(4B):553–560

24. Moran DT, Jafek BW, Rowley JC III. The vomeronasal (Jacobson's) organ in man: ultrastructure and frequency of occurrence. J Steroid Biochem Mol Biol 1991;39(4B):545–552

25. Garcia-Velasco J, Mondragon M. The incidence of the vomeronasal organ in 1000 human subjects and its possible clinical significance. J Steroid Biochem Mol Biol 1991;39(4B):561–563

26. Trotier D, Eloit C, Wassef M, et al. The vomeronasal cavity in adult humans. Chem Senses 2000;25(4):369–380

27. Gaafar HA, Tantawy AA, Melis AA, Hennawy DM, Shehata HM. The vomeronasal (Jacobson's) organ in adult humans: frequency of occurrence and enzymatic study. Acta Otolaryngol 1998;118(3):409–412

28. Won J, Mair EA, Bolger WE, Conran RM. The vomeronasal organ: an objective anatomic analysis of its prevalence. Ear Nose Throat J 2000;79(8):600–605

29. Knecht M, Kühnau D, Hüttenbrink KB, Witt M, Hummel T. Frequency and localization of the putative vomeronasal organ in humans in relation to age and gender. Laryngoscope 2001;111(3):448–452

30. Witt M, Georgiewa B, Knecht M, Hummel T. On the chemosensory nature of the vomeronasal epithelium in adult humans. Histochem Cell Biol 2002;117(6):493–509

31. Foltán R, Sedý J. Behavioral changes of patients after orthognathic surgery develop on the basis of the loss of vomeronasal organ: a hypothesis. Head Face Med 2009;5:5

32. Karlson P, Lüscher M. 'Pheromones': a new term for a class of biologically active substances. Nature 1959;183(4653):55–56

33. Halpern M, Martínez-Marcos A. Structure and function of the vomeronasal system: an update. Prog Neurobiol 2003;70(3):245–318

34. Grammer K, Fink B, Neave N. Human pheromones and sexual attraction. Eur J Obstet Gynecol Reprod Biol 2005;118(2):135–142

35. Meredith M. Human vomeronasal organ function: a critical review of best and worst cases. Chem Senses 2001;26(4):433–445

36. Wysocki CJ, Preti G. Facts, fallacies, fears, and frustrations with human pheromones. Anat Rec A Discov Mol Cell Evol Biol 2004;281(1):1201–1211

37. Gelstein S, Yeshurun Y, Rozenkrantz L, et al. Human tears contain a chemosignal. Science 2011;331(6014):226–230

38. Schaal B. Mammary odor cues and pheromones: mammalian infant-directed communication about maternal state, mammae, and milk. Vitam Horm 2010;83:83–136

39. Boehm T, Zufall F. MHC peptides and the sensory evaluation of genotype. Trends Neurosci 2006;29(2):100–107

40. Porter RH, Cernoch JM, Balogh RD. Odor signatures and kin recognition. Physiol Behav 1985;34(3):445–448

41. Stern K, McClintock MK. Regulation of ovulation by human pheromones. Nature 1998;392(6672):177–179

42. Miller SL, Maner JK. Scent of a woman: men's testosterone responses to olfactory ovulation cues. Psychol Sci 2010;21(2):276–283

43. Boehm U. The vomeronasal system in mice: from the nose to the hypothalamus – and back! Semin Cell Dev Biol 2006;17(4):471–479

44. Jacob S, McClintock MK, Zelano B, Ober C. Paternally inherited HLA alleles are associated with women's choice of male odor. Nat Genet 2002;30(2): 175–179

45. Savic I, Hedén-Blomqvist E, Berglund H. Pheromone signal transduction in humans: what can be learned from olfactory loss. Hum Brain Mapp 2009;30(9):3057–3065

46. Dorries KM, Adkins-Regan E, Halpern BP. Sensitivity and behavioral responses to the pheromone androstenone are not mediated by the vomeronasal organ in domestic pigs. Brain Behav Evol 1997;49(1):53–62

47. Hudson R, Distel H. Pheromonal release of suckling in rabbits does not depend on the vomeronasal organ. Physiol Behav 1986;37(1):123–128

48. Coureaud G, Charra R, Datiche F, et al. A pheromone to behave, a pheromone to learn: the rabbit mammary pheromone. J Comp Physiol A Neuroethol Sens Neural Behav Physiol 2010;196(10):779–790

49. Young JM, Massa HF, Hsu L, Trask BJ. Extreme variability among mammalian V1R gene families. Genome Res 2010;20(1):10–18

50. Kouros-Mehr H, Pintchovski S, Melnyk J, et al. Identification of non-functional human VNO receptor genes provides evidence for vestigiality of the human VNO. Chem Senses 2001;26(9):1167–1174

51. Liman ER, Innan H. Relaxed selective pressure on an essential component of pheromone transduction in primate evolution. Proc Natl Acad Sci U S A 2003;100(6):3328–3332

52. Liberles SD, Horowitz LF, Kuang D, et al. Formyl peptide receptors are candidate chemosensory receptors in the vomeronasal organ. Proc Natl Acad Sci U S A 2009;106(24):9842–9847

53. Hummel T, Schultz S, Witt M, Hatt H. Electrical responses to chemosensory stimulation recorded from the vomeronasal duct and the respiratory epithelium in humans. Int J Psychophysiol 2011; 81(2):116–120

54. Knecht M, Lundström JN, Witt M, Hüttenbrink KB, Heilmann S, Hummel T. Assessment of olfactory function and androstenone odor thresholds in humans with or without functional occlusion of the vomeronasal duct. Behav Neurosci 2003; 117(6):1135–1141

55. Frasnelli J, Lundström JN, Boyle JA, Katsarkas A, Jones-Gotman M. The vomeronasal organ is not involved in the perception of endogenous odors. Hum Brain Mapp 2011;32(3):450–460

56. Rodriguez I, Greer CA, Mok MY, Mombaerts P. A putative pheromone receptor gene expressed in human olfactory mucosa. Nat Genet 2000;26(1): 18–19

57. Shirokova E, Raguse JD, Meyerhof W, Krautwurst D. The human vomeronasal type-1 receptor family—detection of volatiles and cAMP signaling in HeLa/Olf cells. FASEB J 2008;22(5):1416–1425

58. Kelliher KR, Spehr M, Li XH, Zufall F, Leinders-Zufall T. Pheromonal recognition memory induced by TRPC2-independent vomeronasal sensing. Eur J Neurosci 2006;23(12):3385–3390

59. Monti-Bloch L, Jennings-White C, Berliner DL. The human vomeronasal system. A review. Ann N Y Acad Sci 1998;855:373–389

60. Monti-Bloch L. Effect of vomeropherin pregna-4,20-diene-3,6-dione on isolated cells from the human vomeronasal organ. Chem Senses 1997; 22:752

61. Smith TD, Dennis JC, Bhatnagar KP, Garrett EC, Bonar CJ, Morrison EE. Olfactory marker protein expression in the vomeronasal neuroepithelium of tamarins (Saguinus spp). Brain Res 2011; 1375:7–18

62. Munger SD, Leinders-Zufall T, Zufall F. Subsystem organization of the mammalian sense of smell. Annu Rev Physiol 2009;71:115–140

63. Ogura T, Krosnowski K, Zhang L, Bekkerman M, Lin W. Chemoreception regulates chemical access to mouse vomeronasal organ: role of solitary chemosensory cells. PLoS ONE 2010;5(7):e11924

64. Mast TG, Samuelsen CL. Human pheromone detection by the vomeronasal organ: unnecessary for mate selection? Chem Senses 2009;34(6):529–531

65. Price JL. Comparative aspects of amygdala connectivity. Ann N Y Acad Sci 2003;985:50–58

66. Trinh K, Storm DR. Vomeronasal organ detects odorants in absence of signaling through main olfactory epithelium. Nat Neurosci 2003;6(5):519–525

67. Kang N, McCarthy EA, Cherry JA, Baum MJ. A sex comparison of the anatomy and function of the main olfactory bulb medial amygdala projection in mice. Neuroscience 2011;172:196–204

68. Thompson JA, Salcedo E, Restrepo D, Finger TE. Second-order input to the medial amygdala from olfactory sensory neurons expressing the transduction channel TRPM5. J Comp Neurol. 2012;520(8): 1819–1830.

69. Zhuang H, Chien MS, Matsunami H. Dynamic functional evolution of an odorant receptor for sex-steroid–derived odors in primates. Proc Natl Acad Sci U S A 2009;106(50):21247–21251

70. Knecht M, Kittner T, Beleites T, Hüttenbrink KB, Hummel T, Witt M. Morphological and radiologic evaluation of the human nasopalatine duct. Ann Otol Rhinol Laryngol 2005;114(3):229–232

5 Smell and Taste Disorders— Diagnostic and Clinical Work-Up

Antje Welge-Luessen, Donald A. Leopold, Takaki Miwa

Introduction

Smell and taste disorders are common complaints presenting to ear, nose, and throat (ENT) physicians.[1-3] Approximately one-fifth of all adults have some form of olfactory dysfunction,[2,4,5] increasing to 30% or more suffering from functional anosmia over the age of 70 years.[2] These numbers are reflected by 79,000 patients/year in central Europe (Austria, Germany, and Switzerland),[6] and around 200,000 patients/year in the USA,[7] consulting ENT specialists about olfactory disorders.

Taste disorders seem to be less common, affecting around 5% of people[8] if diagnosed by two different psychophysical tests. If, however, only four tastants are applied and the incorrect identification of one of these four is defined as taste disorder, then the prevalence rises to almost 20%.[5] Other epidemiological studies, using questionnaires to evaluate the number of self-perceived taste disorders, report numbers in the range of 0.6%[7] to 0.93%.[9] These numbers increase to 8.7% in patients seeking medical advice.[3] The fact that there are three different nerves on each side, all transmitting taste information, makes this sense more robust than the sense of smell, and less likely to decrease through life.

Even though olfactory receptor cells regenerate throughout life, this regeneration seems to decrease with growing age. Patients suffering from age-related olfactory dysfunction are often not even aware of the disorder,[10] which usually develops gradually and is most likely due to the reduced regenerative capacity of the olfactory receptor cell. In contrast to hearing and visual losses, which are often noticed by spouses, family members, or friends, smell losses usually remain undetected by other persons. This might explain why patients with olfactory disorders, particularly older people, are more likely to encounter hazardous events (e.g., burning food, ingesting spoiled food, fire) than a normosmic control group.[11,12] These hazards have to be especially mentioned when counseling patients with smell loss. The increased risk of these hazards contributes to the loss in quality of life experienced by patients suffering from smell loss. Both the increased risk of hazardous events and the reduction in quality of life are likely to explain why patients with post-traumatic smell loss receive some financial reimbursement from insurance providers (see Chapter 18). With growing age, the sense of taste also decreases, but less than the decline seen in olfaction.[9,13,14]

Making an accurate diagnosis of smell or taste disorder is essential in order to determine appropriate treatment and counseling. The first step is to determine whether the disorder is an olfactory problem, a gustatory problem, or both. As patients do often complain about taste problems or complain simply that, "the food just does not taste the same anymore," it is first necessary to evaluate the kind of chemosensory deficit present.

It has been established for some years now that self-assessment of olfactory function is unreliable.[15] Even in patients complaining of olfactory disorders, self-assessment correlates only moderately with measured olfactory function.[16,17] The use of a validated test that actually measures olfactory ability, gustatory ability, or both is therefore mandatory in all patients seeking advice (see Chapter 6 for smell testing; Chapter 14 for taste testing).

Olfactory Disorders

The vast majority of chemosensory complaints are olfactory, and the patient's history can help to classify the disorder. Smell disorders are classified as sinonasal, postinfectious, post-traumatic, congenital, toxic (including drug-induced disorders), other (postoperative), and idiopathic. The detailed characteristics of each of these disorders are discussed in the following chapters; however, in clinical consultations it is important to differentiate between sinonasal (sometimes called "conductive") and nonsinonasal (sometimes called "neural") disorders within the initial work-up.

Assessment of a patient depends on the situation. In general, one has to distinguish between an asymptomatic patient who has to be evaluated because of a medicolegal reason (e.g., preoperatively [before any endonasal operation] or in the context of a thorough ENT examination [e.g., for an expert opinion]) and a patient presenting with an olfactory complaint. In asymptomatic patients, the use of a validated screening test is recommended (see Chapter 6). It is important to bear in mind that the test has been adapted to cultural factors[18,19] (for details, see Chapter 6). Only if this test reveals any pathological results is further testing required. In Japan, a self-administered odor questionnaire is sometimes used as an instant index.[17]

However, patients seeking medical advice for olfactory disorders have different expectations. They expect not only a diagnosis, but also information concerning prognosis and treatment (or, at least, coping strategies in cases in which therapeutic tools are lacking). To meet these expectations, classification of the disorder is mandatory.

Gustatory Disorders

Like olfactory disorders, gustatory disorders should be classified and measured using a validated test. Unlike preoperative smell testing before endonasal operations, there is currently no consensus about the need for preoperative taste testing in asymptomatic patients undergoing enoral operations such as tonsillectomy or teeth extraction. Whether this approach will change in the future remains to be seen, and is likely to depend on the number of complaints about postoperative taste problems observed in such patients (for details, see Chapter 15).

Nevertheless we do recommend performing a screening taste test in every patient receiving an extensive olfactory test, and vice versa.

Examination of the Patient

History: Olfaction

The importance of a detailed history cannot be overemphasized. Of special importance is the time course of the complaint.

Has the disorder started suddenly or has it developed over a longer period of time? In this context, it is important to remember that the patient should recall a temporal connection to, for example, accidents, intake of medication, or acute infection such as rhinitis or rhinosinusitis. However, the examiner should be cautious not to overinterpret possible causative correlations sometimes offered by patients.

Has the patient ever experienced something like this before? Are there any additional nasal symptoms (discharge, rhinorrhea, postnasal drip, nasal breathing) or concomitant diseases (e.g., thyroid, cardiopulmonary, hepatic, or renal disease, or allergies)? A history of movement disorders (tremor, etc.) or disturbances in memory should also be taken. A family history of Parkinson or Alzheimer disease should be evaluated and considered.

The existence of additional qualitative disturbances, if not mentioned spontaneously, should also be evaluated (see below). The use of a simple history questionnaire as depicted in **Fig. 5.1** (adapted from ref. 20) can be of great help in clinical practice and is recommended. An important question is whether the disorder is continuously present or whether is it fluctuating. Fluctuating disorders point to a sinonasal (conductive) problem. Olfactory distortions most often present in females in the second to fifth decades of life. If a distortion is noted in the teens or twenties, a metabolic disorder should be suspected.[21] It should also be noted whether the distortion is experienced during inhalation or exhalation and whether blocking one or both nostrils can eliminate it.

History: Gustation

Once again, a meticulous history is of great importance. The onset of the disorder—suddenly versus gradually—and any possible causative factors have to be evaluated. Concomitant diseases (renal, liver, other systemic diseases such as autoimmune diseases, etc.) should also be assessed, and a thorough medication history taken. Local factors such as the use of mouth irrigations or saliva problems should be assessed. If possible, the examiner should try to evaluate whether a quantitative or a predominantly qualitative disorder is present; however, qualitative disorders might also be accompanied by quantitative disorders, so a quantitative assessment should always be made. For more details about the history of gustatory disorders, see Chapter 15.

Questionnaire:
History of smell/taste disorder

(self-adhesive label)

Phone (home):

Phone (other):

What kind of problem do you have? *You may check more than one box*	☐ a smell problem ☐ a taste problem concerning aromas (subtle taste perception) ☐ a taste problem concerning the perception of sweet, sour, bitter, or salty
When was the onset of your problem?	☐ less than 3 months ago ☐ 3 to 24 months ago ☐ more than 2 years ago ☐ it has been there as long as I can remember ☐ I don't know
How did the problem start?	☐ slowly ☐ suddenly ☐ I never could smell in all my life ☐ I don't know
How has the situation changed?	☐ there was an improvement ☐ the situation is unchanged ☐ it has become worse
What could have been the cause of your problem?	☐ accident ☐ cold / infection ☐ medication ☐ surgery ☐ breathing through the nose/nasal polyps/sinusitis ☐ dry mouth ☐ dentures ☐ others (please name)
Do you have chronic nasal problems?	☐ no ☐ yes—please indicate: running nose, nasal obstruction, sneezing, allergy, polyps, facial pain ....
Is your condition fluctuating or constant?	☐ fluctuating ☐ constant ☐ I don't know ☐ if fluctuations are dependent on certain circumstances, please describe:
How badly does the problem affect you?	☐ very badly ☐ badly ☐ medium badly ☐ mildly ☐ hardly at all ☐ not at all
How would you describe your nasal patency?	☐ very good ☐ good ☐ bad ☐ very bad ☐ I cannot breathe through the nose at all
The following questions concern **taste** dirorders only	
The taste disorder mainly concerns the perception of:	☐ sweet ☐ sour ☐ salty ☐ bitter ☐ spicy ☐ none of these
Do you suffer from any constant oral sensation?	buning mouth ☐ yes ☐ no bitter taste ☐ yes ☐ no salty taste ☐ yes ☐ no sour taste ☐ yes ☐ no dry mouth ☐ yes ☐ no foreign body sensation ☐ yes ☐ no

Fig. 5.1 History questionnaire. CT, computed tomography; rad.-sinuses, x-rays of the nasal sinuses; MRI, magnetic resonance imaging. (Adapted from Hummel T, Welge-Lüssen A. Riech- und Schmeckstorungen: Physiologie, Pathophysiologie und Therapeutische Ansatze. Stuttgart: Thieme; 2005.)

To be completed by the **physician**	
Weight loss due to problem?	☐ no ☐ yes ....kg/..........years
Medication?	☐ no ☐ yes — which?
Chronic diseases?	☐ no ☐ yes — which? ☐ diabetes ☐ high blood pressure ☐ neoplasia ☐ others: ....
Head surgery?	☐ no ☐ yes — which? ☐ sinuses ☐ nasal septum ☐ nasal ployps ☐ nasal turbinates ☐ palatal tonsils ☐ adenoids ☐ middle ear ☐ left ☐ right ☐ dental surgery: .... ☐ others...
Flu shots?	☐ no ☐ yes – when?
Smoker?	☐ no ☐ yes – extent?
Alcohol?	☐ no ☐ yes – ☐ occasionally ☐ regularly
Diagnostic imaging?	**CT** ☐ no ☐ yes **rad.-sinuses** ☐ no ☐ yes **MRI** ☐ no ☐ yes Findings: ....
Profession?	Specific exposure to gaseous, powdered, or other chemicals? ☐ no ☐ yes If **YES** , which? .... duration (years)? .... hours per day? ....
If idiopathic etiology is suspected:	Parkinson disease among relatives ☐ no ☐ yes Alzheimer disease among relatives ☐ no ☐ yes
Parosmia ☐ no ☐ yes ☐ left ☐ right	☐ daily ☐ not daily ☐ very strong ☐ mild ☐ weight loss due to parosmia ☐ no weight loss
Phantosmia ☐ no ☐ yes ☐ left ☐ right	☐ daily ☐ not daily ☐ very strong ☐ mild ☐ weight loss due to phantosmia ☐ no weight loss

Test results

"Sniffin' Sticks" T: D: I:

Taste Strips (x out of 32): ....

Taste sprays (4 Sprays): ....

Retronasal (x out of 20): ....

Suspected etiology:

☐ post traumatic ☐ post-infectious
☐ sinunasal ☐ idiopathic
☐ toxic ☐ congenital
☐ neurodegenerative ☐ others

Nasal findings

Septal deviation	☐ left	☐ right	☐ none	
Olfactory cleft visible	☐ left	☐ right		
Polyps left:	☐ 0	☐ I	☐ II	☐ III
right	☐ 0	☐ I	☐ II	☐ III

Examiner (name / signature)

Clinical Examination: Olfaction and Gustation

The main focus of the clinical examination is examination of the head and a thorough ENT examination. An anterior rhinoscopy should be followed by an endonasal endoscopy (with or without decongestion) with a narrow 2.7-mm endoscope to evaluate the region of the olfactory cleft. Is it visible? Are polyps present? Is it not completely visible because of high septal deviation? Signs of acute (**Fig. 5.2**) and chronic (**Fig. 5.3**) rhinosinusitis should be evaluated.

After taking a history and performing an endonasal endoscopic examination, the examiner should be able to confirm or exclude an acute or chronic sinonasal etiology. In cases of acute sinonasal disease and concomitant olfactory complaints, the acute infection should be treated appropriately and the patient should be seen again several weeks later. If the olfactory disorder persists after recovery from the acute infection, an olfactory test using a validated tool should be performed. If signs of acute rhinosinusitis are lacking, olfactory testing should also be performed, as depicted in **Fig. 5.4**.

In cases of assumed taste disorder, a careful examination of the oral cavity has to be performed. For details of taste disorder classification, examination, work-up, and therapy, see Chapter 15.

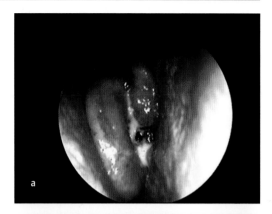

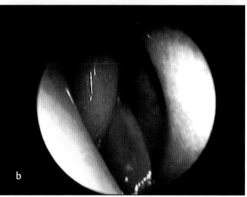

Fig. 5.3a, b Chronic rhinosinusitis.

a Polyps with pus and crusts.

b Polyps only.

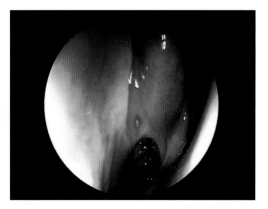

Fig. 5.2 Acute sinusitis, pus inside middle and superior nasal duct.

Quantification of Smell Disorder

The patient's symptoms should be verified using a validated smell test (see Chapter 6). Additionally, a suprathreshold taste test should be included. The results of these tests can be used to classify smell function as normosmic, hyposmic (diminished), or anosmic (completely missing). However, it is important to remember that, for example, the Sniffin' Sticks test uses normative data from a group of healthy individuals aged between 16 and 35 years in order to define absolute normosmia or hyposmia.[22,23] The age of the patient has to be kept in mind when interpreting the test results.

In contrast to these quantitative disorders, qualitative disorders are difficult to measure. Nevertheless, the presence or absence of these, as well as their time course, should be asked when taking

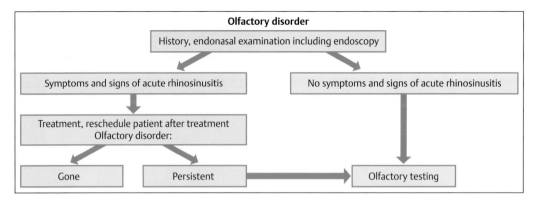

Fig. 5.4 Work-up of olfactory disorder.

the history. According to the existing definitions, qualitative disorders are classified as:

- Parosmia: Disturbed odorant perception in presence of an odorant.
- Phantosmia: Perception of an odorant in the absence of an odorant.
- Pseudosmia: Imaginative reinterpretation of an odorant within the context of strong feelings. Can be of significance within the presence of psychiatric disorders.
- Olfactory intolerance: Exaggerated subjective sensitivity toward odorants.

Additional Work-up

In cases in which olfactory dysfunction due to a suspected sinonasal disorder is confirmed by olfactory testing, further analysis is required. In general, sinonasal olfactory disorders are those in which the etiology lies within the nose or the paranasal sinuses. This can be either inflammatory (chronic rhinosinusitis) or noninflammatory (intranasal tumors, stenosis, scarring). Inflammatory disorders can further be classified as infectious or noninfectious (**Fig. 5.5**). These are discussed in detail in Chapter 7. If the history suggests a sinonasal disorder but the endonasal findings do not correspond with this, computed tomography can be helpful, especially in detecting slight opacification of the olfactory cleft, which sometimes cannot be visualized endoscopically. In cases of suspected sinonasal disorder without clear or distinct signs, it is controversial whether or not to prescribe a short course of decreasing systemic steroids[24] without prior imaging. In these cases in particular, any contraindications for peroral steroids must be ruled out before prescribing the medication.

In cases in which neither history nor clinical examination suggest a sinonasal olfactory disorder, one has to suspect an olfactory disorder that is nonsinonasal. This can be characterized according to **Fig. 5.6**.

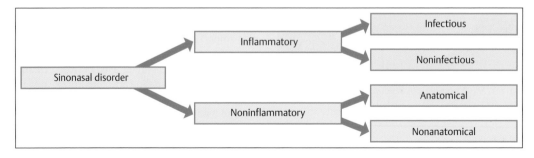

Fig. 5.5 Differentiation of sinonasal disorders.

Postinfectious and post-traumatic disorders can, in most cases, easily be diagnosed from the history. However, patients with severe head trauma may present much later than those with minor trauma because they are not aware of their smell deficit initially. Postinfectious disorders are also diagnosed according to the history, which is typical in such cases. However, sometimes the differentiation of a sinonasal disorder can be difficult (for details see Chapter 9).

Toxic disorders are difficult to diagnose, especially as most patients are exposed to more than one potentially toxic agent. A systematic evaluation of potentially toxic drugs, including all medications, should be included within the history.

Sentences in the history such as, "I cannot recall to have ever smelled" suggest a congenital disorder. Most of these patients present as children or teenagers but they may sometimes present as adults. In these uncommon cases, magnetic resonance tomography (MRT) can reveal aplasia of the olfactory bulb to confirm the diagnosis.[25,26] If the olfactory disorder is not classifiable based on the history and examination, a neurological examination should be performed to rule out early Parkinson disease.[27–30] MRT imaging can also help exclude any intracranial tumors; moreover, MRT can also visualize the olfactory bulb and its volume (for details see Chapter 17).

Diseases such as diabetes mellitus,[31] hypothyroidism, lupus erythematodes, renal disease, liver disease, vitamin A or B_{12} deficits, or Wegener granulomatosis[32] can also be associated with olfactory disorders. In most of these cases, a decrease in olfactory function is apparent,[33,34] rather than complete anosmia.

If all the previously mentioned causes of olfactory disorder have been ruled out and any contraindication to the use of systemic steroids has been excluded, one might try a short course of systemic steroids using a decreasing regimen (e.g., starting with prednisone 60 mg/d) over a period of 14 days, according to the guidance of the Working Group of Olfaction and Gustation.[24] If olfactory function improves, a sinonasal disorder seems likely and it should be investigated further; if, however, olfactory ability remains unchanged, an idiopathic disorder is the most likely diagnosis.

Bearing in mind that only a limited number of therapeutic measures exists, adequate counseling of these patients is very important. Patients should be accurately informed about prognosis and spontaneous recovery rates, especially in cases of postinfectious and post-traumatic disorders (see Chapter 9). Coping mechanisms (e.g., considering dinner as a "social event" rather than concentrating on the experience of the food; checking the expiry date of food; appropriate use of perfume; regular ventilation of homes; regular washing days for clothes; and the purchase of fire/gas detectors) and working conditions should be discussed. While in most cases loss of smell does not affect ability to work, some patients (e.g., food industry workers or gas technicians) might not be able to continue their original work and need special advice.

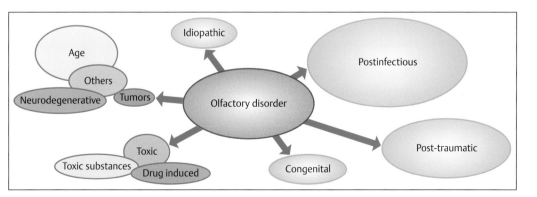

Fig. 5.6 Differentiation of non-sinonasal olfactory disorders.

Summary

A growing number of patients complain about smell and taste disorders. To determine appropriate treatment and provide adequate counseling regarding prognosis, the disorder must be accurately classified. A thorough history—including exact time course of the observed disorder—and standardized olfactory or gustatory testing is mandatory. Additional investigations might be necessary before the disorder can be classified. Only then can therapy be chosen and adequate counseling be provided.

References

1. Landis BN, Konnerth CG, Hummel T. A study on the frequency of olfactory dysfunction. Laryngoscope 2004;114(10):1764–1769
2. Brämerson A, Johansson L, Ek L, Nordin S, Bende M. Prevalence of olfactory dysfunction: the Skövde population-based study. Laryngoscope 2004; 114(4):733–737
3. Deems DA, Doty RL, Settle RG, et al. Smell and taste disorders, a study of 750 patients from the University of Pennsylvania Smell and Taste Center. Arch Otolaryngol Head Neck Surg 1991;117(5):519–528
4. Murphy C, Schubert CR, Cruickshanks KJ, Klein BE, Klein R, Nondahl DM. Prevalence of olfactory impairment in older adults. JAMA 2002; 288(18):2307–2312
5. Vennemann MM, Hummel T, Berger K. The association between smoking and smell and taste impairment in the general population. J Neurol 2008;255(8):1121–1126
6. Damm M, Temmel A, Welge-Lüssen A, et al. Olfactory dysfunctions. Epidemiology and therapy in Germany, Austria and Switzerland. [Article in German] HNO 2004;52(2):112–120
7. Hoffman HJ, Ishii EK, MacTurk RH. Age-related changes in the prevalence of smell/taste problems among the United States adult population. Results of the 1994 disability supplement to the National Health Interview Survey (NHIS). Ann N Y Acad Sci 1998;855:716–722
8. Welge-Lüssen A, Dörig P, Wolfensberger M, Krone F, Hummel T. A study about the frequency of taste disorders. J Neurol 2011;258(3):386–392
9. Hoffman HJ, Cruickshanks KJ, Davis B. Perspectives on population-based epidemiological studies of olfactory and taste impairment. Ann N Y Acad Sci 2009;1170:514–530
10. Nordin S, Monsch AU, Murphy C. Unawareness of smell loss in normal aging and Alzheimer's disease: discrepancy between self-reported and diagnosed smell sensitivity. J Gerontol B Psychol Sci Soc Sci 1995;50(4):187–192
11. Santos DV, Reiter ER, DiNardo LJ, Costanzo RM. Hazardous events associated with impaired olfactory function. Arch Otolaryngol Head Neck Surg 2004;130(3):317–319
12. Miwa T, Furukawa M, Tsukatani T, Costanzo RM, DiNardo LJ, Reiter ER. Impact of olfactory impairment on quality of life and disability. Arch Otolaryngol Head Neck Surg 2001;127(5):497–503
13. Schiffman SS. Taste and smell losses in normal aging and disease. JAMA 1997;278(16):1357–1362
14. Weiffenbach JM, Cowart BJ, Baum BJ. Taste intensity perception in aging. J Gerontol 1986;41(4): 460–468
15. Landis BN, Hummel T, Hugentobler M, Giger R, Lacroix JS. Ratings of overall olfactory function. Chem Senses 2003;28(8):691–694
16. Welge-Luessen A, Hummel T, Stojan T, Wolfensberger M. What is the correlation between ratings and measures of olfactory function in patients with olfactory loss? Am J Rhinol 2005;19(6): 567–571
17. Takebayashi H, Tsuzuki K, Oka H, Fukazawa K, Daimon T, Sakagami M. Clinical availability of a self-administered odor questionnaire for patients with olfactory disorders. Auris Nasus Larynx 2011; 38(1):65–72
18. Saito S, Ayabe-Kanamura S, Takashima Y, et al. Development of a smell identification test using a novel stick-type odor presentation kit. Chem Senses 2006;31(4):379–391
19. Shiga H, Toda H, Kobayakawa T, et al. Usefulness of curry odorant of odor stick identification test for Japanese in olfactory impairment screening. Acta Otolaryngol Suppl 2009;(562):91–94
20. Cornelia H, Landis BN, Frasnelli J, Hummel T. Computerized history of olfactory dysfunction. Chem Senses 2005;30:265–278
21. Leopold DA, Preti G, Mozell MM, Youngentob SL, Wright HN. Fish-odor syndrome presenting as dysosmia. Arch Otolaryngol Head Neck Surg 1990;116(3):354–355
22. Kobal G, Klimek L, Wolfensberger M, et al. Multicenter investigation of 1,036 subjects using a standardized method for the assessment of olfactory function combining tests of odor identification, odor discrimination, and olfactory thresholds. Eur Arch Otorhinolaryngol 2000;257(4):205–211
23. Doty RL, Shaman P, Dann M. Development of the University of Pennsylvania Smell Identification Test: a standardized microencapsulated test of olfactory function. Physiol Behav 1984;32(3): 489–502
24. Riechstörungen—Leitlinie zur Epidemiologie, Pathophysiologie, Klassifikation, Diagnose und Therapie. http://www.awmf.org/leitlinien/detail/ ll/017-050.html
25. Yousem DM, Geckle RJ, Bilker WB, McKeown DA, Doty RL. MR Evaluation of patients with congenital hyposmia or anosmia. Am J Roentgenol 1996;166:439–443
26. Abolmaali ND, Hietschold V, Vogl TJ, Hüttenbrink KB, Hummel T. MR evaluation in patients with isolated anosmia since birth or early childhood. AJNR Am J Neuroradiol 2002;23(1):157–164
27. Müller A, Abolmaali ND, Hummel T, Reichmann H. Riechstörungen—ein frühes Kardinalsymptom des idiopathischen Parkinson-Syndroms. Akt Neurol 2003;30:239–243

28. Müller A, Reichmann H, Livermore A, Hummel T. Olfactory function in idiopathic Parkinson's disease (IPD): results from cross-sectional studies in IPD patients and long-term follow-up of de-novo IPD patients. J Neural Transm 2002;109(5–6):805–811

29. Hawkes C. Olfaction in neurodegenerative disorder. In: Hummel T, Welge-Luessen A, eds. Advances in Oto-Rhino-Laryngology. Basel: Karger-Verlag; 2006:133–151.

30. Hawkes CH, Del Tredici K, Braak H. A timeline for Parkinson's disease. Parkinsonism Relat Disord 2010; 16(2):79–84

31. Naka A, Riedl M, Luger A, Hummel T, Mueller CA. Clinical significance of smell and taste disorders in patients with diabetes mellitus. Eur Arch Otorhinolaryngol 2010;267(4):547–550

32. Göktas Ö, Cao Van H, Fleiner F, Lacroix JS, Landis BN. Chemosensory function in Wegener's granulomatosis: a preliminary report. Eur Arch Otorhinolaryngol 2010;267(7):1089–1093

33. Smith DV, Seiden AM. Olfactory dysfunction. In: Laing DG, Doty RL, Breipohl W, eds. The Human Sense of Smell. Berlin: Springer; 1991:283–305.

34. Murphy C, Doty RL, Duncan HJ. Clinical disorders of olfaction. In: Doty RL, ed. Handbook of Olfaction and Gustation. 2nd ed. New York, Basel: Marcel Dekker; 2003. 461–478.

6 Assessment of Olfaction and Gustation

Thomas Hummel, Cornelia Hummel, Antje Welge-Luessen

Summary

Smell disorders occur frequently. In general, 5 to 6% of the population exhibit functional anosmia. Typically, interviews are insufficient to properly assess patients' symptoms. Structured diagnostic procedures are required to quantify olfactory function. Among diagnostic measures, simple psychophysical instruments are most important, but electrophysiological procedures are widely established as well. In addition, both imaging methods—e.g., volumetric assessment of the olfactory bulb or functional magnetic resonance imaging with gustatory or olfactory stimulation—and immunohistochemical evaluation of biopsy material are available.

Why Assess the Chemical Senses?

Approximately 5% of the population are unable to smell and roughly 20% above the age of 50 years are suffering from significant smell loss,[1] with the main causes being sinonasal disorders[2] or age dependent impairment of olfaction.[3,4]

To evaluate smell disorders, they need first to be quantified. A patient history is important but insufficient because of the discrepancy between self-described and quantified olfactory function in the majority of patients.[5] A similar situation exists with respect to gustatory function.[6] Interestingly, it has been shown that self-description of olfactory performance does not reflect olfactory function per se, but rather nasal airflow! Only if the patient's focus is directed toward their actual olfactory acuity (e.g., by means of a smell test) does rating of their own olfactory sensibility become more accurate.[5] Therefore, assessment of chemosensory performance is indispensable.

> **Note**
>
> Self-ratings of olfaction and gustation correlate poorly with quantified test results. Smell and taste function need to be assessed properly; subjective estimates are of limited value.

Psychophysical methods to evaluate the sense of smell are widely used. Approximately 200 psychophysical testing methods are available but only the most important will be introduced here: First, because many tests are basically very similar and, second, because most of them are unvalidated (see ref. 7). The majority currently assess orthonasal olfaction (with odors entering the nose by sniffing) rather than retronasal olfaction (in which odors reach the nose during eating and drinking). However, significant differences between processing olfactory stimuli from the two pathways have been established,[8,9] which are also present on a clinical level.[10]

Psychophysical tests are based upon interviewing patients and rely upon their cooperation. In cases of insufficient ability to cooperate (e.g., in children or patients with cognitive impairment) or lack of motivation to accomplish the test (e.g., if the aim of the test is to yield an expert medical opinion), findings may be difficult to evaluate. Here, different procedures may be helpful, particularly ones based upon electrophysiological methods, such as recording of olfactory event-related potentials (see below). These procedures, granting a higher degree of objectivity, are technically more demanding than psychophysical tests, and require the investigator's expertise. Owing to their expense, they are primarily used in legal contexts where medical evidence is required. Furthermore, biopsies from the olfactory mucosa, and imaging methods, both structural and functional, yield additional ways of evaluating olfaction or prognosis of smell disorders. However, the practical value of these tools on an intra-individual level has yet to be clarified.

Of course, prior to applying a test or starting an examination, the patient's history has to be ascertained. A detailed introduction to establishing the history of smell and taste disorders may be found in the Guidelines of the German ENT Society (compare with ref. 11).

Tests of Olfaction

Psychophysical Assessment of Orthonasal Olfaction

Short Tests

Several tests are based upon odor naming, because of the ease and comprehensibility of this approach.[12] However, as most of these tools include verbal components, one has to consider the influence of cognition and language on these tests. Short screening tests are able to differentiate between normosmia and hyposmia/anosmia. Their advantage is their short duration; their disadvantage is their comparatively poor validity with respect to detailed results, which renders the short tests unsuitable for medicolegal contexts and—at least on an individual basis—evaluation of the course of therapy.

Cross-Cultural Smell Identification Test

The "Cross-Cultural Smell Identification Test" (CCSIT) is a short test requiring the patient to identify odors from lists of four identifiers.[13] In a multiple forced-choice procedure, 12 odors are tested. Microencapsulated odors are attached to paper, and may be released by rubbing the paper with a pencil. The test has a long shelf-life and is well validated. It may be performed by patients unassisted.

Sniffin' Sticks Screening

The "Sniffin' Sticks," too, allow screening of olfactory function, analogous to the CCSIT. Odors are released from small cylinders with capped points, similar to felt pens. The screening procedure is an identification test and may be performed with either 12 pens[14] or 16 pens in an extended version.[15] The test is well validated and, unlike the CCSIT, may be used repeatedly. Depending on the frequency of application, the pens' shelf-life may be a year or longer. Patients may perform the test by themselves.[16]

> **Note**
> Several well-validated, inexpensive, easy, and quick tests are available for olfactory screening.

European Test of Olfactory Capabilities

The "European Test of Olfactory Capabilities"[17] is based upon 12 odors (**Fig. 6.1a**) in small glass bottles. Two procedures are performed: The first task is to identify one out of four bottles containing an odorant, which then has to be identified from a four-item list in multiple choice mode.

Zürcher Riechtest

The "Zürcher Riechtest"[18] includes eight odors on so-called smell disks; odors have to be identified from three items. The disks are reusable and may be applied by patients unassisted. The test has been validated in a relatively small sample.

Identification Tests with Very Few Odors

Among the identification tests using very few odors are those from the UPSIT family ("University of Pennsylvania Smell Identification Tests"), namely, the "Pocket-Smell-Test" and another tool, both based upon three odors.[19] The "Sniffin' Sticks" family, too, includes short versions with three[20] and five[21] odors, which distinguish normosmic patients from anosmic patients with high specificity at very low scores, occasionally failing, however, to identify an anosmic patient. These tests are primarily useful in contexts requiring a global estimate rather than a detailed olfactory assessment.

Another very simple tool is the "Alcohol-Sniff-Test."[22] The sachet of a disposable, prepackaged alcohol swab is opened and the pad is slowly moved toward the nose; the distance from which the smell is perceived yields a diagnostic clue with respect to olfactory function.

> **Note**
> Humans are typically poor at correctly identifying odors. Basically, this can only be achieved if a list of items to choose from is available. Thus, the mere presentation of a tin of ground coffee or a flask of perfume is, at best, a fragrance-assisted interview, and cannot be considered a smell test.

Psychophysical Tests Assessing Olfaction in a More Extensive Manner

In recent years, both standardized and validated psychophysical tests have been developed to investigate olfactory function in a detailed fashion. Several aspects are assessed, such as perception thresholds of one or more odorants; the ability to discriminate between odors and to identify them; olfactory memory; and the rating of suprathreshold odor concentrations.

University of Pennsylvania Smell Identification Tests

Exclusively an odor identification test, the UPSIT consists of forty microencapsulated odorants embedded in paper, which are released by rubbing ("scratch and sniff," see **Fig. 6.1b**), and identified in multiple forced-choice mode from item lists.[23] Although this disposable tool is the most frequently applied smell identification test worldwide, the original version is somewhat regionally restricted because of intercultural differences in familiarity of odors (e.g., root beer, wintergreen). However, UPSIT versions are available today that have been adapted to a number of languages (www.sensonics.com).

Sniffin' Sticks

"Sniffin' Sticks" permit a more detailed evaluation of the sense of smell[24-26] (**Fig. 6.1c**). They are reusable. The whole test is divided into a threshold, a discrimination, and an identification part, with the last two being suprathreshold tests. The test battery is based upon the notion that different tests assess different dimensions of olfaction.[27,28] In this concept, it is assumed that threshold tests rather reflect peripheral aspects of the olfactory system, as opposed to more advanced, complex processing levels represented in identification and discrimination tasks. However, an absolutely clear-cut separation of these functions cannot be achieved by specific olfactory tests (see ref. 29), as discriminating and memory processes do play an important role in threshold testing, and, conversely, odor intensity is correlated with the activity of olfactory receptor neurons (ORNs).[30]

Threshold testing with Sniffin' Sticks yields the concentration above which an odor is perceived.

Olfactory sensitivity may be tested with n-butanol or phenylethyl alcohol. During this test, patients wear a blindfold to conceal the pens' labels. Concentrations of the odor solutions represent a geometric series, starting at a concentration of 4%, and progressing in a total of 16 steps with a dilution ratio of 1:2 at each step.

Patients are presented with triplets of Sniffin' Sticks. Each triplet consists of one odorous pen and two pens containing an odorless solvent. The sequence of presentation within triplets is random. Patients are required to identify the smelling pen in each triplet. Starting at a low concentration, and continuing with increasing concentrations as long as no correct response is obtained, the first "turning point" is reached when the odorous pen is identified in two succeeding triplets (indicating that the threshold has been passed). At any turning point, the direction of concentration changes is reversed from decreasing to increasing or vice versa, and presentation thus continues until the next failure or success, respectively. The procedure is completed at the seventh turning point, and the mean of the last four turning points is established as the threshold. A similar test, based upon odor flasks, is available in conjunction with the UPSIT. Other methods of odor threshold detection are used (for example, refs. 31–37), but at least some of them appear to be less suitable than Sniffin' Sticks in clinical contexts.[36]

The nonverbal **discrimination** test of the Sniffin' Sticks battery tests the ability to discriminate between odors. Again, patients are blindfolded, and triplets are presented, in this case with suprathreshold concentrations in all pens. In each triplet, two items contain the same odorant, whereas the third one is different, and is required to be detected. Patients are presented with each pen only once. Altogether, 16 triplets are used; the number of correctly identified items represents the discrimination score. This test appears to be strongly affected by cognitive abilities.[28]

Identification is tested as in the UPSIT procedure, with Sniffin' Sticks used rather than microencapsulated odors, and the number of items typically being 16 or 32.[26] Odor identification is influenced by numerous factors (e.g., cognitive abilities, verbal skills, number of items in the multiple choice list, or similarity of these items, etc.).[38,39]

After completion of the entire test battery, the sum of the scores from all three subtests is calcu-

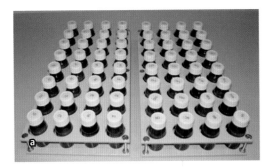

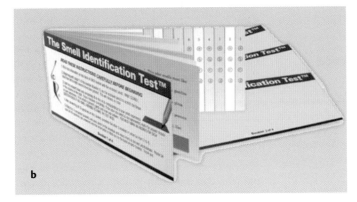

Fig. 6.1a–e Five smell tests are displayed. (Images courtesy of Richard L. Doty, Philadelphia; William S. Cain, San Diego; Moustafa Bensafi, Lyon; Tadashi Ishimaru, Kanazawa.) (From Hummel T, Welge-Lüssen A. Riech- und Schmeckstorungen: Physiologie, Pathophysiologie und Therapeutische Ansatze. Stuttgart: Thieme; 2005.)

a "European Test for Olfactory Capabilities," with eight odorants in eight concentrations, for threshold and identification testing.

b "University of Pennsylvania Smell Identification Test," a so-called scratch-and-sniff test.

c "Sniffin' Sticks" identification subtest with 12 items.

d "Connecticut Chemosensory Clinical Research Centers" test, comes in bottles for assessing butanol threshold and a salt dispenser-like container for the identification task. The table presents verbal descriptors of odors, some of which are presented during odor identification and some of which are not (distractors).

e "T&T olfactometer," with five odorants in eight concentrations, to test thresholds of odor perception and odor identification.

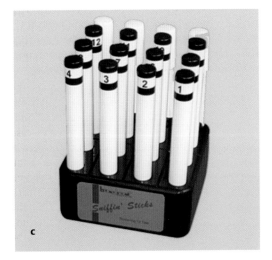

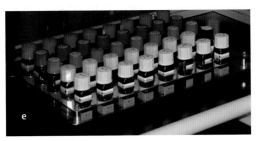

Odor names	
Ammonia	Peanut butter
Baby powder	Pepper (black)
Burnt paper	Rubber
Chocolate	Sardines
Cinnamon	Soap (bar)
Coffee	Tobacco
Garlic	Turpentine
Ketchup	Vicks
Mothballs	Wintergreen
Onion	Woodshavings

lated (**T**hreshold + **D**iscrimination + **I**dentification = TDI score). A TDI score difference of six and above indicates a clinically significant change.[40] For computer assisted test procedure and documentation, free software may be downloaded from: http://www.tu-dresden.de/medkhno/riechen_schmecken/download.htm

> **Note**
>
> Olfactory threshold, discrimination, and identification tests tap into different portions of olfactory function.

Connecticut Chemosensory Clinical Research Center Test

The test developed by the Connecticut Chemosensory Clinical Research Center (**CCCRC-Test**[32]) is available in two parts (**Fig. 6.1d**). The **threshold** is assessed for butanol. Starting at a very low concentration, increasing odorant concentrations are presented, along with a nonodorous sample; patients are asked to identify the sample containing the odorant. The threshold is represented by the concentration that is correctly identified in three to five consecutive trials. In the identification task, patients are presented with eight odorants that have to be identified from a 16-item list. Scores of both subtests are combined to a single score.

> **Note**
>
> Clinically, testing is almost exclusively performed for both nostrils together; monorhinal testing is frequently omitted. This procedure misses lateralized differences in olfactory function (which are frequent; see ref. 41). Such differences may be indicative of lateralized brain lesions (e.g., olfactory meningioma). They may also contain information on the prognosis of the olfactory loss.[42]

T&T Test

The Japanese **T&T Test** (the name refers to the developers of the test, Professor SF Takagi and Professor B Toyoda[43]) is based upon five odors (β-phenylethyl alcohol, methyl cyclopentenolone, isovaleric acid, γ-undecalactone, scatole) in eight concentrations (**Fig. 6.1e**). Presenting samples in increasing concentrations, first the perception threshold (the concentration at which the odor is first perceived), and then the identification threshold (the concentration at which the odor is correctly recognized), is established.

All extensive tests permit differentiation among normosmia, hyposmia, and anosmia (**Table 6.1**). By way of commercial availability and standardized application in several centers, comparability of various investigations could be accomplished.

Table 6.1 Definition of olfactory disorders: quantitative disorders are highlighted in light red, and qualitative disorders in darker red

Diagnosis	Description
Anosmia	Total loss of olfactory function
Functional anosmia	Significantly impaired olfaction, including both total loss and minimal residual perception
Partial anosmia	Significantly reduced sensibility toward one odorant or group of odorants, compared with the general population—without clinical relevance
Hyposmia	Partial loss (frequent, e.g., in old age)
Olfactory intolerance	Subjective hypersensitivity toward odorants, but normal olfactory function
Hyperosmia	Hypernormal olfactory sensitivity (very rare, e.g., in migraine)
Parosmia (synonym, troposmia)	Abnormal perception, with sensory input present
Phantosmia	Abnormal perception, with sensory input absent

> **Note**
>
> Forced-choice procedures are indispensable to avoid patients deciding on the "no smell" option, as this is easy and tempting and will be chosen by several patients, irrespective of whether anything was perceived or not. Only if these patients are requested to concentrate on the presented stimuli using forced-choice tasks, may they realize their perceptive abilities—which often come as a surprise to the patients themselves!

Psychophysical Assessment of Retronasal Olfaction

Retronasal olfaction represents the perception of smell during eating and drinking (**Fig. 6.2a**). As retronasal olfaction occurs virtually exclusively in the context of food and drink intake, it is mostly mistaken for taste perception. This explains why ~60% of patients suffering from only smell disorders complain about loss of smell and taste.[44] Therefore, at least some cursory taste test (sweet, bitter, sour, and salty), ought to be performed along with a smell test in any patient presenting with a taste problem. Frequently, exclusive olfactory disorders are found in these cases, without any impairment of taste function.[44]

To our knowledge, the first clinical test of retronasal olfaction was introduced by **Güttich**,[45] who believed he had found the ideal tool to expose malingerers in medicolegal investigations. The basic idea was that anosmic people would be unable to perceive the "taste" of liquid odorants applied to the mouth (e.g., "cherry in rum"). If an alleged anosmic could still identify the "taste" of the solutions, this would indicate odor perception. The test is, however, unstructured and thus unreliable.[46]

In spite of impaired orthonasal olfaction, some patients are able to identify retronasally presented odors.[47] Aside from that, in disorders such as nasal polyposis or hyperplastic tonsils, discrepancies between ortho- and retronasal olfaction occur. In addition, in a small group of patients, orthonasal smelling was found to be selectively affected, whereas retronasal olfaction was still intact.[48]

The **Aachen "rhinotest"**[49] is a screening test of retronasal smell identification, using six odorous sprays applied to the mouth. Individuals are required to select odor quality from a list of six identifiers (flowery, disgusting, fruity, raisiny, stinging, spicy). This reusable test has a long shelf-life and can be applied by the patients themselves.

In a test developed in Japan, odorants such as prosultiamine (smell of garlic) are administered **intravenously**[50] and the latency at which the odor is perceived (if at all) is assessed. This test is based on the pulmonary exhalation of the odorant.

Another test of retronasal olfaction is the standardized **"taste powder"** tool[47] (**Fig. 6.2b**).

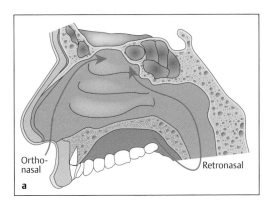
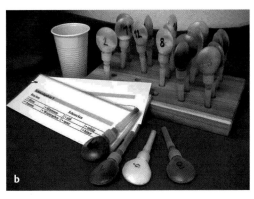

Fig. 6.2a, b Retronasal olfaction. (From Hummel T, Welge-Lüssen A. Riech- und Schmeckstorungen: Physiologie, Pathophysiologie und Therapeutische Ansatze. Stuttgart: Thieme; 2005.)

a Schematic sketch of air flow in ortho- and retronasal olfaction. (Image courtesy of Thomas Beleites, Dresden.)

b Retronasal smell test "taste powders:" Smelling food powders are whiffed onto the tongue by means of powder applicators. Similar to the orthonasal test, patients identify the "taste" in forced-choice mode from a four-item list.

So-called taste powders (20 pulverized food and spice samples, e.g., cinnamon) are applied to the mouth and identified by patients from lists of four items. This relatively simple test may be easily performed anywhere with powders purchased from a grocery. It is suitable to validate complaints of complete olfactory loss with (nearly) unimpaired gustation and vice versa.[48] Recently, another test of retronasal sensitivity has been introduced,[51] which is based on aromatized sorbitol candies.

> **Note**
>
> Ortho- and retronasal olfaction may be selectively affected. Therefore, separate testing of both pathways is worthwhile.

Electrophysiological Procedures to Assess Olfaction

Olfactory Event-related Potentials

Electroencephalography (EEG)-based **olfactory event-related potentials (ERP)**[52,53] is a method to validate smell disorders quantitatively. It has become a routine technique in many countries. Prerequisites of the stimulating device (olfactometer), apart from precise duration, concentration, and steep rise of the chemical stimuli, are constant flow, temperature, and humidity of the air stream (**Fig. 6.3**).

Stimulus durations of 200 milliseconds at intervals of 30 to 40 seconds are recommended, with an airflow of 7 to 8 L/min (but see also ref. 54). Typically, 16 to 80 stimuli (optimally 80) are used to calculate an average ERP.[55] An essential requirement of olfactory ERP is a sufficiently steep rising edge of the stimuli. At the olfactometer's outlet, air temperature should approximate body temperature, and air humidity should be 70 to 80%. Chemical stimulation must not be accompanied by any mechanical, thermal, or acoustic phenomena, as these are likely to elicit evoked responses that interfere with the olfactory response.[53] Olfactory ERPs have been shown to be generated in areas of the brain including the amygdala, the insula, and the orbitofrontal cortex.[56]

Only "pure" olfactory stimulants such as hydrogen sulfide ("rotten eggs"), vanillin, or phenylethyl alcohol ("rose fragrance") should be used to elicit olfactory ERPs. In addition, a trigeminal stimulant should be applied separately for control purposes (e.g., odorless carbon dioxide). For clinical evaluation of smell disorders, olfactory ERPs should be obtained from at least three recording positions, with the patient's eyes open. The main ERP recordings are a negative deflection at latencies between 200 and 700 milliseconds, and a positive peak at latencies between 300 and 800 milliseconds. In cases in which olfactory ERPs are obtained, it can be assumed that olfactory function is present.[55,57,58] This is of particular significance in contexts where expert medical opinions are required.[53]

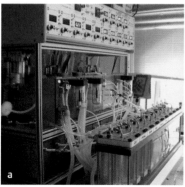 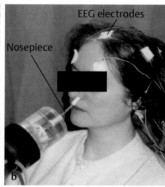 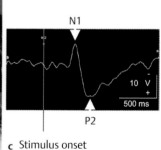

Fig. 6.3a–c Olfactory evoked potentials. (From Hummel T, Welge-Lüssen A. Riech- und Schmeckstorungen: Physiologie, Pathophysiologie und Therapeutische Ansatze. Stuttgart: Thieme; 2005.)

a Stimulating device to obtain olfactory-evoked potentials (OEP): Olfactometer OM6b (Burghart instruments, Wedel).

b Subject with olfactometer outlet and electroencephalography (EEG) electrodes during OEP recording.

c Typical OEP after stimulation with phenylethyl alcohol (rose fragrance); main peaks marked N1 and P2. In anosmic patients no such OEP is obtained.

Electro-olfactogram

Peripheral mucosal potentials (so-called **electro-olfactograms**) can be obtained in humans from the olfactory epithelium.[52,59,60] However attractive this method is in an experimental context, its clinical value is decreased by the fact that it is not recordable in all patients, even in those with a normal sense of smell,[30] and that there are situations where it can be recorded even though the stimulus is not perceived.[61,62]

Contingent Negative Variation

The so-called **contingent negative variation (CNV)** is a negative deflection in the EEG occurring when an event is expected. This phenomenon is also exploited in the assessment of olfactory function.[63] In a so-called S1–S2 paradigm, patients are acquainted with a sequence whereby an olfactory stimulus (S2) is preceded by another (e.g., acoustic) stimulus (S1). After presentation of S1, CNV develops in anticipation of S2 and collapses at occurrence of S2. CNV continuation after S2 indicates that the smell was not perceived. Alternatively, the olfactory stimulus could also be S1; if subjects do not perceive the odor, no CNV will develop. This technique requires the patient's cooperation. Furthermore, the occurrence of a CNV depends on several psychological variables, meaning that it does not occur in every person.[64]

Others

General EEG shifts following the presentation of olfactory stimuli have also been used to validate smell disorders. However, cases have been reported where, although odors were perceived, no EEG reaction could be obtained.[65] With advanced EEG amplifiers and software this method may experience a revival (Huart, personal communication). Another method tested for its prognostic value in olfactory disorders is measurement of **trigeminal ERPs** after intranasal stimulation with carbon dioxide,[66] but large, prospective studies have not yet been conducted. The **psychogalvanic skin reaction** ("lie detector test") has also been used to test olfactory function in a medicolegal context.[67]

Investigation of Reactions Following Olfactory Stimulation

Gudziol and Wächter were able to show that respiratory changes after olfactory stimulation are clinically significant in terms of the distinction between hyposmia and anosmia.[68] This method is also applicable in medicolegal contexts. Based on the same reaction—smell-induced changes in respiration—but requiring less technical expenditure, is the so-called Compu-Sniff test[69] (**Fig. 6.4**), which assesses sniffing parameters in relation to the presence or absence of odors. As these procedures are nonverbal, they also appear to be suitable for testing children.

Both **pupillary**[70,71] and **wink reflexes**[72] have also been tested; these procedures, however, remain of pure experimental interest and are not clinically applied.

Functional Magnetic Resonance Imaging

In functional magnetic resonance imaging (fMRI), the so-called BOLD (Blood Oxygenation Level–Dependent) effect is assessed in response to olfactory or gustatory stimuli[73] (**Fig. 6.5**). As the effects reflect regional blood flow changes in the brain, and thus, indirectly, changes of neuronal activation, it permits assessment of both cerebral activation and the location where it occurs. In the last decade, this technique has gained widespread currency and yielded a multitude of new findings.[74,75] However, it is questionable whether it is useful in clinical practice, because of high interindividual variability. In addition, it seems that even anosmic patients exhibit some random brain activation.

> **Note**
>
> Olfactory ERPs are particularly significant in medicolegal contexts, and have been studied in much more detail than other nonpsychophysical instruments validating olfactory function.

Volumetric Assessment of the Olfactory Bulb

Plasticity of the olfactory bulb (OB) is outstanding among the central nervous system.[76] It is ensured

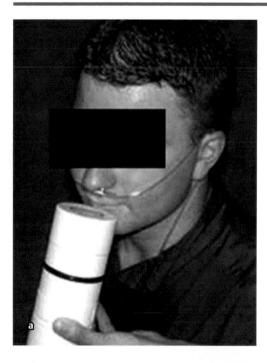

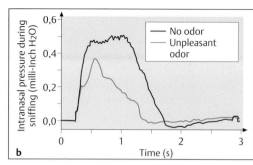

Fig. 6.4a, b Compu-Sniff test. (Images courtesy of Robert Frank, Cincinnatti.) (From Hummel T, Welge-Lüssen A. Riech- und Schmeckstorungen: Physiologie, Pathophysiologie und Therapeutische Ansatze. Stuttgart: Thieme; 2005.)

a Subject with nasal probe (connected to a piezo pressure transducer) containing odorant to be released upon sniffing.

b Results (pressure–time diagrams; sampling rate 100 Hz) of no odor and unpleasant odor: perception of unpleasant smell significantly changes sniffing behavior.

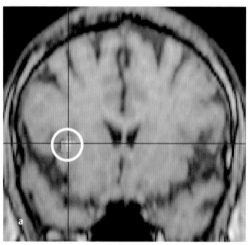

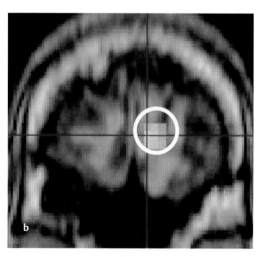

Fig. 6.5a, b Functional magnetic resonance imaging: Typical cerebral activation of insula (**a**) and orbito-frontal cortex (**b**) after gustatory stimulation with sucrose and citric acid in a healthy subject (see ref. 73).

by continuous neurogenesis, which itself seems to be dependent on peripheral neuronal activity.[77] Anatomical changes in the OB may be gauged from structural magnetic resonance images (circularly polarized coil, T2-weighted, frontal constructive interference in steady-state precession sequences acquired in three-dimensional mode; resolution less than $0.2 \times 0.5 \times 0.7$ mm³). As expected, the OB is hypo- or aplastic in patients with congenital anosmia[78]; this is also expedient as a diagnostic criterion. In addition, a flattening of the olfactory sulcus is characteristic in these patients.[79,80] Patients suffering from postinfectious or posttraumatic olfactory deficits have smaller OB volumes than normosmic subjects.[81] Moreover, OB volumes correlate with the degree of olfactory impairment,[82] and with intraindividual changes in sense of smell[83,84] (**Fig. 6.6**). Therefore, OB volum-

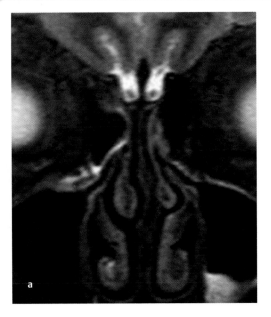

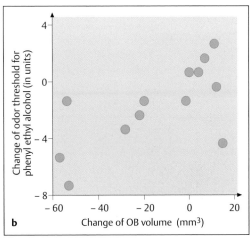

Fig. 6.6a, b Assessment of olfactory bulb volume. (From Hummel T, Welge-Lüssen A. Riech- und Schmeckstorungen: Physiologie, Pathophysiologie und Therapeutische Ansatze. Stuttgart: Thieme; 2005.)

a Cranial magnetic resonance imaging cross section (frontal plane) from a healthy subject, with both olfactory bulbs (OBs) marked by white circles.

b Dependency of OB volume on threshold changes for phenylethyl alcohol (rose fragrance); modified from ref. 83.

etry is considered a possible tool to estimate individual prognosis in olfactory disorders.

Biopsies from the Olfactory Mucosa

Morphological examinations can assess the presence of peripheral ORNs, and gain information about peripheral conditions causing smell disorders.[85,86]

Biopsies can correlate the most frequent olfactory disorders with their histopathological findings. **(1) Post-traumatic** alterations are associated with disorganization and thickening of the olfactory epithelium, and a small number of degenerated cells.[87] **(2) Postviral anosmia** biopsies often show reduced numbers of ORNs and, occasionally, squamous epithelial metaplasia.[88] **(3)** In smell disorders caused by **sinonasal** conditions, olfactory epithelium is normal in the early stages[89,90] but may demonstrate squamous epithelial metaplasia or fibrosis in chronic cases. Potentially, biopsy of the olfactory mucosa appears reasonable to evaluate idiopathic smell disorders. However, nonspecific alterations occur relatively frequently even in normosmic subjects, particularly in old age, which often renders the relationship between biopsy findings and functional conditions inconclusive.[91]

> **Note**
> Biopsies are highly valuable in experimental contexts, but are of limited value in the evaluation of olfactory disorders in individual patients.

How to Evaluate Parosmia and Phantosmia

The diagnoses "parosmia" and "phantosmia" are solely based upon the patient's report.[92] They may be graded using the following system:

- Frequency of occurrence: daily = 1 point, otherwise = 0 points
- Intensity: very strong = 1 point, otherwise = 0 points
- Social effects (e.g., weight loss, significant change of habits): yes = 1 point, no = 0 points

The sum score represents the degree of the disorder. Findings to support the diagnosis of qualitative smell disorders are low scores in smell identification tests[93] and small OB volumes compared with patients with unimpaired olfaction.[81,82] The latter may indicate decreased numbers of OB interneurons, resulting in reduced lateral inhibition, which, in turn, may generate qualitative olfactory dysfunction.

> **Note**
>
> Objective methods to validate parosmia and phantosmia are lacking. These disorders are established solely based upon the patient's history.

Assessment of Taste Function

Taste stimuli are processed via three cranial nerves: The facial nerve, glossopharyngeal nerve, and vagal nerve. Taste receptors are present in the mouth, oropharynx, and pharyngeal portion of the epiglottis (and also in the gut![94]). In addition, the vagal nerve contributes sensations of temperature, texture, and irritation. The brainstem, thalamus, orbitofrontal cortex, and insula are essentially involved in taste processing. Gustatory sensitivity decreases with age—if less so than olfactory sensitivity—and, as in olfaction, is greater in women than men.

After establishing the patient's history and performing a basic clinical examination (see Chapter 5), a specific taste test is applied, either to the entire oral cavity or in a localized fashion, using both natural and electrical stimulation. Local testing yields more detailed results, permitting, for example, the detection of lateralized taste dis-

orders, whereas whole-mouth testing simulates everyday taste experience.

Particularly in cases of dysgeusia (e.g., bitter or metallic tastes), subjective reports of taste sensations are highly significant, as no quantitative method is currently available to assess these types of disorders (**Table 6.2**).

Psychophysical Whole-mouth Tests

In **whole-mouth testing**, small amounts of taste substances (e.g., drops or sprays) are applied. Patients distribute the sample in the oral cavity, disgorge it after a few seconds, and rinse their mouth with water. Suprathreshold testing may be performed with so-called **taste sprays**, using the natural substances sucrose (1 g in 10 g aqua; sweet), citric acid (0.5 g in 10 g aqua; sour), sodium chloride (0.75 g in 10 g aqua; salty), and quinine hydrochloride (0.005 g in 10 g aqua; bitter). This suprathreshold procedure is a simple screening tool that tests a patient's ability to identify taste qualities.

Another frequently used method is the **three drops test**.[95] Drops (volume: < 0.1 mL) of either water or a taste solution are administered in groups of three, with each group consisting of two water and one taste drop, applied successively in a random sequence. The first group contains the lowest concentration of the tastant. Patients are asked to identify the tasting drop within each group. The test aims to assess the taste threshold, which is established as the concentration identified three times in a row (for standard values, please see ref. 96). Further taste tests have been

Table 6.2 Definition of gustatory disorders: quantitative disorders are highlighted in light red, and qualitative disorders in dark red

Diagnosis	Description
Ageusia	Total loss of gustatory function
Functional ageusia	Significantly impaired gustation, including both total loss and minimal residual perception
Partial ageusia	Reduced sensitivity toward one taste quality
Hypogeusia	Reduced sensitivity, compared with young, healthy subjects
Hypergeusia	Increased sensitivity, compared with young, healthy subjects
Parageusia	Abnormal perception, with sensory input present
Phantogeusia	Abnormal perception, with sensory input absent

suggested, including "taste tablets," which dissolve in the oral cavity to release taste substances,[97] or wafers impregnated with taste substances[98]; however, these tests are not commercially available. Recent developments are based on soluble material impregnated with tastant.[99]

Note

Any taste test should be accompanied by a brief smell test and vice versa, as patients are prone to mistake aromas for taste sensations, and therefore complain about taste problems instead of smell problems.

Psychophysical Taste Tests Applied To Several Oral Sites (Local Taste Tests)

Among local taste tests, the **two-alternative forced-choice** procedure is widely used. Patients are asked to decide which of two stimuli, presented, for example, on the left and right side, elicits a taste sensation. This method may also be used to assess taste thresholds. **Fig. 6.7** illustrates local taste tests.

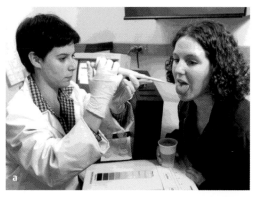

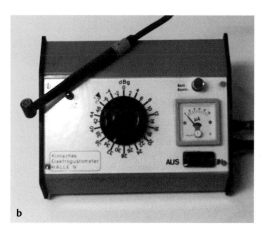

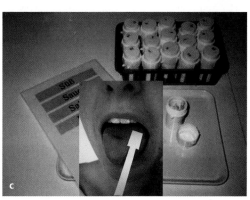

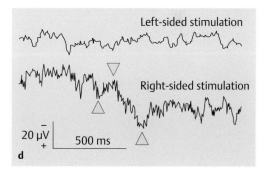

Fig. 6.7a–d Taste tests. (From Hummel T, Welge-Lüssen A. Riech- und Schmeckstorungen: Physiologie, Pathophysiologie und Therapeutische Ansatze. Stuttgart: Thieme; 2005.)

a Local testing with adequate stimulus: application of a taste solution to one side of the tongue with a pipette.

b Electrogustometer "Halle IV," with stimulating electrode, to be placed upon tongue or palate.

c Taste strips with sweet, sour, salty, and bitter tastes in four concentrations each, to be placed upon the tongue's left or right side, with the patient being required to indicate the perceived taste in a list.

d Example of gustatory-evoked potentials after stimulation with acetic acid vapor in a patient with left-sided ageusia: clear evoked potential after stimulation of the right side (bottom curve, with arrows indicating peaks) as opposed to the left side (top curve, no evoked response).

Local Taste Tests Using Adequate Stimuli

Adequate taste stimuli may be applied using either liquid taste solutions or so-called taste strips,[100-102] which consist of strips of filter paper impregnated with taste substances. Liquid taste solutions may be dabbed on with cotton swabs,[103] or applied by means of a pipette[104] or soaked pieces of filter paper.[105] Usually, identification thresholds of each gustatory area are assessed using increasing concentrations of taste substances. Patients are instructed to keep their tongues immobile in a slightly protruded position until they have indicated the perceived taste by pointing to the respective descriptor on a board; after that, they rinse their mouths with water. The tongue's extended position during testing is essential to avoid distribution of the tastant outside the tested regions; as soon as the tongue is moved into the mouth, tastants will inevitably spread throughout the oral cavity, thwarting local testing.

Advantages of the taste strips are their long shelf-life, the option of lateralized testing, and availability of several concentrations of tastants. Normative data have been established.[106] The procedure is highly reliable and has been successfully used in several clinical studies (e.g., refs. 107, 108).

In another variety of tests quantifying gustation, intensity estimates of different concentrations of taste solutions are obtained either using a rating scale ranging from "weak" through to "strong" or, in a cross-modal approach, by comparison with variable volumes of a 1,000-Hz sound.[103]

> **Note**
>
> When taste testing the anterior two-thirds of the tongue, the tongue must remain protruded until the patient has indicated the perceived taste quality.

Electrogustometry

Electrogustometry, first introduced in the 19th century, has been established as a reliable procedure to assess gustatory function.[109] Perception thresholds are obtained by direct current stimulation with 1.5 to 400 µA in monopolar (anodal) or bipolar (coaxial) mode. It is important to compare left- and right-sided function.

Electrogustometry is simple and provides quick evidence of nerve lesions, but there are also several drawbacks: the method does not permit differentiation between taste qualities in gustatory disorders; accompanying trigeminal sensations may occur at higher stimulus intensities; and correlation between electrical and chemosensory taste testing is weak.[110] Nevertheless, electrogustometry may have a specific value in separating ageusia from hypogeusia.[111]

"Objective" Tests

Recordings of **gustatory-evoked potentials** are available in very few specialized centers (compare olfactory ERP). Gustatory stimuli are applied either to the whole oral cavity or in a lateralized fashion. At present, the method is primarily used in experimental and medicolegal contexts.[112]

Occasionally, **fMRI** in response to gustatory stimulation (see above) may be performed,[73] but its value as a diagnostic tool in individual cases is yet to be demonstrated (**Fig. 6.5**).

> **Note**
>
> Few centers offer "objective" techniques to assess taste disorders, such as gustatory ERPs or gustatory fMRI.

Assessment of Morphological Changes

Two methods to assess morphological changes are available: biopsy (e.g., ref. 113) and contact endoscopy (e.g., ref. 114). In the latter, the tongue's epithelium is dyed with methylene blue and a fiber optic scope is placed on the mucosa, where cells are discernible at 60 to 150 × magnification. Thus, for example, in patients with a transected chorda tympani, fewer and flatter fungiform papillae are found in the ipsilateral epithelium than in the contralateral epithelium[114] (**Fig. 6.8**). In addition, vascular meshes beneath the epithelium are visible even without dye. Currently, however, this technique is not widely available.

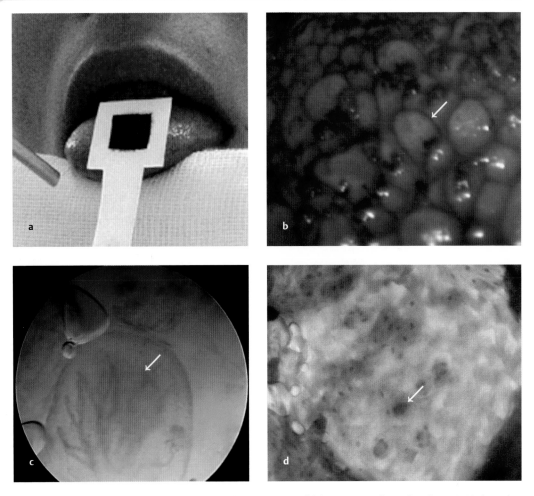

Fig. 6.8a–d Contact endoscopy. (Images courtesy of Tino Just, Rostock.) (From Hummel T, Welge-Lüssen A. Riech- und Schmeckstorungen: Physiologie, Pathophysiologie und Therapeutische Ansatze. Stuttgart: Thieme; 2005.)

a Partial dying of the tongue prior to contact endoscopy.

b Arrow indicates a fungiform papilla (fpap).

c Arrow indicates vascular architecture of fpap.

d Surface of an fpap (same region, dyed with methylene blue); arrow indicates pore of a taste bud.

Investigation of the Intranasal Trigeminal System

No standardized and clinically validated psycho-physical tests are available to assess the chemo-sensory function of the trigeminal nerve. In experimental contexts, "lateralization" of trigeminal stimuli[115–118] is exploited: Unlike pure olfactory stimuli, nasal sensations such as tingling, burning, stinging, or tickling—elicited in addition to smells by many odorants and mediated by the trigeminal nerve—may be localized. Thus, after unilateral pre-sentation of a bimodal olfactory/trigeminal stimulant such as menthol, the stimulated nostril can be identified, whereas this would be extremely difficult with a specific olfactory stimulant such as vanillin.[115]

In addition, threshold assessment of trigeminal stimuli, and intensity estimates in the supra-threshold range, may be performed.[119] Another, experimental, approach aims to record reflexive physiological effects (e.g., nasal secretion or respiration) induced by trigeminal stimulation (overview in ref. 120).

"Chemosomatosensory ERP" is also used to assess the trigeminal system.[121,122] Typically, odorless carbon dioxide is chosen as a stimulant which, at concentrations above 30%, and at 200-millisecond stimulus duration, elicits burning, stinging sensations. Possibly, these trigeminal ERPs may also convey prognostic information concerning smell disorders[66] (compare Minovi et al 2007[123]). Another method of investigating the trigeminal system is to record potentials from the respiratory mucosa (negative mucosa potential),[124] a sophisticated technique currently used only in research (e.g., refs. 125–127).

> **Note**
>
> Few methods—and these mainly in experimental contexts—are available to assess trigeminal chemosensory function. However, it may be assumed that olfactory disorders are accompanied by reduced trigeminal sensitivity[128]—an important aspect, particularly with respect to medicolegal evidence (see Chapter 18).

Summary and Outlook

To thoroughly evaluate patients' symptoms, detailed investigation of chemosensory function is required. The availability of standardized procedures to assess smell and taste seems to be of the utmost importance in the development of new strategies to cure chemosensory dysfunction.

References

1. Landis BN, Hummel T. New evidence for high occurrence of olfactory dysfunctions within the population. Am J Med 2006;119(1):91–92
2. Damm M, Temmel A, Welge-Lüssen A, et al. Damm M, Temmel A, Welge-Lüssen A, et al. Olfactory dysfunctions. Epidemiology and therapy in Germany, Austria and Switzerland. [Article in German] HNO 2004;52(2):112–120
3. Doty RL, Shaman P, Applebaum SL, Giberson R, Siksorski L, Rosenberg L. Smell identification ability: changes with age. Science 1984;226(4681):1441–1443
4. Mackay-Sim A, Johnston AN, Owen C, Burne TH. Olfactory ability in the healthy population: reassessing presbyosmia. Chem Senses 2006;31(8):763–771
5. Landis BN, Hummel T, Hugentobler M, Giger R, Lacroix JS. Ratings of overall olfactory function. Chem Senses 2003;28(8):691–694
6. Soter A, Kim J, Jackman A, Tourbier I, Kaul A, Doty RL. Accuracy of self-report in detecting taste dysfunction. Laryngoscope 2008;118(4):611–617
7. Doty RL, Laing DG. Psychophysical measurement of human olfactory function, including odorant mixture assessment. In: Doty RL, ed. Handbook of Olfaction and Gustation. 2nd ed. New York: Marcel Dekker; 2003:203–228.
8. Small DM, Gerber JC, Mak YE, Hummel T. Differential neural responses evoked by orthonasal versus retronasal odorant perception in humans. Neuron 2005;47(4):593–605
9. Scott JW, Acevedo HP, Sherrill L, Phan M. Responses of the rat olfactory epithelium to retronasal air flow. J Neurophysiol 2007;97(3):1941–1950
10. Hummel T, Heilmann S, Landis BN, et al. Perceptual differences between chemical stimuli presented through the ortho- or retronasal route. Flavor Fragr J 2006;21:42–47
11. Förster G, Damm M, Gudziol H, et al. Olfactory dysfunction. Epidemiology, pathophysiological classification, diagnosis and therapy. [Article in German] HNO 2004;52(8):679–684
12. Gudziol H, Förster G. Medicolegal screening of olfactory function. [Article in German] Laryngo-rhinootologie 2002;81(8):586–590
13. Doty RL, Marcus A, Lee WW. Development of the 12-item cross-cultural smell identification test (CC-SIT). Laryngoscope 1996;106(3 Pt 1):353–356
14. Hummel T, Konnerth CG, Rosenheim K, Kobal G. Screening of olfactory function with a four-minute odor identification test: reliability, normative data, and investigations in patients with olfactory loss. Ann Otol Rhinol Laryngol 2001;110(10):976–981
15. Hummel T, Sekinger B, Wolf SR, Pauli E, Kobal G. 'Sniffin' sticks': olfactory performance assessed by the combined testing of odor identification, odor discrimination and olfactory threshold. Chem Senses 1997;22(1):39–52
16. Mueller CA, Grassinger E, Naka A, Temmel AF, Hummel T, Kobal G. A self-administered odor identification test procedure using the "Sniffin' Sticks". Chem Senses 2006;31(6):595–598
17. Thomas-Danguin T, Rouby C, Sicard G, et al. Development of the ETOC: a European test of olfactory capabilities. Rhinology 2003;41(3):142–151
18. Simmen D, Briner HR. Olfaction in rhinology—methods of assessing the sense of smell. Rhinology 2006;44(2):98–101
19. Jackman AH, Doty RL. Utility of a three-item smell identification test in detecting olfactory dysfunction. Laryngoscope 2005;115(12):2209–2212
20. Hummel T, Pfetzing U, Lötsch J. A short olfactory test based on the identification of three odors. J Neurol 2010;257(8):1316–1321
21. Mueller C, Renner B. A new procedure for the short screening of olfactory function using five items from the "Sniffin' Sticks" identification test kit. Am J Rhinol 2006;20(1):113–116
22. Davidson TM, Murphy C. Rapid clinical evaluation of anosmia. The alcohol sniff test. Arch Otolaryngol Head Neck Surg 1997;123(6):591–594
23. Doty RL, Shaman P, Dann M. Development of the University of Pennsylvania Smell Identification Test:

a standardized microencapsulated test of olfactory function. Physiol Behav 1984;32(3):489–502

24. Kobal G, Hummel T, Sekinger B, Barz S, Roscher S, Wolf SR. "Sniffin' Sticks": screening of olfactory performance. Rhinology 1996;34(4):222–226

25. Hummel T, Kobal G, Gudziol H, Mackay-Sim A. Normative data for the "Sniffin' Sticks" including tests of odor identification, odor discrimination, and olfactory thresholds: an upgrade based on a group of more than 3,000 subjects. Eur Arch Otorhinolaryngol 2007;264(3):237–243

26. Haehner A, Mayer AM, Landis BN, et al. High test-retest reliability of the extended version of the "Sniffin' Sticks" test. Chem Senses 2009;34(8):705–711

27. Lötsch J, Reichmann H, Hummel T. Different odor tests contribute differently to the evaluation of olfactory loss. Chem Senses 2008;33(1):17–21

28. Hedner M, Larsson M, Arnold N, Zucco GM, Hummel T. Cognitive factors in odor detection, odor discrimination, and odor identification tasks. J Clin Exp Neuropsychol 2010;32(10):1062–1067

29. Doty RL, McKeown DA, Lee WW, Shaman P. A study of the test-retest reliability of ten olfactory tests. Chem Senses 1995;20(6):645–656

30. Knecht M, Hummel T. Recording of the human electro-olfactogram. Physiol Behav 2004;83(1):13–19

31. Stevens JC, Cain WS, Burke RJ. Variability of olfactory thresholds. Chem Senses 1988;13:643–653

32. Cain WS, Gent JF, Goodspeed RB, Leonard G. Evaluation of olfactory dysfunction in the Connecticut Chemosensory Clinical Research Center. Laryngoscope 1988;98(1):83–88

33. Kobal G, Palisch K, Wolf SR, et al. A threshold-like measure for the assessment of olfactory sensitivity: the "random" procedure. Eur Arch Otorhinolaryngol 2001;258(4):168–172

34. Linschoten MR, Harvey LO Jr, Eller PM, Jafek BW. Fast and accurate measurement of taste and smell thresholds using a maximum-likelihood adaptive staircase procedure. Percept Psychophys 2001;63(8):1330–1347

35. Walker JC, Hall SB, Walker DB, Kendal-Reed MS, Hood AF, Niu XF. Human odor detectability: new methodology used to determine threshold and variation. Chem Senses 2003;28(9):817–826

36. Lötsch J, Lange C, Hummel T. A simple and reliable method for clinical assessment of odor thresholds. Chem Senses 2004;29(4):311–317

37. Cometto-Muñiz JE, Cain WS, Abraham MH, Gil-Lostes J. Concentration-detection functions for the odor of homologous n-acetate esters. Physiol Behav 2008;95(5):658–667

38. Gudziol V, Hummel T. The influence of distractors on odor identification. Arch Otolaryngol Head Neck Surg 2009;135(2):143–145

39. Negoias S, Troeger C, Rombaux P, Halewyck S, Hummel T. Number of descriptors in cued odor identification tests. Arch Otolaryngol Head Neck Surg 2010;136(3):296–300

40. Gudziol V, Lötsch J, Hähner A, Zahnert T, Hummel T. Clinical significance of results from olfactory testing. Laryngoscope 2006;116(10):1858–1863

41. Welge-Lüssen A, Gudziol V, Wolfensberger M, Hummel T. Olfactory testing in clinical settings—is there additional benefit from unilateral testing? Rhinology 2010;48(2):156–159

42. Gudziol V, Paech I, Hummel T. Unilateral reduced sense of smell is an early indicator for global olfactory loss. J Neurol 2010;257(6):959–963

43. Kondo H, Matsuda T, Hashiba M, Baba S. A study of the relationship between the T&T olfactometer and the University of Pennsylvania Smell Identification Test in a Japanese population. Am J Rhinol 1998;12(5):353–358

44. Deems DA, Doty RL, Settle RG, et al. Smell and taste disorders, a study of 750 patients from the University of Pennsylvania Smell and Taste Center. Arch Otolaryngol Head Neck Surg 1991;117(5):519–528

45. Güttich H. Gustatorische Riechprüfung mit Riechstoffen und Mischreizschmeckstoffen. Arch Ohren Nasen Kehlkopfheilkd 1961;178:327–330

46. Hummel T, Rosenheim K, Knecht M, Heilmann S, Mürbe D, Hüttenbrink KB. Gustatory olfactory function test with the Güttich technique: an evaluation of the clinical value. [Article in German] Laryngorhinootologie 1999;78(11):627–631

47. Heilmann S, Strehle G, Rosenheim K, Damm M, Hummel T. Clinical assessment of retronasal olfactory function. Arch Otolaryngol Head Neck Surg 2002;128(4):414–418

48. Landis BN, Frasnelli J, Reden J, Lacroix JS, Hummel T. Differences between orthonasal and retronasal olfactory functions in patients with loss of the sense of smell. Arch Otolaryngol Head Neck Surg 2005;131(11):977–981

49. Kremer B, Klimek L, Mösges R. Clinical validation of a new olfactory test. Eur Arch Otorhinolaryngol 1998;255(7):355–358

50. Nakashima T, Kidera K, Miyazaki J, Kuratomi Y, Inokuchi A. Smell intensity monitoring using metal oxide semiconductor odor sensors during intravenous olfaction test. Chem Senses 2006; 31(1):43–47

51. Renner B, Mueller CA, Dreier J, Faulhaber S, Rascher W, Kobal G. The candy smell test: a new test for retronasal olfactory performance. Laryngoscope 2009;119(3):487–495

52. Kobal G. Elektrophysiologische Untersuchungen des menschlichen Geruchssinns. Stuttgart: Thieme Verlag; 1981.

53. Hummel T, Klimek L, Welge-Lüssen A, et al. Chemosensory evoked potentials for clinical diagnosis of olfactory disorders. [Article in German] HNO 2000;48(6):481–485

54. Kassab A, Schaub F, Vent J, Hüttenbrink KB, Damm M. Effects of short inter-stimulus intervals on olfactory and trigeminal event-related potentials. Acta Otolaryngol 2009;129(11):1250–1256

55. Lötsch J, Hummel T. The clinical significance of electrophysiological measures of olfactory function. Behav Brain Res 2006;170(1):78–83

56. Lascano AM, Hummel T, Lacroix JS, Landis BN, Michel CM. Spatio-temporal dynamics of olfactory processing in the human brain: an event-related source imaging study. Neuroscience 2010; 167(3):700–708

57. Rombaux P, Bertrand B, Keller T, Mouraux A. Clinical significance of olfactory event-related potentials related to orthonasal and retronasal olfactory testing. Laryngoscope 2007;117(6):1096–1101

58. Yang L, Wei Y, Yu D, Zhang J, Liu Y. Olfactory and gustatory function in healthy adult Chinese subjects. Otolaryngol Head Neck Surg 2010;143(4):554–560

59. Ottoson D. Analysis of the electrical activity of the olfactory epithelium. Acta Physiol Scand Suppl 1955;35(122):1–83

60. Getchell TV. Electrogenic sources of slow voltage transients recorded from frog olfactory epithelium. J Neurophysiol 1974;37(6):1115–1130

61. Rawson NE, Brand JG, Cowart BJ, et al. Functionally mature olfactory neurons from two anosmic patients with Kallmann syndrome. Brain Res 1995;681(1–2):58–64

62. Hummel T, Mojet J, Kobal G. Electro-olfactograms are present when odorous stimuli have not been perceived. Neurosci Lett 2006;397(3):224–228

63. Mrowinski D, Scholz G. Objective olfactometry by recording simultaneously olfactory evoked potentials and contingent negative variation. Chem Senses 1996;21:487

64. Lorig TS, Roberts M. Odor and cognitive alteration of the contingent negative variation. Chem Senses 1990;15:537–545

65. Perbellini D, Scolari R. Electroencephalo-olfactometry. Clinical contribution. [Article in Italian] Ann Laringol Otol Rinol Faringol 1966;65(4):421–429

66. Rombaux P, Mouraux A, Keller T, Hummel T. Trigeminal event-related potentials in patients with olfactory dysfunction. Rhinology 2008;46(3):170–174

67. Asaka H. The studies on the objective olfactory test by galvanic skin response (reflex). [Article in Japanese] Nippon Jibiinkoka Gakkai Kaiho 1965;68:100–112

68. Gudziol H, Wächter R. Are there olfactory evoked alterations of breathing patterns? [Article in German] Laryngorhinootologie 2004;83(6):367–373

69. Frank RA, Gesteland RC, Bailie J, Rybalsky K, Seiden A, Dulay MF. Characterization of the sniff magnitude test. Arch Otolaryngol Head Neck Surg 2006;132(5):532–536

70. Sneppe R, Gonay P. Objective, quantitative and qualitative evaluation of the sense of smell. [Article in French] Electrodiagn Ther 1973;10(1):5–17

71. Schneider CB, Ziemssen T, Schuster B, Seo HS, Haehner A, Hummel T. Pupillary responses to intranasal trigeminal and olfactory stimulation. J Neural Transm 2009;116(7):885–889

72. Ichihara M, Komatsu A, Ichihara F, Asaga H, Hirayoshi K. Test of smell based on the wink response. [Article in Japanese] Jibiinkoka 1967;39(9):947–953

73. Hummel C, Frasnelli J, Gerber J, Hummel T. Cerebral processing of gustatory stimuli in patients with taste loss. Behav Brain Res 2007;185(1):59–64

74. Gottfried JA. Smell: central nervous processing. Adv Otorhinolaryngol 2006;63:44–69

75. Small DM. Central gustatory processing in humans. Adv Otorhinolaryngol 2006;63:191–220

76. Ortega-Perez I, Murray K, Lledo PM. The how and why of adult neurogenesis. J Mol Histol 2007;38(6):555–562

77. Lledo PM, Gheusi G, Vincent JD. Information processing in the mammalian olfactory system. Physiol Rev 2005;85(1):281–317

78. Yousem DM, Geckle RJ, Bilker W, McKeown DA, Doty RL. MR evaluation of patients with congenital hyposmia or anosmia. AJR Am J Roentgenol 1996;166(2):439–443

79. Abolmaali ND, Hietschold V, Vogl TJ, Hüttenbrink KB, Hummel T. MR evaluation in patients with isolated anosmia since birth or early childhood. AJNR Am J Neuroradiol 2002;23(1):157–164

80. Huart C, Meusel T, Gerber J, Duprez T, Rombaux P, Hummel T. The depth of the olfactory sulcus is an indicator of congenital anosmia. AJNR Am J Neuroradiol 2011;32(10):1911–1914

81. Mueller A, Rodewald A, Reden J, Gerber J, von Kummer R, Hummel T. Reduced olfactory bulb volume in post-traumatic and post-infectious olfactory dysfunction. Neuroreport 2005;16(5):475–478

82. Rombaux P, Mouraux A, Bertrand B, Nicolas G, Duprez T, Hummel T. Retronasal and orthonasal olfactory function in relation to olfactory bulb volume in patients with posttraumatic loss of smell. Laryngoscope 2006;116(6):901–905

83. Haehner A, Rodewald A, Gerber JC, Hummel T. Correlation of olfactory function with changes in the volume of the human olfactory bulb. Arch Otolaryngol Head Neck Surg 2008;134(6):621–624

84. Gudziol V, Buschhüter D, Abolmaali N, Gerber J, Rombaux P, Hummel T. Increasing olfactory bulb volume due to treatment of chronic rhinosinusitis—a longitudinal study. Brain 2009; 132(Pt 11):3096–3101

85. Holbrook EH, Leopold DA, Schwob JE. Abnormalities of axon growth in human olfactory mucosa. Laryngoscope 2005;115(12):2144–2154

86. Witt M, Bormann K, Gudziol V, et al. Biopsies of olfactory epithelium in patients with Parkinson's disease. Mov Disord 2009;24(6):906–914

87. Hasegawa S, Yamagishi M, Nakano Y. Microscopic studies of human olfactory epithelia following traumatic anosmia. Arch Otorhinolaryngol 1986; 243(2):112–116

88. Yamagishi M, Fujiwara M, Nakamura H. Olfactory mucosal findings and clinical course in patients with olfactory disorders following upper respiratory viral infection. Rhinology 1994;32(3):113–118

89. Jafek BW, Murrow B, Michaels R, Restrepo D, Linschoten M. Biopsies of human olfactory epithelium. Chem Senses 2002;27(7):623–628

90. Doty RL, Haxel BR. Objective assessment of terbinafine-induced taste loss. Laryngoscope 2005; 115(11):2035–2037

91. Hummel T, Witt M, Reichmann H, Welge-Luessen A, Haehner A. Immunohistochemical, volumetric, and functional neuroimaging studies in patients with idiopathic Parkinson's disease. J Neurol Sci 2010;289(1–2):119–122

92. Leopold D. Distortion of olfactory perception: diagnosis and treatment. Chem Senses 2002; 27(7):611–615

93. Nordin S, Murphy C, Davidson TM, Quiñonez C, Jalowayski AA, Ellison DW. Prevalence and assessment of qualitative olfactory dysfunction in different age groups. Laryngoscope 1996;106(6): 739–744

94. Katz DB, Nicolelis MA, Simon SA. Nutrient tasting and signaling mechanisms in the gut. IV. There is more to taste than meets the tongue. Am J Physiol Gastrointest Liver Physiol 2000;278(1):G6–G9

95. Henkin RI, Gill JR, Bartter FC. Studies on taste thresholds in normal man and in patients with adrenal cortical insufficiency: the role of adrenal cortical steroids and serum sodium concentration. J Clin Invest 1963;42(5):727–735

96. Gudziol H, Hummel T. Normative values for the assessment of gustatory function using liquid tastants. Acta Otolaryngol 2007;127(6):658–661

97. Ahne G, Erras A, Hummel T, Kobal G. Assessment of gustatory function by means of tasting tablets. Laryngoscope 2000;110(8):1396–1401

98. Hummel T, Erras A, Kobal G. A test for the screening of taste function. Rhinology 1997;35(4):146–148

99. Smutzer G, Lam S, Hastings L, et al. A test for measuring gustatory function. Laryngoscope 2008; 118(8):1411–1416

100. Mueller C, Kallert S, Renner B, et al. Quantitative assessment of gustatory function in a clinical context using impregnated "taste strips". Rhinology 2003; 41(1):2–6

101. Nordin S, Brämerson A, Bringlöv E, Kobal G, Hummel T, Bende M. Substance and tongue-region specific loss in basic taste-quality identification in elderly adults. Eur Arch Otorhinolaryngol 2007;264(3): 285–289

102. Grüngreiff K, Abicht K, Kluge M, et al. Clinical studies on zinc in chronic liver diseases. Z Gastroenterol 1988;26(8):409–415

103. Bartoshuk LM. Clinical evaluation of the sense of taste. Ear Nose Throat J 1989;68(4):331–337

104. Pingel J, Ostwald J, Pau HW, Hummel T, Just T. Normative data for a solution-based taste test. Eur Arch Otorhinolaryngol 2010;267(12):1911–1917

105. Tomita H. Methods in taste examination. In: Surjan L, Bodo G, eds. Proceedings of the XIIth ORL World Congress, Budapest, Hungary, 1981. Amsterdam, Oxford: Excerpta Medica; 1982:627.

106. Landis BN, Welge-Luessen A, Brämerson A, et al. "Taste Strips"—a rapid, lateralized, gustatory bedside identification test based on impregnated filter papers. J Neurol 2009;256(2):242–248

107. Konstantinidis I, Chatziavramidis A, Printza A, Metaxas S, Constantinidis J. Effects of smoking on taste: assessment with contact endoscopy and taste strips. Laryngoscope 2010;120(10):1958–1963

108. Weiland R, Macht M, Ellgring H, Gross-Lesch S, Lesch KP, Pauli P. Olfactory and gustatory sensitivity in adults with attention-deficit/hyperactivity disorder. Atten Defic Hyperact Disord 2011; 3(1):53–60

109. Neumann CE. Die Electricität als Mittel zur Untersuchung des Geschmacksinnes im gesunden und kranken Zuständen und die Geschmacksfunction der Chorda tympani. Königsberger medicinische Jahrbücher. 1864;4:1–22.

110. Stillman JA, Morton RP, Hay KD, Ahmad Z, Goldsmith D. Electrogustometry: strengths, weaknesses, and clinical evidence of stimulus boundaries. Clin Otolaryngol Allied Sci 2003;28(5):406–410

111. Tomita H, Ikeda M. Clinical use of electrogustometry: strengths and limitations. Acta Otolaryngol Suppl 2002;546(546):27–38

112. Kobal G. Gustatory evoked potentials in man. Electroencephalogr Clin Neurophysiol 1985;62(6):449–454

113. Astbäck J, Fernström A, Hylander B, Arvidson K, Johansson O. Taste buds and neuronal markers in patients with chronic renal failure. Perit Dial Int 1999;19(Suppl 2):S315–S323

114. Just T, Pau HW, Witt M, Hummel T. Contact endoscopic comparison of morphology of human fungiform papillae of healthy subjects and patients with transected chorda tympani nerve. Laryngoscope 2006;116(7):1216–1222

115. Kobal G, Van Toller S, Hummel T. Is there directional smelling? Experientia 1989;45(2):130–132

116. Hummel T, Roudnitzky N, Kempter W, Laing DG. Intranasal trigeminal function in children. Dev Med Child Neurol 2007;49(11):849–853

117. Porter J, Craven B, Khan RM, et al. Mechanisms of scent-tracking in humans. Nat Neurosci 2007; 10(1):27–29

118. Frasnelli J, Hummel T, Berg J, Huang G, Doty RL. Intranasal localizability of odorants: influence of stimulus volume. Chem Senses 2011;36(4): 405–410

119. Frasnelli J, Hummel T. Intranasal trigeminal thresholds in healthy subjects. Environ Toxicol Pharmacol 2005;19(3):575–580

120. Hummel T. Assessment of intranasal trigeminal function. Int J Psychophysiol 2000;36(2):147–155

121. Hummel T, Kobal G. Olfactory event-related potentials. In: Simon SA, Nicolelis MAL, eds. Methods and Frontiers in Chemosensory Research. Boca Raton, FL: CRC Press; 2001:429–464.

122. Stuck BA, Frey S, Freiburg C, Hörmann K, Zahnert T, Hummel T. Chemosensory event-related potentials in relation to side of stimulation, age, sex, and stimulus concentration. Clin Neurophysiol 2006;117(6):1367–1375

123. Minovi A, Hummel T, Ural A, Draf W, Bockmühl U. Predictors of the outcome of nasal surgery in terms of olfactory function. Eur Arch Otorhinolaryngol 2008;265(1):57–61

124. Kobal G. Pain-related electrical potentials of the human nasal mucosa elicited by chemical stimulation. Pain 1985;22(2):151–163

125. Scheibe M, Zahnert T, Hummel T. Topographical differences in the trigeminal sensitivity of the human nasal mucosa. Neuroreport 2006; 17(13):1417–1420

126. Cain WS, Lee NS, Wise PM, et al. Chemesthesis from volatile organic compounds: Psychophysical and neural responses. Physiol Behav 2006;88(4–5): 317–324

127. Meusel T, Negoias S, Scheibe M, Hummel T. Topographical differences in distribution and responsiveness of trigeminal sensitivity within the human nasal mucosa. Pain 2010;151(2):516–521

128. Gudziol H, Schubert M, Hummel T. Decreased trigeminal sensitivity in anosmia. ORL J Otorhinolaryngol Relat Spec 2001;63(2):72–75

7 Sinonasal Olfactory Disorders

Michael Damm, Randy M. Leung, Robert C. Kern

Summary

Sinonasal olfactory dysfunction has a high prevalence in the general population. Within the otorhinolaryngological patient population, sinonasal diseases are responsible for about three-quarters of olfactory dysfunction. The underlying causes are most frequently inflammatory diseases of the nose or the paranasal sinuses (75%), which are defined and characterized in this section. It is assumed that most sinonasal diseases affect the olfactory epithelium secondarily. Current information about the pathophysiology and treatment strategies of sinonasal diseases is included in this chapter because improvement in olfactory dysfunction is usually achieved by improvement of the underlying disease.

Introduction and Epidemiolgy

Rhinitis and rhinosinusitis are broad terms that refer to conditions characterized by inflammation of mucosa of the nose and paranasal sinuses, typically subdivided on the basis of a temporal profile into acute, recurrent acute, or chronic rhinosinusitis.[1–3] It is now widely accepted that in cases of rhinitis, the paranasal sinuses are commonly affected as well.[4] However, separate definitions for the different entities exist. Rhinitis is defined according to the consensus report of the International Rhinitis Management Working Group[5] as an inflammation of the lining of the nose, and is characterized by nasal symptoms including anterior or posterior rhinorrhea, sneezing, nasal blockage, or itching of the nose. These symptoms occur on two or more consecutive days for more than 1 hour on most days.[5] Considering the etiology, we can distinguish between infectious and noninfectious, and between inflammatory and noninflammatory, subtypes of rhinitis (**Table 7.1**).[6] Allergies and acute viral infections of the upper respiratory tract are the most common causes of rhinitis. Viral rhinitis is the most prevalent disease affecting humans.[7] Allergic rhinitis (AR) is the most common form of noninfectious rhinitis, the lifetime prevalence of AR being above 20%.[8] Several other noninfectious conditions can cause similar symptoms: hormonal imbalance, physical agents, anatomical anomalies, and the use of certain drugs.[6] Olfactory impairment in rhinitis is usually reversible, but on many occasions the loss of olfaction persists.[9] Persistent postviral or postinfectious olfactory dysfunction has been attributed in particular to influenza-like infections.[10] If it follows one isolated acute infection of the upper respiratory tract, it should be classed as postviral (postinfectious) olfactory dysfunction rather than rhinitis (see Chapter 8). Other differential diagnoses of rhinitis are condensed in **Table 7.2**.

Acute rhinosinusitis (ARS) is described as the presence of drainage accompanied by nasal obstruction or facial pain/pressure. ARS is most commonly preceded by a viral upper respiratory tract infection (URTI); the US adult population suffers from an average of 2.18 URTIs per person per year, of which an estimated 0.5 to 2% develop into acute bacterial rhinosinusitis.[11,12]

The criteria for an ARS episode should include a total duration of greater than 10 days, so it cannot to be confused with a viral respiratory infection, and less than 4 weeks to distinguish it from chronic rhinosinusitis (CRS). Recurrent acute rhinosinusitis (RARS) is defined by four or more episodes of bacterial ARS per year with complete resolution of symptoms between episodes—although the literature has diagnostic ranges from two to four per year. CRS is defined as more than 12 weeks of symptoms without an intervening symptom-free period,[13] and is estimated to affect 13% of the US population, or 32 million adults.[14] This temporal classification system says very little about the etiology of CRS, which remains idiopathic in the overwhelming majority of cases. A very small fraction, however, are associated with systemic diseases such as Wegener granulomatosis, sarcoidosis, or cystic fibrosis, and these are beyond the scope of this chapter.

Rhinosinusitis is defined according to the Rhinosinusitis Task Force (RTF)[15] and the European Position Paper on Rhinosinusitis and Nasal Polyps

Table 7.1 Classification of rhinitis

	Infectious	Noninfectious
Inflammatory	• Acute viral rhinitis	• Allergic rhinitis
	• Acute bacterial rhinitis	• Occupational (synonym: work-related rhinitis; either an allergic reaction or an irritant response [toxic rhinitis])
	• Primary atrophic rhinitis (attributed to infection with *Klebsiella ozaenae*)	• Drug-induced rhinitis (e.g., aspirin-exacerbated respiratory disease)
	• Secondary atrophic rhinitis[b] (e.g., total turbinectomy; superinfection is uniformly present)	• NARES[a]
	• Hyperplastic adenoids	• Idiopathic rhinitis (e.g., due to local immunological inflammation)
Noninflammatory		• Idiopathic rhinitis (e.g., parasympathetic/sympathetic dysregulation)
		• Drug induced (e.g., side effects of ACE inhibitors or reserpine)
		• Hormonal rhinitis (e.g., during last trimester of pregnancy)
		• Emotional rhinitis (e.g., stress or sexual arousal)
		• Food-induced rhinitis (gustatory rhinitis; e.g., "hot food" stimulation of nerve fibers)
		• Cocaine sniffing

[a] Nonallergic rhinitis with eosinophilia syndrome.
[b] Related to granulomatous diseases (e.g., sarcoid, leprosy, rhinoscleroma).
ACE, angiotensin-converting enzyme.

Table 7.2 Differential diagnosis of rhinitis

Inflammatory conditions	**Anatomical factors**
• Chronic rhinosinusitis with or without nasal polyps	• Septal deviation
	• Turbinate hyperplasia
	• Choanal atresia
Tumors	**Granulomas**
Benign (e.g., inverting papilloma, fibroma, neurilemoma, ossifying fibroma, osteoma)	• Vasculitidae (Wegener granulomatosis, Churg–Strauss syndrome)
Malignant (e.g., squamous cell carcinoma, adenocarcinoma, lymphoma, melanoma, esthesioneuroblastoma)	• Sarcoidosis
	• Infectious
	• Malignant—midline destructive granuloma
Pseudotumors	**Genetic disease**
• Adenoidal hyperplasia, mucoceles	• Ciliary defects
	• Cystic fibrosis
Others	
• Cerebrospinal rhinorrhea	
• Foreign bodies	

(EPOS) guideline documents.[13] In terms of symptoms, diagnosis requires at least two symptoms of nasal obstruction/blockage/congestion, purulent nasal discharge (anterior or posterior), facial pain/pressure, and hyposmia. The EPOS guidelines (**Table 7.3**) go one step further and stipulate that at least one symptom must be obstruction/blockage/congestion or nasal discharge. The guidelines for the diagnosis of CRS include both subjective and objective criteria. Although the sensitivity of symptoms is high, the specificity is low. Positive computed tomography (CT) scans with Lund–Mackay scores (**Table 7.4**) of 4 or more are found in only 20 to 36% of patients meeting symptom criteria for CRS.[16–18] Therefore, the diagnosis of CRS should be accompanied by objective evidence in the form of endoscopic or radiographic correlation. Specifically, endoscopic evidence of CRS may take the form of middle meatal edema, polyps, or purulence. CT evidence of CRS is characterized by air–fluid levels, thickened mucosa, or polyps, within the sinuses. These objective CT or endoscopic findings are important as they typically divide CRS into two broad subtypes: chronic rhinosinusitis without nasal polyps (CRSsNP) and chronic rhinosinusitis with nasal polyps (CRSwNP), which will be discussed in more detail below.

Even though the clinical pictures of rhinitis and rhinosinusitis are merging, the diseases will be discussed separately within this chapter to cover different time courses, etiologies, and therapy of the olfactory disorder.

Acute Viral Rhinitis—Acute Bacterial Rhinosinusitis

Clincal Course

Acute viral rhinitis (common cold) is defined as a as sudden onset, acute inflammation of the upper airway lasting less than 10 days.[6] Common initial symptoms/signs are burning sensations located in the nose or nasopharynx, consistent with an underlying viral infection. The cardinal symptoms of acute viral rhinitis are nasal obstruction/blockage, nasal discharge (anterior/postnasal drip), hyposmia or anosmia, and, depending on the clinical course, general symptoms. The nasal symptom–sign complex for rhinovirus and influenza occurs within 3 days after exposure; that for respiratory syncytial viruses (RSV) is delayed by as much as 7 days.[7] The systemic symptoms of fever, headache, malaise, myalgia, and anorexia are related to the effects of cytokines released from immune cells, and these responses develop rapidly in the first days of infection when the virus is detected by the immune system. The local symptoms of nasal con-

Table 7.3 Definition of rhinosinusitis according to the EPOS (European Position Paper on Rhinosinusitis and Nasal Polyps) guidelines

Inflammation of the nose and the paranasal sinuses characterized by two or more symptoms, one of which should be either nasal blockage/obstruction/congestion or nasal discharge (anterior/posterior nasal drip): ± facial pain/pressure ± reduction or loss of smell
AND/EITHER Endoscopic sign of: • Polyps and/or • Mucopurulent discharge primarily from middle meatus and/or edema/mucosal obstruction primarily in middle meatus
AND/OR Computed tomography changes • Mucosal changes within the osteomeatal complex and/or sinuses
Chronic rhinosinusitis with or without nasal polyps is defined as: Presence of two or more symptoms one of which should be either nasal blockage/obstruction/congestion or nasal discharge (anterior/posterior nasal drip): ± facial pain/pressure ± reduction or loss of smell for > 12 weeks

Table 7.4 Lund–Mackay score (computed tomography scoring system)

Sinus system	Left	Right
Maxillary (0,1,2)		
Anterior ethmoids (0,1,2)		
Posterior ethmoids (0,1,2)		
Sphenoid (0,1,2)		
Frontal (0,1,2)		
Osteomeatal complex (0 or 2[a])		
Total points		

0, no abnormalities; 1, partial opacification; 2, total opacification.
Maximum score: 12 / side
[a] 0, not occluded; 2, occluded

gestion and rhinorrhea are dependent on the generation of inflammatory mediators such as prostaglandins and bradykinin.[19] Headache and purulent secretion indicate bacterial rhinosinusitis.

Pathophysiology

Acute viral rhinitis/rhinosinusitis is an inflammatory process of the nose and the paranasal sinuses, caused mostly by infection with rhinoviruses, RSV, adenoviruses, influenza viruses, parainfluenza viruses, coronaviruses, and others.[7,20] The viral infection frequently begins in the nasal/nasopharyngeal mucosa and, upon detection by the host, invokes two interactive and temporally overlapping defense systems: A generalized, innate immune response and a virus-specific, adaptive immune response. Both systems include inflammatory pathways that facilitate and actively recruit antiviral proteins and effector cells to the site of infection.[7] Rhinoviruses account for 30 to 50% of all colds, and coronaviruses are the second most common agent, accounting for 10 to 15% of colds.[19] These infections do not usually cause a substantial destruction of olfactory epithelium. Nasal obstruction due to mucosal swelling with hypersecretion is partly responsible for the typical temporary olfactory disorder that accompanies these viral URTIs. Nasal congestion in viral rhinitis is caused by the dilation of large veins in the nasal epithelium (venous sinuses) in response to the generation of vasodilator mediators of inflammation such as bradykinin, and swelling of mucous membranes that block odor transport toward the olfactory mucosa. The nasal discharge associated with viral rhinitis is a complex mix of elements derived from glands, goblet cells, plasma cells, and plasma exudates from capillaries, with the relative contributions from these different sources varying with the time course of the infection and the severity of the inflammatory response.[19] Moreover, numerous proinflammatory cytokines/chemokines and other mediators (e.g., histamine, leukotrienes, prostaglandins) have been reported to be involved in the inflammatory regulation of viral rhinitis and might contribute to the olfactory disorder. However, appropriate studies supporting this hypothesis are lacking.

If the clinical course is prolonged (more than 7 to 10 days) or complicated (e.g., purulent nasal secretion), bacterial superinfection should be assumed. Some of the main pathogens are *Streptococcus pneumoniae* or *pyogenes*, *Haemophilus influenzae*, *Staphylococcus aureus*, or *Moraxella catarrhalis*.[21] Overall, however, only ~1% of viral respiratory infections lead to acute bacterial rhinosinusitis.[13] Pathologically, swelling of the nasal mucosa promotes blockade of the osteomeatal complex in the middle meatus, followed by subsequent impairment of ventilation and drainage of the sinuses, and bacterial superinfection. Other nonswelling-induced mechanisms, such as enhanced bacterial adhesion during the viral replication phase, also promote superinfection (e.g., between influenza A virus infections and streptococci).

At the initial inflammatory phase there is overexpression of interleukin-6 (IL-6), IL-8, and intercellular adhesion molecule (ICAM). A possible source of these cytokines and ICAM is airway epithelial cells. The CXC-chemokine IL-8 has potent chemotactic properties for neutrophils, which are capable of releasing proteases and cytokines (e.g., IL-8, tumor necrosis factor α) as effector cells in ARS.[13] These proinflammatory mediators also activate T-helper (T_h) cells, and mediate the migration of macrophages into the inflamed tissue. IL-1β, IL-12, and other proinflammatory cytokines are upregulated to initiate and maintain cellular defense. As these inflammatory processes involve the olfactory epithelium, olfactory disorders associated with ARS may also be a result of infiltration of the olfactory epithelium with inflammatory cells, of interaction with the involved inflammatory mediators, or of a direct infection-related functional impairment (e.g., virulence factors or immunomodulatory bacterial products).

Olfactory Dysfunction

Olfactory dysfunction is temporary and mild or moderate in most patients with acute viral rhinitis or acute bacterial rhinosinusitis (ABRS), and typically olfactory function mirrors the clinical course of the respiratory disease. Akerlund et al[9] studied olfactory thresholds and nasal mucosal changes in patients with experimentally induced common colds. They found that individuals with an induced coronavirus 229E rhinitis had impaired olfaction and that the change in smelling ability correlated to the nasal congestion but not to the nasal discharge. Hummel et al[22] found the following effects on olfaction after the onset of viral rhinitis: a transient increase in olfactory

threshold; a decrease of odor intensity rating; and a decrease in the N1 peak of chemosensory event-related potential (CSERP) amplitude to olfactory and trigeminal stimuli. They also studied the effect of nasal decongestion with oxymetazoline during the cold and reported that N1 CSERP amplitudes to olfactory stimuli—but not olfactory thresholds or trigeminal CSERP—exhibited a significant increase. Hummel et al[22] concluded from this observation that viral rhinitis has a small effect on olfactory function that may be independent of nasal congestion. To summarize, it appears that the temporary olfactory dysfunction associated with viral rhinitis results mainly from conductive causes owing to nasal blockage, but an inflammatory interaction with the olfactory epithelium or central olfactory structures also appears possible. The endonasal regions that have been shown to influence the olfactory performance are depicted in **Fig. 7.1**.

Treatment

Temporary hyposmia or anosmia, occurring during acute viral infection of the upper respiratory tract, is thought not to require specific therapy. Usually, viral rhinitis is treated symptomatically with drugs such as topical antihistamines, topical anticholinergic drops, decongestants, and antiphlogistic drugs. However, their effects on olfactory function remain unclear.

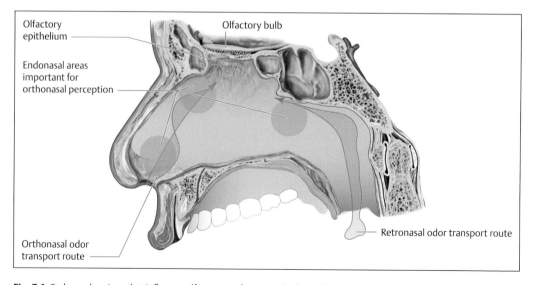

Fig. 7.1 Endonasal regions that influence olfactory performance (indicated in orange). (From Hummel T, Welge-Lüssen A. Riech- und Schmeckstorungen: Physiologie, Pathophysiologie und Therapeutische Ansatze. Stuttgart: Thieme; 2005.)

ABRS resolves without antibiotic treatment in most cases. Antibiotic or anti-inflammatory therapy should be considered in patients suffering from repeated severe episodes of ABRS with significant prolonged olfactory dysfunction. Antibiotic therapy should target the main pathogens. First-line therapy at most centers is usually amoxicillin, or a macrolide antibiotic in patients allergic to penicillin, because of the low cost, ease of administration, and low toxicity of these agents. If patients fail to respond to the initial course of treatment, an alternative antibacterial agent should be considered. Ideally, a nasal swab test should be conducted before initiating an alternative regimen.

Decongestants, mucolytic agents, and nasal or oral steroids are in widespread use is adjuvant therapies. While the evidence for treatment with decongestants and mucolytics mainly results from clinical experience, several studies have documented positive effects of flunisolide, budesonide, and mometasone on ABRS symptoms. If local decongestants are used, they should be placed on cotton as so-called *high inlay* in the middle meatus.[13] The efficacy of antibiotics or adjuvant drugs on olfactory disorders in ABRS has not been systematically evaluated.

Allergic Rhinitis

Clincal Course

AR is a symptomatic nasal hypersensitivity reaction caused by allergen-induced immunoglobulin E (IgE)-mediated inflammation of the mucous membrane.[6]

According to the World Health Organization (WHO), AR is subdivided, based on the duration of symptoms, into "intermittent" (symptoms on < 4 days per week or on < 4 weeks per year) and "persistent" (symptoms on > 4 days per week and on > 4 weeks per year).[6,23] The severity of symptoms in untreated patients should be quantified, according to the Allergic Rhinitis and its Impact on Asthma (ARIA) guidelines, as "mild" (mild symptoms, no impact on social life, school, and work) or "moderate to severe" (severe symptoms, restriction of life quality, school, and work). The symptoms of AR are caused by the interaction of inflammatory mediators with glandular, vascular, or neurogenic

structures of the nose. Nasal secretions result from an increase of plasma exudates or secretions of submucosal glands and goblet cells, triggered by parasympathetic innervations or by increased transmitter release (e.g., vasoactive intestinal peptide, the main source may be also T_h2 lymphocytes). Sneezing is a consequence of trigeminal nerve fiber stimulation by histamine, bradykinin, or various neuropeptides. Acute nasal blockage is caused by dilation and filling of venous sinusoids triggered by parasympathetic transmitters. The long-term decrease in nasal breathing is thought to result from thickening of the vascular connective tissue due to infiltration with inflammatory cells, organized edema, and fibrosis. However, airway remodeling appears to be less extensive in the nasal mucosa than in the bronchial mucosa.[8,23]

Pathophysiology

The immune response in AR involves the release of inflammatory mediators as well as the activation and recruitment of cells to the nasal mucosa. In AR, different stages of the disease can be distinguished. During sensitization, antigen-presenting cells play a crucial role. Dendritic cells take up the allergen and migrate to the mucosa-associated lymphoid tissue and neck lymph nodes, where they prime naïve CD4+ T-lymphocytes (T_h0 cells) that bear receptors for the specific antigen. The nasal mucosa in AR is characterized by the presence of a high percentage of activated T_h2 cells releasing IL-4, IL-5, and IL-13. IL-4 and IL-13 then act on B-cells to promote production of antigen-specific IgE antibodies. Allergen-specific IgE becomes fixed to high affinity IgE receptors (FcεRI) on the membranes of mast cells and basophils. Mast cells are not only effector cells of the immediate phase response, but also play a role in ongoing allergic inflammation. Eosinophils are both increased in numbers and activated in the nasal mucosa of symptomatic allergic patients. T-cells, macrophages, fibroblasts, and other cells are also present. Once the patient is sensitized to the specific allergen, subsequent exposure leads to a cascade of events that result in the symptoms of AR. The allergic response can be divided into two phases: The immediate response (within minutes after allergen exposure) and the late-phase response (4 to 8 hours after allergen exposure).[23]

Olfactory Dysfunction

Olfactory dysfunction has been reported in ~23 to 88% of patients with AR.[24,25] In AR, there is usually a temporary quantitative olfactory dysfunction with periods of reduced or abrogated olfactory sensitivity during allergen exposure.[26] In subjects with grass pollen allergies, performance in olfactory identification and discrimination tests is not different from nonallergic controls if tested out of the season, but a significant decrease in odor threshold and odor identification has been reported from the seventh day of the allergy season in untreated patients.[27] In persistent AR, patients have a more stable, moderate loss of smell, with a higher impairment in those with self-reported hyposmia and moderate-to-severe rhinitis.[28] Patients with dust mite rhinitis performed worse than healthy controls in odor identification, odor threshold, and odor discrimination testing during the winter season, when high allergen exposure may be expected.[25]

There are three reasons for olfactory disorder in AR: (1) Conductive olfactory dysfunction (due to swelling of nasal mucous membranes or massive hypersecretion); (2) changes in olfactory mucus (qualitative or quantitative); and (3) direct effects of mucosal inflammation on the olfactory cleft. With few exceptions (e.g., upregulation of eosinophil cationic protein), the interactions between immunoinflammatory or neurogenic mediators and the olfactory epithelium are widely unknown in AR.[23,27,29] Infiltration of the olfactory cleft mucosa with eosinophils has been described in humans with seasonal AR,[29] and a significant relationship between olfactory threshold and eosinophil levels in blood and nasal discharge has been reported.[30] It is therefore thought that the most important causes of olfactory dysfunction in AR are infiltration by inflammatory cells and upregulation of immunological mediators, altering the function of neurogenic olfactory structures.

Treatment

Although the general consensus is that allergen avoidance should lead to an improvement in symptoms, a systematic review of dust mite allergen avoidance has shown that single measures are not effective in reducing symptoms of AR. The role of allergen avoidance for the improvement of olfactory disorders is not yet clear.[13,23]

Topical steroids have been used successfully to improve odor threshold, odor identification, and odor discrimination.[26,29] Topical steroids are superior to antihistamines in treatment of nasal congestion in seasonal AR, and particularly in the improvement of olfactory function.[31] However, using conventional drops or spray devices, most of the drug is deposited in the anterior third of the nasal cavity, and has no direct effect on the olfactory region.[32,33] To achieve better deposition of the drug at or near the olfactory cleft, nasal drops can be administered in the so-called head-down-forward position,[33] or sprays with prolonged applicators or cannulae should be used (**Fig. 7.2**).[34] **Fig. 7.2a** shows a reshaped spray cannula (for Xylocaine® pump spray, AstraZeneca GmbH, Wedel, Germany) on a self-made budesonide pump spray. **Fig. 7.2b** depicts the cannula inserted in the right nasal cavity directly below the olfactory cleft. Patients can be trained with video endoscopy to locate the head of the spray cannula correctly. Additionally, oral steroids can be used in therapy-refractory rhinitis, especially as a so-called short-term oral steroid trial in severe cases. The short-term administration of topical decongestants may provide additive effects as a trailblazer for other anti-inflammatory drugs in patients with severe nasal blockage.

Leukotriene receptor antagonists play no role today in the treatment of sinonasal olfactory disorders. Specific immunotherapy (SIT) addresses the cause of allergic diseases and should be used early in the course of the disease when indicated.[6,23] The effect of SIT on olfactory dysfunction has not been systematically evaluated. Surgical intervention may be used to improve severe nasal obstruction (e.g., in patients with massive septal deviation or turbinate hyperplasia).[6,23]

Other forms of rhinitis are classified as idiopathic rhinitis (IR), which is an umbrella term suggested by the ARIA–WHO Working Group for rhinitis with an unknown pathogenesis.[6,8,23] Olfactory function was reportedly poorer in "nonallergic rhinitis" patients than in seasonal or perennial AR patients.[35,36] The poorly understood pathophysiology of IR does not currently allow a precise hypothesis for sinonasal olfactory disorders. However, it is likely that the modified release of neurotransmitters in neurogenic inflammation affects the olfactory and trigeminal systems in IR.[37] Treatment consists of topical steroids (budesonide 400 or 800 mg/d, or fluticasone 200 or 400 mg/d) or topical antihistamine (azelastine 1.1 mg/d).[8]

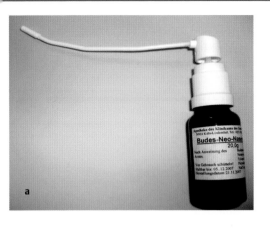

Fig. 7.2a,b Administration of nasal spray to the olfactory cleft.

a Self-made spray device with long cannula.

b Endoscopic view into the right nasal cavity: the spray cannula is located directly below the olfactory cleft.

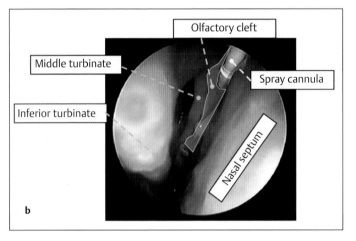

Nonallergic rhinitis with eosinophilia syndrome is characterized by the presence of nasal eosinophilia (nasal cytology analysis showing greater than 20% eosinophils) and perennial symptoms of sneezing, itching, and rhinorrhea in the absence of demonstrable allergy.[6] Anosmia is a prominent feature not shared with AR. Treatment consists mainly of intranasal corticosteroids with or without the addition of second-generation antihistamines or leukotriene receptor antagonists as an adjuvant.[38]

Atrophic Rhinitis

Primary atrophic rhinitis is characterized by progressive atrophy of the nasal mucosa and underlying bone. Ciliated epithelium is replaced by stratified squamous epithelium. The nasal cavity is widened and is filled with stinking crusts that are black or dark green and dry. It has been attributed to infection with *Klebsiella ozaenae*, although its role as a primary pathogen has not been determined.[6] The condition produces nasal obstruction, a persistent hyposmia or anosmia, and an unpleasant odor. It must be distinguished from secondary atrophic rhinitis, which is associated with specific conditions such as syphilis, lupus, leprosy, rhinoscleroma, granulomatous disease, excessive nasal surgery, and radiation therapy.[6,39,40] The sensory loss of atrophic rhinitis may be related to atrophy of nerves in the nasal cavity.

Treatment of atrophic rhinitis can be either medical or surgical, including nasal irrigation with saline, local antibiotics, or narrowing of nasal cavities by, for example, medial displacement of the lateral wall of the nose.[39,40]

Chronic Rhinosinusitis

Clinical Course

According to the definition, symptoms of rhinosinusitis include facial pain and pressure, nasal obstruction, drainage, and hyposmia. While viral URTIs have an established although unknown incidence of olfactory loss (see Chapter 8), neither ARS nor RARS have a significant association with olfactory loss. CRS, on the other hand, is associated with olfactory deficits, but literature on the outcome of its treatment has focused on relief of obstruction and pain/pressure symptoms with relatively little data on either the incidence of smell loss in CRS or improvement post treatment. More recent studies, which have focused on this issue, demonstrated that olfactory dysfunction occurs in over 60% of patients with CRS,[2,41] even though 8 to 25% of these patients are not aware of their olfactory deficit.[42,43] Nasal polyposis, asthma, acetylsalicylic acid intolerance, and revision surgery are risk factors for hyposmia and anosmia in patients with CRS.[1,44] Furthermore, the degree of olfactory dysfunction correlates with the burden of inflammatory disease on endoscopy and CT. The diagnosis, as mentioned in the introduction, is made according to RTF[15] and EPOS guidelines,[13] the latter of which also distinguishes acute from recurrent and chronic rhinosinusitis. Endoscopically, two different forms, CRSsNP and CRSwNP, can be distinguished. The etiology of both forms remains unclear and significant overlap can exist, but they can be distinguished to a degree by the pattern of inflammation and clinical course. Specifically, CRSwNP is associated with a T_h2 pattern of inflammation and more pronounced symptoms of obstruction and smell loss than CRSsNP. CRSsNP exhibits a T_h1 pattern of inflammation and more pronounced complaints of drainage and facial pressure.[45] While both forms can cause smell loss, the presence of nasal polyps carries an odds ratio of 2.38 for risk of hyposmia.[1]

Pathophysiology

Biopsy of the olfactory mucosa demonstrates inflammatory changes in CRS, suggesting that direct damage to the receptor epithelium contributes to olfactory dysfunction in CRS patients (**Fig. 7.3**). Moreover, there appears to be a correlation between the intensity of the inflammation in the olfactory mucosa on biopsy and the presence of olfactory dysfunction.[46,47] More recently, Yee et al identified three patterns of mucosal change associated with CRS.[48] While many patients demonstrated normal olfactory neuroepithelium, several distinct histological patterns were described, apparently reflecting local pathological responses to various degrees of chronic inflammation. The *goblet cell hyperplasia* pattern is characterized by the presence of goblet cells intermixed with olfactory supporting cells with preservation of the underlying neuronal layers within the olfactory epithelium. Under normal circumstances, goblet cells are typically found in the respiratory epithelium only, and not the olfactory epithelium. The *squamous metaplasia* pattern is characterized by a change of the apical layers to thick squamous

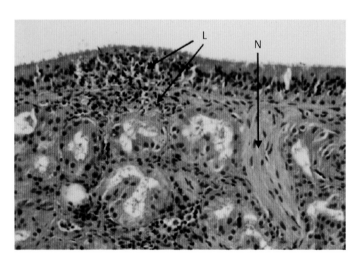

Fig. 7.3 High power hematoxylin and eosin–stained olfactory mucosa in chronic rhinosinusitis. Note the presence of inflammatory infiltrate within the olfactory epithelium. N, olfactory nerve bundles; L, lymphocytic infiltrate.

layers extending into the olfactory epithelium. Severe squamous metaplasia is characterized by sloughing of apical layers with transformation into a continuous squamous layer. This pattern is also characterized by hyperproliferation of basal layers. The squamous change has been hypothesized to be a protective response to injury, irritation, and chronic inflammation, but this may actually inhibit recovery of sensory epithelium. Finally, the *erosive pattern* can range from mild loss of apical cell layers and some supporting cells, to severe erosion with preservation of only a few layers of basal cells, to complete erosion with exposed basement membrane. This pattern is presumed to result from the local activity of degradative enzymes released from inflammatory cells, rendering the epithelium vulnerable to mechanical stresses and sloughing. It is postulated that these patterns represent a spectrum of disease intensity. Given a decreasing prevalence of eosinophils, macrophages, and neutrophils from erosion, to squamous metaplasia, to goblet cell hyperplasia, it is possible that this may represent a sequence of damage followed by repair. However, whether this represents an orderly progression of change remains unclear. Lastly, it should be borne in mind that olfactory mucus has vastly different ion concentrations from surrounding respiratory mucus. Maintenance of this ionic milieu is critical for olfactory transduction along the apical surface of the sensory epithelium.[49,50] Although this topic has not been properly studied, chronic inflammation is likely to alter these concentrations with secondary, negative effects on olfaction. Most likely, olfactory deficits in patients with CRS are the summation of diminished airflow, damage to the epithelium, and alterations to the local ionic microenvironment.

Medical Treatment

The medical treatment of CRS depends on its phenotype. For CRSsNP, treatment should include oral antibiotic therapy for more than 2 weeks as well as intranasal steroids and nasal saline douches. There are no clear data on the efficacy of oral steroids, but they are included in guideline recommendations in some countries (e.g., Germany), and they are commonly prescribed for unresponsive patients, in particular those with significant concomitant AR. The use of oral prednisone, in addition to antibiotics, is particularly common in patients with CRSsNP who present with significant olfactory deficits. The choice of antibiotic should be directed against organisms isolated on culture when possible, but, when purulent secretions are not identified, a broad spectrum antibiotic with coverage for gram-positive, gram-negative, and some anaerobic coverage should be initiated.[51]

CRSwNP is typically more responsive to corticosteroid treatment, and current recommendations include the use of steroids (both oral and intranasal) as well as nasal saline douches. Steroid therapy has been shown to reverse olfactory dysfunction, although effects tend to be incomplete and transient. Seiden and Duncan performed a retrospective study of patients with hyposmia/anosmia as a primary symptom.[52] After a "pulse dose" of oral steroids, they found that 83% (30/36) improved, while only 25% (13/52) of those treated with topical steroids noticed improvement. Complete failure to respond to oral corticosteroids with even transient improvement should suggest the possibility of additional contributions to olfactory loss beyond nasal polyposis. The use of antibiotics is not currently in the guideline recommendations for CRSwNP, although Van Zele et al recently conducted a double-blind, randomized, placebo-controlled trial where patients with recurrent polyposis after surgery or massive polyposis received placebo (n = 19), methylprednisolone taper (n = 14), or doxycycline (n = 14) for 20 days.[53] They found that doxycycline provided lasting reduction in polyp size and reduction in postnasal drip for the duration of the 12-week study period. Unfortunately, doxycycline did not provide any significant change in smell loss. Methylprednisolone provided a more dramatic improvement initially, but these changes—including reduced hyposmia—returned to baseline levels within 1 to 2 months.[53] It has to be kept in mind that only subjective ratings were obtained. These are known to be rather unreliable and tend to reflect nasal breathing rather than measured olfactory function.[54]

Oral antihistamine may also be beneficial in allergic patients postoperatively to prevent recurrence, but has no impact on polyp size and no documented effect on hyposmia. Oral leukotriene antagonists may have some benefit in the treatment of polyps. Parnes and Chuma followed an uncontrolled cohort of 36 patients with CRSwNP who were given zafirlukast or zileuton in addition to standard medical therapy over a mean of 7.4 months.[55] Twenty-four patients noticed some symptomatic improvement including rated, but not measured, olfactory acuity. However, this is within the range of expected improvement from standard medical therapy, making it difficult to attribute the change to the addition of leukotriene antagonists. Prospective randomized controlled trials are needed. These medications are not currently recommended as a standard part of therapy.

If patients improve with medical therapy, maintenance regimens including intranasal steroids are prescribed, but long standing improvement, particularly in olfactory loss, can be problematic.[56] Patients with either form of CRS who fail to improve with medical therapy, or require high-dose oral corticosteroids to control symptoms, may be candidates for surgical therapy. A preoperative CT should be obtained to facilitate surgical planning and to confirm the diagnosis (if not already identified via endoscopy).

Surgical Treatment of Chronic Rhinosinusitis

In cases of medical failure, endoscopic sinus surgery (ESS) is the current gold standard approach to addressing CRS symptoms, including hyposmia. An attempt should be made to address the affected sinuses conservatively, without disruption of other sinus mucosa or outflow tracts.[57,58] As mentioned earlier, CRSwNP has a much higher incidence of associated smell loss than CRSsNP and cases of more severe olfactory deficits are only rarely the result of CRSsNP alone. Surgical goals are potentially different for the two phenotypes as CRSsNP is widely believed to be related to mechanical outflow obstruction at the osteomeatal complex, while CRSwNP probably reflects a more primary mucosal inflammatory process, developing independently of ventilation status. As such, newer, minimally invasive balloon dilatational techniques, which are fundamentally geared toward establishing sinus ventilation alone, may not be adequate for management of CRSwNP. Actual studies of balloon dilatation alone for the management of CRSwNP are lacking, however. Standard ESS ventilates the sinus cavities and removes inflamed sinonasal tissue (including polyps), reducing the inflammatory burden as well as improving airflow to the olfactory cleft. Postoperatively, intranasal steroids have increased access to the nasal and olfactory mucosa, presumably enhancing efficacy. The limitation of ESS for the management of CRSwNP is polyp recurrence. Studies indicate that around 20% of patients will require repeat ESS within 5 years to maintain symptom control.[59]

Moreover, hyposmia may be the most difficult symptom to control, as smell loss is often the first sign of polyp regrowth. Hence, a combination of intermittent oral corticosteroid bursts may be required post ESS to maintain olfactory sensation at normal levels. The clinician must weigh the long-term side effects of this regimen versus quality of life issues in the individual patient. Several studies have specifically focused on sinus surgery to maintain olfactory sensation in CRSwNP. Jafek et al[60] first reported two patients who had nasal polyps and anosmia. Both patients had undergone polypectomy and suffered recurrence of their polyps. Following revision surgery, both patients remained anosmic, ultimately necessitating oral corticosteroid regimens to maintain long-term improvement of anosmia. The requirement for combined treatment (surgery and corticosteroids) was the first suggestion that olfactory loss in CRSwNP was more complex than simple mechanical blockage of airflow to the olfactory cleft. More recently, Stevens studied 24 patients who had polyps with anosmia and underwent sinus surgery.[61] Half of the patients remained anosmic after surgery and were unresponsive to nasal steroids, but most of these patients' sense of smell was restored with oral steroids. In this series, the patients who had improvement and those who did not were similar, all having preoperative diffuse sinonasal polyposis. The effectiveness of oral corticosteroids in restoring olfactory function reinforced the work of Jafek's group, suggesting a direct effect on the olfactory neuroepithelium. Further studies focusing primarily on surgical effects have also documented improvement in olfaction, albeit incomplete. Lund and Scadding[62] in a series of 50 patients followed over a mean of 2.3 years, found significant improvement of visual analog and University of Pennsylvania Smell Identification Test (UPSIT) scores; however the average UPSIT score of 25 remained in the markedly hyposmic range. Klimek et al[63] evaluated 31 patients with hyposmia and CRSwP immediately prior to surgery and at six times postoperatively. They found that improvement to mild hyposmia occurred at 3 months postoperatively with olfactory decline to preoperative states between 3 to 6 months postoperatively. Rowe-Jones and Mackay[64] followed 115 patients with CRS prospectively, evaluating the effects of surgery and postoperative oral prednisone tapered over 3 weeks with amoxicillin/clavulinic acid. They found improvement in 87% subjectively, and 82%

by visual analog scale. Delank and Stoll[43] measured odorant detection thresholds for CRS patients undergoing ESS and found that despite a 70% rate of postoperative olfactory improvement, only 25% of hyposmics and 5% of anosmics reached normal olfactory thresholds. Pade and Hummel[65] examined 387 patients preoperatively and 206 patients post sinus surgery using the "Sniffin' Sticks" test battery, and were only able to measure an increase in olfactory function in 48 patients while 140 did not show any change in their olfactory function. It has to be pointed out that it is of great importance to measure olfactory function rather than evaluate olfactory function using a visual analog scale as has commonly been done, especially in earlier studies. These data concerning olfactory self-assessment are rather unreliable. The flowchart (**Fig. 7.4**) summarizes the work-up and possible therapeutic options in CRS.

Conclusion

CRS, typically the polypoid form, is associated with smell loss as a major complaint. The pathology probably involves diminished access of odorants to the olfactory cleft as well as direct inflammation of the neuroepithelium. Medical therapy including oral corticosteroids is standard, with surgery (ESS) offered to those who fail to improve or require excessive corticosteroids to control symptoms. Physicians and patients should understand that smell loss may be the most difficult of all CRS symptoms to treat long term, often necessitating combined ESS and medical therapy. Studies indicate that long-term oral corticosteroids may be necessary as well, to maintain olfactory sensation in the normosmic range.

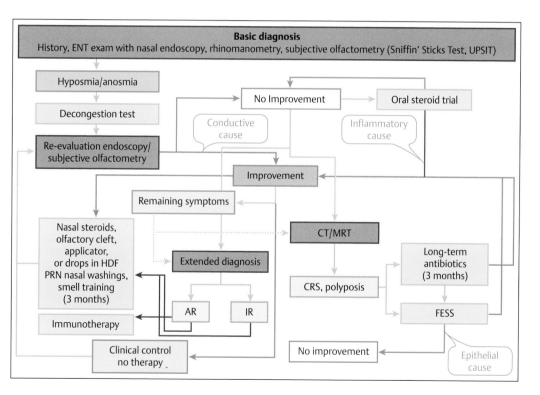

Fig. 7.4 Treatment algorithm for sinonasal olfactory disorders. AR, allergic rhinitis; CRS, chronic rhinosinusitis; CT, computed tomography; ENT, ear, nose, and throat; FESS, functional endoscopic sinus surgery; HDF, head-down-forward position; IR, idiopathic rhinitis; MRT, magnetic resonance tomography; PRN, as needed; UPSIT, University of Pennsylvania Smell Identification Test. Olfactory cleft applicator: see Fig. 7.2a.

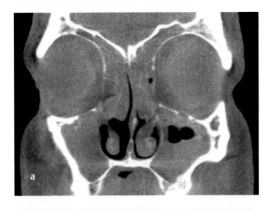

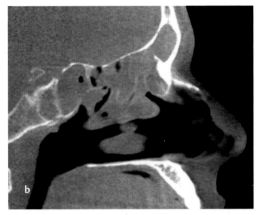

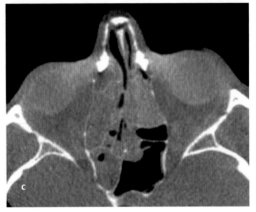

Fig. 7.5a–c CT of a patient with nasal polyps involving and nearly obstructing all sinuses on coronal (**a**), sagittal (**b**), and axial (**c**) images.

Case Study

A 37-year-old man was referred for evaluation of the gradual onset of nasal symptoms over the past 5 months. He was severely hyposmic but his other CRS symptoms were described as relatively mild, including nasal obstruction, facial pressure, and increased sneezing. His wife noticed that he had started snoring more often. He denied any symptoms of purulent discharge, Eustachian tube dysfunction, or history of asthma. He had been treated with intranasal corticosteroids without much improvement.

He was otherwise generally healthy with no known allergies. Skin prick testing was positive to trees, dust mites, cats, dogs, and cockroaches. He did not smoke or drink alcohol. He worked as a financial director.

A complete head and neck examination was performed, yielding only edematous inferior turbinates. Flexible nasal endoscopy demonstrated nasal polyps originating from his middle meatus, and occupying 50% of his nasal airway bilaterally.

CT demonstrated the presence of polyps in all of his sinuses (**Fig. 7.5**) and a course of oral and nasal steroids was initiated. His symptoms improved only minimally, and he agreed to ESS with polypectomy.

His pathology revealed nasal polyps with marked eosinophilia.

Postoperatively, he was able to obtain significant improvement on maintenance therapy with fluticasone propionate only. His UPSIT scores increased from 23/40 (severe microsomia) to 36/40 (normal) at 6 months postsurgery.

References

1. Litvack JR, Fong K, Mace J, James KE, Smith TL. Predictors of olfactory dysfunction in patients with chronic rhinosinusitis. Laryngoscope 2008; 118(12):2225–2230
2. Damm M, Quante G, Jungehuelsing M, Stennert E. Impact of functional endoscopic sinus surgery on symptoms and quality of life in chronic rhinosinusitis. Laryngoscope 2002;112(2):310–315

3. Klimek L, Hummel T, Moll B, Kobal G, Mann WJ. Lateralized and bilateral olfactory function in patients with chronic sinusitis compared with healthy control subjects. Laryngoscope 1998;108(1 Pt 1):111–114

4. Alho OP. Nasal airflow, mucociliary clearance, and sinus functioning during viral colds: effects of allergic rhinitis and susceptibility to recurrent sinusitis. Am J Rhinol 2004;18(6):349–355

5. International Rhinitis Management Working Group. International consensus report on the diagnosis and management of rhinitis. Allergy 1994; 49(19, Suppl)1–34

6. Bousquet J, Khaltaev N, Cruz AA, et al; World Health Organization; GA(2)LEN; AllerGen. Allergic Rhinitis and its Impact on Asthma (ARIA) 2008 update (in collaboration with the World Health Organization, GA(2)LEN and AllerGen). Allergy 2008;63(Suppl 86):8–160

7. Doyle WJ, Skoner DP, Gentile D. Nasal cytokines as mediators of illness during the common cold. Curr Allergy Asthma Rep 2005;5(3):173–181

8. Damm M. Idiopathic rhinitis. [Article in German] Laryngorhinootologie 2006;85(5):361–377, quiz 378–379

9. Akerlund A, Bende M, Murphy C. Olfactory threshold and nasal mucosal changes in experimentally induced common cold. Acta Otolaryngol 1995; 115(1):88–92

10. Konstantinidis I, Haehner A, Frasnelli J, et al. Post-infectious olfactory dysfunction exhibits a seasonal pattern. Rhinology 2006;44(2):135–139

11. Takkouche B, Regueira-Méndez C, García-Closas R, Figueiras A, Gestal-Otero JJ. Intake of vitamin C and zinc and risk of common cold: a cohort study. Epidemiology 2002;13(1):38–44

12. Monto AS. Epidemiology of viral respiratory infections. Am J Med 2002;112(Suppl 6A):4S–12S

13. Fokkens W, Lund V, Mullol J; European Position Paper on Rhinosinusitis and Nasal Polyps group. European position paper on rhinosinusitis and nasal polyps 2007. Rhinol Suppl 2007; (20):1–136

14. Pleis JR, Ward BW, Lucas JW. Summary health statistics for U.S. adults: National Health Interview Survey, 2009. Vital Health Stat 2010;10(249):1–207

15. Rosenfeld RM. Clinical practice guideline on adult sinusitis. Otolaryngol Head Neck Surg 2007;137(3):365–377

16. Stankiewicz JA, Chow JM. A diagnostic dilemma for chronic rhinosinusitis: definition accuracy and validity. Am J Rhinol 2002;16(4):199–202

17. Bhattacharyya N, Lee LN. Evaluating the diagnosis of chronic rhinosinusitis based on clinical guidelines and endoscopy. Otolaryngol Head Neck Surg 2010;143(1):147–151

18. Hwang PH, Irwin SB, Griest SE, Caro JE, Nesbit GM. Radiologic correlates of symptom-based diagnostic criteria for chronic rhinosinusitis. Otolaryngol Head Neck Surg 2003;128(4):489–496

19. Eccles R. Understanding the symptoms of the common cold and influenza. Lancet Infect Dis 2005;5(11):718–725

20. Linden M, Greiff L, Andersson M, et al. Nasal cytokines in common cold and allergic rhinitis. Clin Exp Allergy 1995;25(2):166–172

21. Payne SC, Benninger MS. *Staphylococcus aureus* is a major pathogen in acute bacterial rhinosinusitis: a meta-analysis. Clin Infect Dis 2007; 45(10):e121–e127

22. Hummel T, Rothbauer C, Barz S, Grosser K, Pauli E, Kobal G. Olfactory function in acute rhinitis. Ann N Y Acad Sci 1998;855:616–624

23. Bousquet J, Van Cauwenberge P, Khaltaev N; Aria Workshop Group; World Health Organization. Allergic rhinitis and its impact on asthma. J Allergy Clin Immunol 2001; 108(5, Suppl):S147–S334

24. Cowart BJ, Flynn-Rodden K, McGeady SJ, Lowry LD. Hyposmia in allergic rhinitis. J Allergy Clin Immunol 1993;91(3):747–751

25. Moll B, Klimek L, Eggers G, Mann W. Comparison of olfactory function in patients with seasonal and perennial allergic rhinitis. Allergy 1998; 53(3):297–301

26. Stuck BA, Blum A, Hagner AE, Hummel T, Klimek L, Hörmann K. Mometasone furoate nasal spray improves olfactory performance in seasonal allergic rhinitis. Allergy 2003;58(11):1195–1216

27. Klimek L, Eggers G. Olfactory dysfunction in allergic rhinitis is related to nasal eosinophilic inflammation. J Allergy Clin Immunol 1997;100(2):158–164

28. Guilemany JM, García-Piñero A, Alobid I, et al. Persistent allergic rhinitis has a moderate impact on the sense of smell, depending on both nasal congestion and inflammation. Laryngoscope 2009; 119(2):233–238

29. Sivam A, Jeswani S, Reder L, et al. Olfactory cleft inflammation is present in seasonal allergic rhinitis and is reduced with intranasal steroids. Am J Rhinol Allergy 2010;24(4):286–290

30. Rydzewski B, Pruszewicz A, Sulkowski WJ. Assessment of smell and taste in patients with allergic rhinitis. Acta Otolaryngol 2000;120(2):323–326

31. Hilberg O. Effect of terfenadine and budesonide on nasal symptoms, olfaction, and nasal airway patency following allergen challenge. Allergy 1995;50(8):683–688

32. Scheibe M, Bethge C, Witt M, Hummel T. Intranasal administration of drugs. Arch Otolaryngol Head Neck Surg 2008;134(6):643–646

33. Benninger MS, Hadley JA, Osguthorpe JD, et al. Techniques of intranasal steroid use. Otolaryngol Head Neck Surg 2004;130(1):5–24

34. Damm M. Sinunasale Dysosmien. In: Hummel T, Welge-Lüssen A, eds. Riech- und Schmeckstörungen Physiologie, Pathophysiologie und therapeutische Ansätze. Stuttgart: Thieme; 2009: 61–76.

35. Di Lorenzo G, Pacor ML, Amodio E, et al. Differences and similarities between allergic and nonallergic rhinitis in a large sample of adult patients with rhinitis symptoms. Int Arch Allergy Immunol 2011;155(3):263–270

36. Simola M, Malmberg H. Sense of smell in allergic and nonallergic rhinitis. Allergy 1998;53(2):190–194

37. Hummel T, Scheibe M, Zahnert T, Landis BN. Impact of nonallergic rhinitis on chemosensory function. Clin Allergy Immunol 2007;19:389–400

38. Ellis AK, Keith PK. Nonallergic rhinitis with eosinophilia syndrome and related disorders. Clin Allergy Immunol 2007;19:87–100

39. Botelho-Nevers E, Gouriet F, Lepidi H, et al. Chronic nasal infection caused by *Klebsiella rhinoscleromatis* or *Klebsiella ozaenae*: two forgotten infectious diseases. Int J Infect Dis 2007;11(5):423–429

40. Hildenbrand T, Weber RK, Brehmer D. Rhinitis sicca, dry nose and atrophic rhinitis: a review of the literature. Eur Arch Otorhinolaryngol 2011; 268(1):17–26

41. Litvack JR, Mace JC, Smith TL. Olfactory function and disease severity in chronic rhinosinusitis. Am J Rhinol Allergy 2009;23(2):139–144

42. Nordin S, Monsch AU, Murphy C. Unawareness of smell loss in normal aging and Alzheimer's disease: discrepancy between self-reported and diagnosed smell sensitivity. J Gerontol B Psychol Sci Soc Sci 1995;50(4):187–192

43. Delank KW, Stoll W. Olfactory function after functional endoscopic sinus surgery for chronic sinusitis. Rhinology 1998;36(1):15–19

44. Katotomichelakis M, Riga M, Davris S, et al. Allergic rhinitis and aspirin-exacerbated respiratory disease as predictors of the olfactory outcome after endoscopic sinus surgery. Am J Rhinol Allergy 2009;23(3):348–353

45. Georgalas C, Videler W, Freling N, Fokkens WJ. Global Osteitis Scoring Scale and chronic rhinosinusitis: a marker of revision surgery. Clin Otolaryngol 2010;35(6):455–461

46. Kern RC. Chronic sinusitis and anosmia: pathologic changes in the olfactory mucosa. Laryngoscope 2000;110(7):1071–1077

47. Kern RC, Conley DB, Haines GK III, Robinson AM. Treatment of olfactory dysfunction, II: studies with minocycline. Laryngoscope 2004;114(12): 2200–2204

48. Yee KK, Pribitkin EA, Cowart BJ, et al. Neuropathology of the olfactory mucosa in chronic rhinosinusitis. Am J Rhinol Allergy 2010;24(2):110–120

49. Kern RC, Kerr TP, Getchell TV. Ultrastructural localization of Na+/K(+)-ATPase in rodent olfactory epithelium. Brain Res 1991;546(1):8–17

50. Fong KJ, Kern RC, Foster JD, Zhao JC, Pitovski DZ. Olfactory secretion and sodium, potassium-adenosine triphosphatase: regulation by corticosteroids. Laryngoscope 1999;109(3):383–388

51. Braunstahl GJ, Overbeek SE, Kleinjan A, Prins J-B, Hoogsteden HC, Fokkens WJ. Nasal allergen provocation induces adhesion molecule expression and tissue eosinophilia in upper and lower airways. J Allergy Clin Immunol 2001;107(3):469–476

52. Seiden AM, Duncan HJ. The diagnosis of a conductive olfactory loss. Laryngoscope 2001;111(1):9–14

53. Van Zele T, Gevaert P, Holtappels G et al. Oral steroids and doxycycline: two different approaches to treat nasal polyps. J Allergy Clin Immunol 2010;125(5):1069–1076.e4

54. Landis BN, Hummel T, Hugentobler M, Giger R, Lacroix JS. Ratings of overall olfactory function. Chem Senses 2003;28(8):691–694

55. Parnes SM, Chuma AV. Acute effects of antileukotrienes on sinonasal polyposis and sinusitis. Ear Nose Throat J 2000;79(1):18–20, 24–25

56. van Camp C, Clement PA. Results of oral steroid treatment in nasal polyposis. Rhinology 1994;32(1): 5–9

57. Kennedy DW. Functional endoscopic sinus surgery. Technique Arch Otolaryngol 1985;111(10): 643–649

58. Kennedy DW, Zinreich SJ, Rosenbaum AE, Johns ME. Functional endoscopic sinus surgery. Theory and diagnostic evaluation. Arch Otolaryngol 1985; 111(9):576–582

59. Hopkins C, Slack R, Lund V, Brown P, Copley L, Browne J. Long-term outcomes from the English national comparative audit of surgery for nasal polyposis and chronic rhinosinusitis. Laryngoscope 2009;119(12):2459–2465

60. Jafek BW, Moran DT, Eller PM, Rowley JC III, Jafek TB. Steroid-dependent anosmia. Arch Otolaryngol Head Neck Surg 1987;113(5):547–549

61. Stevens MH. Steroid-dependent anosmia. Laryngoscope 2001;111(2):200–203

62. Lund VJ, Scadding GK. Objective assessment of endoscopic sinus surgery in the management of chronic rhinosinusitis: an update. J Laryngol Otol 1994;108(9):749–753

63. Klimek L, Moll B, Amedee RG, Mann WJ. Olfactory function after microscopic endonasal surgery in patients with nasal polyps. Am J Rhinol 1997;11(4):251–255

64. Rowe-Jones JM, Mackay IS. A prospective study of olfaction following endoscopic sinus surgery with adjuvant medical treatment. Clin Otolaryngol Allied Sci 1997;22(4):377–381

65. Pade J, Hummel T. Olfactory function following nasal surgery. Laryngoscope 2008;118(7):1260–1264

8 Postinfectious and Post-traumatic Olfactory Disorders

Carl Philpott, Ron DeVere

Etiology, Prevalence, and Pathophysiology

Postinfectious Olfactory Disorders

The common cold, while a minor inconvenience for most, remains a scourge of modern medicine, with treatments limited to over-the-counter remedies. All of us can probably recall having had a cold where our sense of smell and the pleasure of eating was lost for a few days. However, for an unfortunate minority, this disturbance in olfactory function persists long after the nasal congestion and rhinorrhea have abated. Estimates of the prevalence of olfactory disorders of any cause suggest that ~5% of the population is affected.[1-4] Postinfectious olfactory disorders are believed to account for 11 to 40% of cases[5,6] with the higher figures likely to represent the prevalence in specialist centers. Extrapolation of the lower figures suggests that an estimated 1.7 million people in the USA and 330,000 people in the UK are suffering from postinfectious olfactory disorder at any one time. Viruses that give rise to the common cold are thought to be the pathological agents responsible for postinfectious olfactory loss. These include rhinoviruses (30 to 50%), parainfluenza virus (5%), coronavirus (10 to 15%), influenza virus (5 to 15%), coxsackie virus (<5%), adenoviruses (<5%), and respiratory syncytial viruses (10%). However, there are over 200 viruses in total that can cause upper respiratory tract infections (URTIs).[7] When Wang et al set out to study the most likely culprit of this disparate band of viruses, they found that parainfluenza virus was present in 88% of patients with postviral olfactory loss compared with 9% of controls[8]; Sugiura et al had similar findings.[9,10] However, another study published the same year by Suzuki et al showed that at least four viruses were identified in biopsies from patients with postviral olfactory loss and parainfluenza virus only accounted for 1 of the 24 cases examined. Other identified viruses included Epstein–Barr virus, rhinovirus, and coronavirus.[11] The mechanism by which the virus wreaks its havoc usually involves hijacking of the cellular apparatus, but the exact details may depend on the actual virus implicated. Rhinovirus, for instance, causes a selective neutrophil and monocyte recruitment to occur. The ensuing inflammatory cascade includes an increase in bradykinin, cytokine, chemokine, and soluble intercellular adhesion molecule-1 concentrations.[12] The response in an immunocompetent individual involves T-lymphocyte activation, allowing the viral pathogen to be eliminated.

With specific respect to the olfactory apparatus, these viruses appear to cause partial loss of receptors in the olfactory epithelium. Ultrastructurally, previous studies of olfactory epithelial biopsy specimens have revealed a decrease in the number of olfactory receptor cells and nerve bundles, with squamous metaplasia occurring in a few cases.[13] This reduction in ciliated olfactory receptors means there is a lack of dendrites and vesicles at the epithelial surface and, therefore, a decrease in the area available for odor molecule detection.[14] Studies of patients with congenital anosmia have shown that the number of olfactory receptors in the neuroepithelium is likely to reflect the severity of the loss.[15] It is unclear why an individual may be susceptible to the viral agents, but, as the age range of affected patients is typically after the fourth decade of life, there is weight behind the argument of a cumulative effect of the virus(es) on the olfactory epithelium. This may explain why some patients do not recover their olfactory ability, especially as the regenerative ability of the olfactory epithelium denudes with advancing age.[16]

It is by virtue of this partial loss of receptors that patients typically complain of hyposmia rather than anosmia, but, more importantly, they frequently describe various forms of dysosmia.[17] Decreased olfactory input to the OBs (1–3) downregulates dopaminergic interneurons (arrows), which may affect transmission from the olfactory nerve to the bulb and subsequent processing of those signals from the bulb (solid/dotted lines) (**Fig. 8.1**). As all inflammatory edema associated with the initial viral URTI should have dissipated

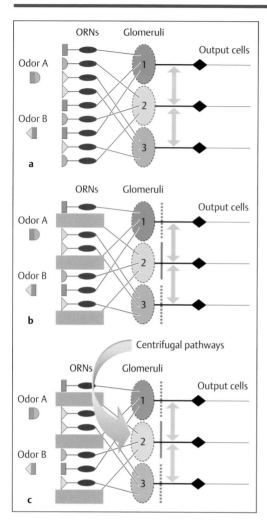

Fig. 8.1a–c Effects of viral insult. ORNs, olfactory receptor neurons.

a   Olfactory receptors.

b   Viral injury to olfactory epithelium.

c   Central modulation of damaged neuroepithelium.

assessing patients with postinfectious olfactory loss should bear in mind that these patients may have a multifactorial etiology implicated in their disorder.

Beyond the peripheral theory described above, central theories have also been mooted for the qualitative disorders that encompass parosmias. However, in the presence of the postinfectious disorder, viral receptor damage is strongly believed to be the key culprit. In fact, it is largely due to the fact that postinfectious and post-traumatic disorders account for most parosmia, and that some degree of olfactory function is preserved, that the peripheral theory is the most popular. Certainly OB volume has been shown to be decreased in parosmic versus nonparosmic patients, indicating possible decreased and incorrect rewiring between the neuroepithelium and the OB.[18,19] Functional magnetic resonance imaging studies have shown the impact that the addition of parosmia to hyposmia can have upon central olfactory processing.[20] The anterior cingulate gyrus, thalamus, and orbitofrontal cortex showed more activation in patients with only hyposmia, adding further weight to the theory of decreased signal traffic between the neuroepithelium and the OB. It should be remembered, when discussing the mechanism of viral impact on the olfactory epithelium, that the olfactory system is a portal of entry for viruses to invade the central nervous system and so central effects of viruses cannot be discounted.[21,22]

- At least 10% of olfactory disorders are due to viral URTIs.
- Rhinoviruses are the most common infective agent.
- Postinfectious olfactory loss typically occurs after the fourth decade of life.

after the initial event, postinfectious disorders are considered to be sensorineural olfactory disorders (SNODs) and are not caused by pathology in the nasal cavity, olfactory cleft, or the paranasal sinuses; that is to say, airflow into the olfactory cleft is normal both orthonasally and retronasally. That does not, of course, mean that postinfectious olfactory disorders are exclusive from those secondary to chronic rhinosinusitis; indeed the viral URTI may have been the precursor to acute bacterial rhinosinusitis that then fails to resolve; there may also be septal deviation. The physician

Post-traumatic Olfactory Disorders

The clinical term *post-traumatic anosmia* (PTA) is commonly used to describe olfactory impairment following a head injury. The injury can include direct injury to the face and nasal structures or any part of the skull. The reported incidence varies from 5%[23] to 66%,[24] but this extreme difference is because of the inclusion of specialized smell centers that have a high incidence of referrals. The important point is that PTA is not an uncommon cause of olfactory impairment and it should be clinically pursued as a cause in any patient presenting with olfactory loss or taste impairment. Of cases of olfactory loss presenting to a physician, 17 to 24%[3] are due to head or facial trauma.[25,26] Olfactory loss due to head trauma can be divided into four mechanisms as discussed below, and can be the result of any combinations of these.

> Head or facial trauma is responsible for 17 to 24% of all cases of smell loss presenting to a physician.

Direct Injury to the Nose and Face with or without Nasal and Facial Fractures

Head trauma associated with direct facial and nasal injuries, with or without fractures, often results in edema and mucosal hematoma of the nasal passages, which can lead to olfactory impairment by preventing odors from reaching the olfactory cleft and olfactory receptors (conductive disorder) (**Fig. 8.2**). This same trauma can cause injury to the olfactory receptors directly, or later on by scarring of the olfactory epithelium and possible development of rhinosinusitis.[24] With time, as the edema and possible hematoma subside, the conductive block improves, with possible recovery of olfactory function. However, injury to the olfactory receptors at the onset or secondary to scar tissue, or presence of rhinosinusitis, can lead to longer term

olfactory loss. The incidence of olfactory loss in facial and nasal fractures varies from 11 to 60%.[27,28] It is hard at times to isolate the pathophysiology of olfactory loss specifically, because injuries to the face and nose (e.g., fracture of the nasal skeleton) may not only cause a blockage of the nose, but also produce direct impairment of the olfactory organ and indirect injury to olfactory nerves owing to the acceleration and deceleration of the head when the nasal trauma occurs.

Direct Injury to Any Part of the Skull without Contusion or Hemorrhage into the Brain

In direct skull injury, acceleration and deceleration forces shift the brain forward and backward very rapidly, and the olfactory nerves, passing through the cribriform plate of the anterior cranial fossa en route to the OB, get sheared or stretched (**Fig. 8.3**). Some studies have suggested that occipital head trauma is more likely to cause olfactory injury than trauma to other areas.[29] In a series of 168 post-traumatic anosmia cases, it was found that injury to the occiput and the sides of the head was more likely to cause greater olfactory nerve damage than frontal head injuries.[24] It is believed that the frontal sinus may be somewhat protective in helping to decrease the force of the blow. Fractures of the cribriform plate were relatively rare. In this mechanism of olfactory loss, biopsy of the neuroepithelium in the olfactory cleft has found degeneration of the olfactory vesicles and cilia.[30] Other studies of the histopathology of post-traumatic anosmia have confirmed similar findings to postinfectious changes, with disorganization of the olfactory epithelium as well as damage to olfactory nerve fibers and changes in the OB.[14,31]

> Injuries to the occipital and temporal regions of the head are more likely to cause smell impairment than frontal injuries.

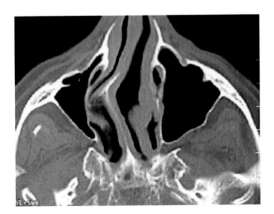

Fig. 8.2 Septal deviation contributing to conductive olfactory deficit.

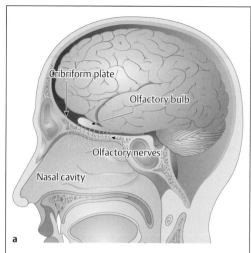

The olfactory nerves are shown passing through the cribriform plate into the nasal cavity.

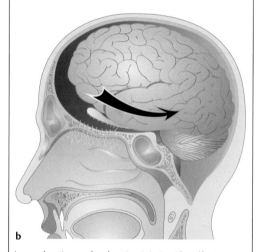

In acceleration or deceleration injuries, the olfactory bulb is pulled toward the back of the skull, leading to stretching and tearing of the olfactory nerves.

Fig. 8.3 Shearing of olfactory fibers.

Direct Injury to Any Part of the Skull with Contusion or Hemorrhage into the Brain

PTA can occur in mild, moderate, or severe head injury because of contusions to the OB and the brain, or intraparenchymal brain hemorrhage. Contusions of the OB and the orbitofrontal pole

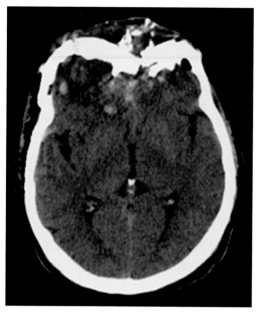

Fig. 8.4 Frontal lobe contusions associated with depressed fracture. (From Jallo J, Loftus CM. Neurotrauma and Critical Care of the Brain. New York, Stuttgart: Thieme; 2009: 108.)

of the brain are the most common injuries associated with olfactory loss in this category (**Fig. 8.4**).[32] Injuries to other areas of the brain (e.g., the anterior piriform cortex, amygdala, and temporal lobe regions) lead to loss of olfactory discrimination and odor identification because olfactory nerve fibers leave the OB and synapse in all these areas.[33] The reason that head trauma particularly affects the frontal and temporal lobe is that, during acceleration and deceleration, the brain slides over the rough base of the anterior and middle cranial fossae as it hits the front part of the inside of the skull (**Fig. 8.5**). The clue to involvement of these cerebral regions is that memory and other areas of cognitive function, including behavior, are often impaired.

> The frontal and temporal lobes are the most commonly injured regions of the brain in head and facial trauma, because the brain slides over the rough bone of the anterior and middle cranial fossae.

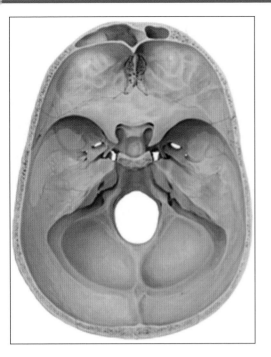

Fig. 8.5 Skull base viewed from above. (From Schünke et al. Thieme Atlas of Anatomy: Head and Neuroanatomy ©. Thieme; 2010. Illustration by Karl Wesker.)

Typical Clinical Findings

Postinfectious Olfactory Disorders

As outlined above, patients with postinfectious olfactory disorders experience, in the first instance, the usual symptoms of the common cold, including nasal congestion, rhinorrhea, coryza, pyrexia, and general malaise. Symptoms of olfactory disturbance will become apparent as the illness progresses. Other symptoms may also develop, such as facial pressure, otalgia, dental pain, and postnasal drip, indicating a wider picture of acute viral rhinosinusitis. A duration of 10 days or more is currently accepted as the demarcation between a viral and a bacterial etiology for acute rhinosinusitis. Unfortunately, it is only when all the other symptoms have subsided, and the loss of olfactory perception persists, that the problem becomes apparent. Patients will initially assume that the symptom will eventually disappear and hence there is often a delay in presentation to a physician (closing the ideal window of opportunity for early intervention, if this does indeed exist). However, a sense of apathy and lack of knowledge or interest among many physicians encountering patients with olfactory disorders means that patients are often dismissed, and, even among those who make it to secondary care, a further level of apathy prevents many from receiving a satisfactory assessment of their problem.

Along with hyposmia/anosmia, it is likely that about two-thirds of patients will suffer from parosmia (a distorted olfactory sensation; usually unpleasant). Conversely, of patients suffering from parosmia, 40 to 80% have a viral URTI as the preceding cause.[17,34] This symptom in itself can become more disabling than the actual loss of olfactory ability, with over half of patients saying that it has a negative impact on their quality of life.[17]

A history for a patient presenting with olfactory loss following the presence of other upper respiratory tract symptoms should clarify whether the onset of the olfactory disturbance coincided with that of the other symptoms. If there is any doubt that the URTI was associated with the onset of olfactory disturbances, consideration should be given to other potential causes, which may modify subsequent investigations. Obviously, if other symptoms of rhinological origin are still present, then it is likely that active and continuing sinonasal disease is present and needs to be thoroughly evaluated as indicated in Chapter 7. A significant problem with the delay between development of the disorder and presentation to a physician with an interest in olfaction is that patients often find it difficult to remember the onset of symptoms. Some patients may, however, remember the cold as being "more severe" than previous URTIs. Typically, patients are aged between 40 and 70 years old, and women appear to be afflicted more often than men. The highest incidence occurs in March and May, following peaks of URTI bouts in the community.

The duration of olfactory disturbances after a viral URTI can vary widely, although approximately one-third of patients is expected to spontaneously recover normal function within 3 years. The disturbing symptoms of parosmia have been separately reported to disappear in 29% of affected patients after a mean duration of about a year. Interestingly, the presence of parosmia from the outset of the disturbance has been shown in a recent study to be less likely to lead to an anosmic outcome in the long term than parosmia that develops later.[35]

> All symptoms disappear after the URTI clears except the reduced olfactory function.
>
> At least 50% of sufferers will also have parosmia.
>
> One-third of patients experiences spontaneous recovery within 3 years.

Post-traumatic Olfactory Disorders

In mild-to-moderate head injuries without facial or nasal fractures or cerebral complications, complaints of altered smell or taste are usually noticed early after the injury (2 days to 1 week). In one study, 25 patients with post-traumatic anosmia presented within 7 days of the head injury.[36] In another study, it was reported that 83% of patients presented with smell loss immediately (1 to 5 days) after trauma, while 17% noted deficits 3 weeks to 4 months after injury.[37] The reason for these differences is that traumatic anosmia can be associated with hospitalization, memory and cognitive impairment, and behavior problems, if cerebral hemorrhage or contusions occur. In addition, hospitalization for fractured bones and other organ complications can prolong recovery and recognition of smell loss. The nature and severity of smell impairment in traumatic olfactory loss shows strong similarities in many studies. The incidence of anosmia varies from 60 to 80%, with hyposmia occurring in 20 to 25%.[24,38–40]

> Smell loss after mild head trauma is recognized 1 to 5 days after injury in 85% of cases. In 17% of injuries, smell loss may not be recognized for up to 3 weeks, particlarly in more severe head trauma associated with memory loss and longer hospitalization.

Parosmia is not uncommon in post-traumatic olfactory loss. The incidence of post-traumatic parosmia varies from 14 to 35%.[23,24,41] These differences are probably due to history taking and the fact that many patients recover early and may be missed. Does the occurrence of parosmia correlate with olfactory loss? One study found that it was more common in hyposmia than anosmia.[24] It appears to be more common with frontal and tem-

poral lobe injury than injuries to other brain areas, occurring in 45 to 50% of such cases.[42] Fortunately from a prognostic perspective, parosmia shows gradual spontaneous improvement in the majority of cases. In an 8-year study, it improved or disappeared in 15 to 42% of cases.[24]

> Post-traumatic parosmia occurs in 14 to 35% of cases. It is more common in patients with hyposmia than anosmia, and gradually improves spontaneously in the majority of cases.

Investigations

Initial investigation should first involve a cursory endoscopic examination of the nose to assess two things: presence or absence of signs of persisting sinonasal disease, such as mucosal congestion, mucopus, polyps, or anatomical deviances that may contribute to ongoing symptoms; and visualization of the olfactory cleft to ensure that it is free of any disease process (especially neoplasia, which may have been masquerading as a common cold). One should carefully ask about and look for a postnasal drip or clear rhinorrhea, which could represent a cerebrospinal fluid leak due to a fracture of the anterior cranial skull base or adjacent ethmoid sinuses[43]; this can be confirmed through testing for β2-transferrin and magnetic resonance (MR) cisternography. Imaging of the facial and nasal structures, sinuses, and cribriform plate for identification of fractures and nasal airflow obstruction is best achieved via computed tomography (CT) (without contrast). Detailed imaging of the brain and skull base to assess olfactory system structures (OB and tracts, gyrus rectus, and medial temporal lobe) that are commonly injured in post-traumatic anosmia is best achieved by MR imaging (MRI) (**Fig. 8.6**).[36]

A detailed olfactory and gustatory history should be taken about the occurrence and nature of any head trauma and about the common complaint of secondary taste impairment due to loss of flavor. This is very important because it may contribute information to the degree of post-traumatic olfactory loss and prognosis. Taste impairment may be accompanied by weight loss or decreased appetite. The presence of dysosmia, such as phantosmia or parosmia, should be established. Its presence can seriously impair appetite and quality

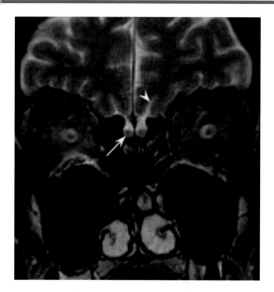

Fig. 8.6 Coronal view of olfactory bulbs (arrow) and olfactory sulcus (arrowhead) on fast spin-echo T2-weighted magnetic resonance image. (From Binder D, Sonne DC, Fischbein NJ. Cranical Nerves: Anatomy, Pathology, Imaging. Stuttgart, New York: Thieme; 2010:3).

confirm the severity of loss.[50–52] Typically, CSERPs will be preserved but OERPs may be absent or present depending on the degree of loss, and will tend to show good correlation with psychophysical test results that distinguish hyposmia and anosmia.[53] CSERPs may, however, show a reduced response, indicating crossover between olfactory and trigeminal processing (**Fig. 8.7**).[54,55] The presence of OERPs is considered to be a good prognostic sign for eventual recovery.[56]

- A psychophysical test of olfaction and endoscopic examination of the nose, including the olfactory clefts, should be the minimum level of assessment.
- CT or MRI may be appropriate in selected cases, especially with head injuries.

Thorough standardized smell and taste testing should be performed in all symptomatic cases. OERPs and CSERPs should be considered in facilities where these are available, to confirm the severity of the olfactory loss.

of life.[44,45] If seen by a neurologist, a detailed cognitive and neurological exam should be performed. There is evidence that gustatory thresholds can be decreased in post-traumatic anosmia, and primary taste testing with threshold measurements should be performed.[46]

Pyschophysical testing should be the minimum standard to quantify the degree of olfactory loss, but the qualitative disorders of parosmia and cacosmia are very difficult to quantify by these means. Nonetheless, a validated olfactory test should be used to rank the patient's disorder (see Chapter 6). A comprehensive test, such as the "Sniffin' Sticks",[47] allows an accurate assessment of this, but it is time consuming and other test kits may be more practical if time constraints or other resource limitations are present. The choice of test kit may also be influenced by cultural considerations in terms of the odor choices available. If time and financial constraints dictate limited testing, then a threshold test will give the most reliable assessment as an individual component, as has been demonstrated in at least two studies.[48,49]

Higher level testing, such as olfactory event-related potentials (OERPs) and chemosensory event-related potentials (CSERPs), can be performed where facilities allow, and may serve to

Treatment, Prognosis, and Case Reports

Postinfectious Hyposmia

High-quality evidence to support the various treatment options for postinfectious hyposmia is lacking. However, it is generally accepted that a course of oral steroids and topical steroids should be tried in an attempt to promote recovery of olfactory function, based on one trial that does show good evidence,[57] and other contributory studies.[58–61] Zinc, in a conventional form, has probably been discounted[62] (and, in fact, has even been associated with the development of olfactory disturbances[63]), but zinc nanoparticles may hold some promise for future progress.[64] The role of topical steroids in addition to oral steroids has been suggested to be useful in patients with a good initial response to oral steroids.[65]

Several treatment options have been investigated to date, either specifically for postinfectious loss or more generally for SNODs. First α-lipoic acid was investigated on the premise that its antioxidant effects and release of nerve growth factor would promote neuroepithelial regeneration. A study of patients receiving 600 mg per day for an

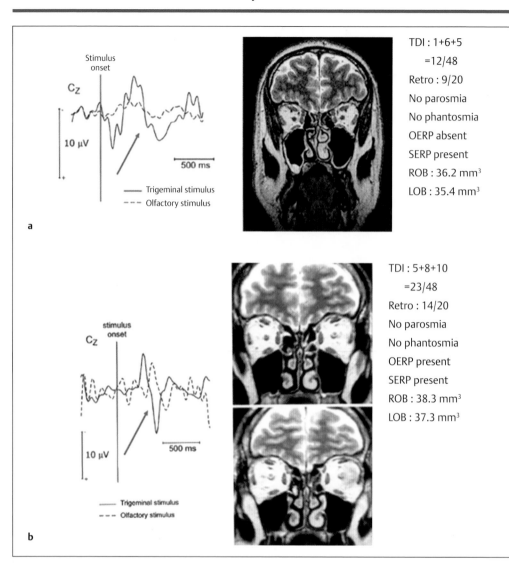

TDI : 1+6+5
=12/48
Retro : 9/20
No parosmia
No phantosmia
OERP absent
SERP present
ROB : 36.2 mm^3
LOB : 35.4 mm^3

TDI : 5+8+10
=23/48
Retro : 14/20
No parosmia
No phantosmia
OERP present
SERP present
ROB : 38.3 mm^3
LOB : 37.3 mm^3

Fig. 8.7a–c Olfactory event-related potentials (OERPs) and sensory event-related potentials (SERPs). LOB, left olfactory bulb; ROB, right olfactory bulb; TDI, threshold, discrimination, and identification score. (Figures courtesy of Dr. Philippe Rombaux, University of Louvain, Brussels, Belgium.)

a   Post-infection OERPs and SERPs in anosmia.

b   Post-infectious olfactory loss OERPs and SERPs in hyposmia.

average of 4.5 months showed a mixed response, with a significant overall improvement in function as judged by the "Sniffin' Sticks" test.[66] However, to date, there has been no double-blind, placebo-controlled trial to confirm this, but notable findings included a decrease in parosmias and a tendency for younger patients to fare better than those over the age of 60 years.

Pentoxifylline is another oral medication that has been subjected to a non-randomized con-trolled trial. It is a peripheral vasodilator indicated for use in peripheral vascular disease. It is a non-specific phosphodiesterase inhibitor, and its mechanism of action in olfactory loss is believed to be due to an increase in the activation of odor-sensing cells in the nose caused by an increase in the concentration of cyclic adenosine mono-phosphate (cAMP). Another study to investigate its use in sudden-onset sensorineural hearing loss provided anecdotal evidence that olfactory

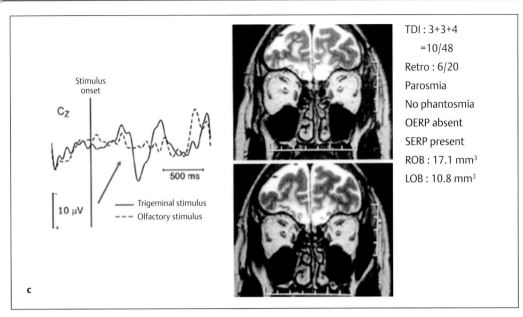

TDI : 3+3+4

=10/48

Retro : 6/20

Parosmia

No phantosmia

OERP absent

SERP present

ROB : 17.1 mm³

LOB : 10.8 mm³

◁ continued

c Post-traumatic olfactory loss OERPs and SERPs.

performance improved.[67] This study was actually for patients receiving an intravenous formulation, rather than the oral form of the drug. Similarly, theophylline, another non-specific phosphodiesterase inhibitor, was evaluated in an open trial of 312 patients, of which 31% had a postinfectious loss.[68] Unfortunately, although they showed a 50% improvement using doses of up to 800 mg per day, the results were stratified by olfactory severity rather than by cause and it was not conducted as a double-blind, randomized controlled trial. However, it is a further hint that modifying the concentration of cAMP may have a role in treatment.[69]

Sodium citrate douches were investigated as a topical means of treating patients with SNODs, as reported by Panagiotopoulos et al in 2005.[70] The theory for this treatment is based on the ability of the citrate anion to absorb free calcium ions in the nasal mucus layer overlying the olfactory neuroepithelium. This would lead to a change in the calcium ion gradient between the mucus layer and the cytoplasm of the primary olfactory neurons, thus reducing calcium uptake into these cells through cyclic nucleotide-gated channels.[71] The result is to prolong the duration of odor molecules binding to epithelial receptors, thereby prolonging the generated action potential (i.e., decreasing adaptation at the receptor level). This theory has

also been shown to work in an animal experimental model. The study group was made up of 31 patients with a mixture of SNODs, of which postinfectious causes accounted for ~60%. Significant improvement in olfactory performance was noted between 15 and 55 minutes after application of the citrate douche. Improvements were seen in nearly all of the subjects both on psychophysical testing ("Sniffin' Sticks") and on subjective reporting. As far as any potential pitfalls in this treatment are concerned, nearly half the group reported nasal itching, although it was only a temporary phenomenon. Again, this study was limited in its applicability by its design and is under further investigation in a double-blind trial by the author. This does, however, give hope of a portable solution to postinfectious hyposmia, which could potentially be applied prior to times of specific olfactory need (such as eating).

Caroverine, like pentoxifylline, is a medication licensed for use in another anatomical location that has been applied to SNODs. It is an antispasmodic, currently available in some European countries as Spasmium (PHAFAG Pharma, Graz, Austria), indicated for irritable bowel disease. As an N-methyl-D-aspartate antagonist, it is believed that its mechanism of action lies in reduction of feedback inhibition in the OB. Quint et al in 2002 reported a proof of concept study where they compared it with zinc sulfate over a course of 4 weeks. Again, this was a mixed group of subjects, with postinfectious olfactory losses accounting for 38 of the 77 patients studied. This subgroup appeared to derive the most benefit.[72]

A recent study from Korea investigated the addition of ginkgo biloba to oral and topical steroids for postinfectious olfactory loss and found that there was a 37% improvement in threshold test scores and 33% improvement in identification test scores, the latter being significantly better than patients receiving steroids alone.[58]

Beyond potential medical treatments, acupuncture has a small evidence base for helping patients with postinfectious hyposmia improve olfactory testing scores. Vent et al studied a small group of 30 patients receiving either weekly 30-minute sessions of acupuncture for 10 weeks or Vitamin B complex orally for 12 weeks.[73] Smell training has also been shown to be of benefit in these patients, albeit small, and has the advantage of being non-invasive and free of side effects.[74] This usually involves asking patients to actively sniff twice a day from bottles of each of the following odors in turn: clove, lemon, rose, and eucalyptus. This process should be repeated for a minimum of 12 weeks.[75]

Summary of Treatment Options for Postinfectious Hyposmia

- Oral steroid trial followed by topical steroids are a first-line measure.
- Non-steroidal pharmacological options:
  - Pentoxifylline
  - Caroverine
  - Theophylline
  - Sodium citrate
  - α-lipoic acid
- Homeopathic options:
  - Ginko biloba
  - Acupuncture
- Smell training

Post-traumatic Anosmia

Treatment of PTA can be divided into acute (within 30 days of trauma) and chronic (greater than 1 month after trauma). In the acute phase, nasal contusion, edema, or fracture, with or without hematoma formation, is treated by an ear, nose, and throat physician. This treatment improves or resolves olfactory loss primarily as a result of conduction block. If the acute phase resolves and olfactory loss is still present, there has probably been injury to the olfactory nerve cells or their pathway to or from the OB.

Olfactory loss due to injury of the olfactory receptors, nerves, OB, or brain can occur in any combination in head trauma. Oral prednisone has been tried in several post-traumatic anosmia studies, mostly in Asian countries. However, these studies have not included matched controls. The largest study enrolled 116 patients with post-traumatic olfactory loss.[76] Patients with nasal trauma confirmed by nasal endoscopy were eliminated. Steroids were given a mean of 10 months after the injury (range 3 to 21 months). The steroids were given as follows: prednisone 15 mg four times daily for 3 days, 10 mg four times daily for 3 days, and 5 mg twice daily for 3 days. Mean follow-up was 5.5 months. Olfactory function was measured using the phenylethylalcohol (PEA) odor detection threshold test (various concentrations of PEA were sniffed and compared with a control bottle with no PEA); 16% of patients improved, and 84% did not. In the group that responded, the improvement occurred in a mean of 1 month (range 1 to 6.5 months). The improvement did not correlate with severity of the head injury and 75% of those with an improvement were aware of it. The conclusion of this very large study suggested that high-dose, short-term oral steroids may improve olfactory acuity without any significant side effects. Further studies with controls are needed, but in the meantime, because post-traumatic olfactory loss causes significant impairment in quality of life, safety, and enjoyment of eating, it may be worthwhile trying this treatment until a further, definitive study is performed. How steroids benefit olfactory loss is not understood, but they may possibly contribute to neural regeneration.[77]

Post-traumatic anosmia responded to a 10-day, tapering course of high-dose steroids within the first 10 months of treatment in 16% of cases (Asian studies only). More studies, here and in other countries, are needed to duplicate these results.

Parosmia

Dealing with qualitative disorders is challenging, as it is difficult to assess the impact of this form of dysfunction. As previously mentioned, dysosmia can be very debilitating and lead to decreased appetite, weight loss, and depression. In light of this, several treatment options have been proposed, in addition to any findings noted above.[66] These are designed to reduce the overall functionality of the olfactory apparatus in order to reduce the potential for the odor molecule interaction that results in the unpleasant sensation. Options include hypertonic saline nasal drops, the continued use of topical decongestants to induce rhinitis medicamentosa, a nose clip (in the case of chemotherapy-induced severe parosmia[78]), topical cocaine hydrochloride to induce anesthesia to the olfactory neurons,[79,80] gabapentin acting centrally,[80] and, in severe cases, stripping the olfactory neuroepithelium along the cribriform plate.[81]

Patient Food Education

In the majority of patients with olfactory loss, loss of flavor and enjoyment of eating is a major complaint, often more so than the loss of smell. This leads to loss of appetite, weight loss in most, and secondary depression. Fortunately, the primary taste system (which is responsible for sensations of sweet, sour, bitter, salty, and the savory broth flavor known as monosodium glutamate [MSG] or umami) and the trigeminal sensory nerves (which are responsible for texture, temperature, and spice sensations) are usually normal. This information should be pointed out to the patient. Adding small amounts of low sodium MSG to chicken, steak, and other meats, with or without spicy condiments such as salsa, Worcester sauce, or A1 steak sauce or equivalent, can improve enjoyment of eating by enriching the "taste" of these foods. Drinking cold grapefruit or orange juice (sour and sweet are preserved in olfactory loss) with pulp can increase the enjoyment and taste of a drink in the place of milk, coffee, or water, which are likely to have little, no, or altered taste. Using recipes that emphasize normal tastants and trigeminal sensory function have been very helpful in providing the same meal for the patient with olfactory impairment and the rest of the family. This can improve eating enjoyment for all.[82]

> Education in changes in food preparation is the mainstay of treatment for post-traumatic anosmia with secondary impaired flavor loss. Emphasizing spared normal taste (sweet, sour, bitter, salty, and umami) and texture, temperature, and spice recognition will help improve enjoyment of eating.

Prognosis

Patients with postinfectious olfactory loss, in the absence of definitive proof for a modifying agent, between 32 and 66% of patients are likely to recover, the latter being reported 3 years after the onset of olfactory loss.[41,83,84] In fact, it has been suggested that the number of patients with ongoing olfactory loss lasting for more than 3 years is only 19%, and, given that there may well be a significant number of patients who experience spontaneous recovery before seeking medical advice, the overall figure may be smaller still.[85] This certainly allows the treating physician to give some ray of hope to the patient who presents with a postinfectious quantitative loss.

The prognosis of PTA has been studied for many years. One study found that the majority of patients who improve do so within 3 months of injury.[32] Another study found that of 66 patients followed from 1 month to 13 years after post-traumatic olfactory loss, 36% improved, 44% showed no change, and 18% worsened. Only three patients recovered normal olfaction. Two were studied 10 years after the injury and the other had a very mild smell loss.[24] In a similar study 10 years earlier, 33% showed olfactory improvement and 27% worsened.[86] Many studies on this subject suffer from the lack of standardized smell tests. Also, subjective improvement has not been taken into account. In the study previously mentioned involving 66 patients,[24] 21% said they improved but only 13% showed smell testing evidence of improvement. What was also interesting in the same study was that, of 38 patients who reported no change in their smell, 29% actually had a better score on their UPSIT smell test. One of the longest follow-up studies of 542 patients with different causes of olfactory loss, including 106 with PTA, was recently published.[87] Patients with PTA were tested on two different occasions between 3 months and 24 years apart (median 3 years). The time between the olfactory loss and the onset of the first smell test was a median of 44 months (range 1 to 476 months). The second smell test was performed at a median of 40 months (range 3 to 189 months). Of 69 patients who were totally anosmic, 44% experienced some improvement, 4.5% improved to absolute normal, and 7% improved to age-adjusted normal. In 26 patients who were hyposmic, 42% experienced some improvement and 27% returned to age-adjusted normal. This study found, most importantly, that over time 35 to 50% of people improve, reflecting the regenerative capability of the olfactory nerve epithelium. The overall conclusion of this very long and detailed follow-up study was that olfactory improvement depends on three main factors:

1. The time between the onset of post-traumatic olfactory loss and baseline smell testing directly correlated with improvement: The longer the period, the better the improvement. This suggests that greater olfactory improvement occurred relatively soon after the injury with subsequent improvement after this period being very slow or not all.
2. The severity of olfactory dysfunction at the initial testing: Hyposmic patients were twice as likely to improve into the normal range.
3. The age of the patient at the time of the head injury and olfactory loss: People older than 74 years had less recovery overall than those less than 74 years old. This was likely to be due to aging factors of the olfactory mucosa and occlusion of the olfactory foramina of the cribriform plate, pinching off axons of the olfactory receptor cells.[16] Also, neurodegenerative diseases such as Alzheimer disease and Parkinson disease are more common in the elderly and can also impair the OB and other pathways.[88]

> Post-traumatic olfactory loss improves overall in 35 to 50% of cases over a 3-year period. Improvement is more likely to occur in individuals with hyposmia rather than anosmia, and in those younger than 74 years.

Conclusion

Both postinfectious and post-traumatic olfactory disorders have the potential to cause significant functional disturbances of both quantitative and qualitative olfaction. This chapter highlights some of the potential therapeutic options, but the authors acknowledge that there is still much work to be done in finding more effective solutions for these conditions.

References

1. Brämerson A, Johansson L, Ek L, Nordin S, Bende M. Prevalence of olfactory dysfunction: the Skövde population-based study. Laryngoscope 2004; 114(4):733–737
2. Landis BN, Konnerth CG, Hummel T. A study on the frequency of olfactory dysfunction. Laryngoscope 2004;114(10):1764–1769
3. Murphy C, Schubert CR, Cruickshanks KJ, Klein BE, Klein R, Nondahl DM. Prevalence of olfactory impairment in older adults. JAMA 2002; 288(18):2307–2312
4. Wysocki CJ, Gilbert AN. National Geographic Smell Survey. Effects of age are heterogenous. Ann N Y Acad Sci 1989;561:12–28
5. Damm M, Temmel A, Welge-Lüssen A, et al. Olfactory dysfunctions. Epidemiology and therapy in Germany, Austria and Switzerland. [Article in German] HNO 2004;52(2):112–120
6. Welge-Lüssen A, Wolfensberger M. Olfactory disorders following upper respiratory tract infections. Adv Otorhinolaryngol 2006;63:125–132
7. Eccles R. Understanding the symptoms of the common cold and influenza. Lancet Infect Dis 2005; 5(11):718–725
8. Wang JH, Kwon HJ, Jang YJ. Detection of parainfluenza virus 3 in turbinate epithelial cells of postviral olfactory dysfunction patients. Laryngoscope 2007;117(8):1445–1449
9. Sugiura M, Aiba T, Mori J, Nakai Y. An epidemiological study of postviral olfactory disorder. Acta Otolaryngol Suppl 1998;538:191–196
10. Konstantinidis I, Haehner A, Frasnelli J, et al. Post-infectious olfactory dysfunction exhibits a seasonal pattern. Rhinology 2006;44(2):135–139
11. Suzuki M, Saito K, Min WP, et al. Identification of viruses in patients with postviral olfactory dysfunction. Laryngoscope 2007;117(2):272–277
12. van Kempen M, Bachert C, Van Cauwenberge P. An update on the pathophysiology of rhinovirus upper respiratory tract infections. Rhinology 1999; 37(3):97–103
13. Yamagishi M, Fujiwara M, Nakamura H. Olfactory mucosal findings and clinical course in patients with olfactory disorders following upper respiratory viral infection. Rhinology 1994;32(3):113–118
14. Moran DT, Jafek BW, Eller PM, Rowley JC III. Ultrastructural histopathology of human olfactory dysfunction. Microsc Res Tech 1992;23(2):103–110
15. Jafek BW, Gordon AS, Moran DT, Eller PM. Congenital anosmia. Ear Nose Throat J 1990;69(5):331–337
16. Loo AT, Youngentob SL, Kent PF, Schwob JE. The aging olfactory epithelium: neurogenesis, response to damage, and odorant-induced activity. Int J Dev Neurosci 1996;14(7–8):881–900

17. Portier F, Faulcon P, Lamblin B, Bonfils P. Signs and symptoms, etiologies and clinical course of parosmia + in a series of 84 patients. [Article in French] Ann Otolaryngol Chir Cervicofac 2000; 117(1):12–18

18. Mueller A, Rodewald A, Reden J, Gerber J, von Kummer R, Hummel T. Reduced olfactory bulb volume in post-traumatic and post-infectious olfactory dysfunction. Neuroreport 2005;16(5): 475–478

19. Rombaux P, Mouraux A, Bertrand B, Nicolas G, Duprez T, Hummel T. Olfactory function and olfactory bulb volume in patients with postinfectious olfactory loss. Laryngoscope 2006;116(3):436–439

20. Levy LM, Henkin RI, Lin CS, Finley A. Rapid imaging of olfaction by functional MRI (fMRI): identification of presence and type of hyposmia. J Comput Assist Tomogr 1999;23(5):767–775

21. Charles PC, Walters E, Margolis F, Johnston RE. Mechanism of neuroinvasion of Venezuelan equine encephalitis virus in the mouse. Virology 1995; 208(2):662–671

22. Reiss CS, Plakhov IV, Komatsu T. Viral replication in olfactory receptor neurons and entry into the olfactory bulb and brain. Ann N Y Acad Sci 1998; 855:751–761

23. Sumner D. Post-traumatic anosmia. Brain 1964; 87:107–120

24. Doty RL, Yousem DM, Pham LT, Kreshak AA, Geckle R, Lee WW. Olfactory dysfunction in patients with head trauma. Arch Neurol 1997;54(9):1131–1140

25. Temmel AF, Quint C, Schickinger-Fischer B, Klimek L, Stoller E, Hummel T. Characteristics of olfactory disorders in relation to major causes of olfactory loss. Arch Otolaryngol Head Neck Surg 2002; 128(6):635–641

26. Murphy C, Schubert CR, Cruickshanks KJ, Klein BE, Klein R, Nondahl DM. Prevalence of olfactory impairment in older adults. JAMA 2002; 288(18):2307–2312

27. Zusho H. Posttraumatic anosmia. Arch Otolaryngol 1982;108(2):90–92

28. Symonds C. Discussion on differential diagnosis and treatment of post-contusional states. Proc R Soc Med 1942;35(9):601–614

29. Sumner D. Disturbance of the sense of smell and taste after head injuries. In: Vinken P, Bruyn G, eds. Handbook of Clinical Neurology. Amsterdam: North Holland Publishing Co; 1975:1–25.

30. Jafek BW, Eller PM, Esses BA, Moran DT. Post-traumatic anosmia. Ultrastructural correlates. Arch Neurol 1989;46(3):300–304

31. Costanzo RM, Takaki M. Post traumatic olfactory loss. In: Hummel T, Welge-Lussen A, eds. Taste and Smell: An Update. New York: Karger; 2006:99–107.

32. Costanzo RM, Zasler N. Head trauma. In: Getchell T, Doty RL, Bartoshuk L, Snow J, eds. Smell and Taste in Health and Disease. New York: Raven Press; 1991:711–730.

33. Levin HS, High WM, Eisenberg HM. Impairment of olfactory recognition after closed head injury. Brain 1985;108(Pt 3):579–591

34. Bonfils P, Avan P, Faulcon P, Malinvaud D. Distorted odorant perception: analysis of a series of 56 patients with parosmia. Arch Otolaryngol Head Neck Surg 2005;131(2):107–112

35. Hummel T, Lötsch J. Prognostic factors of olfactory dysfunction. Arch Otolaryngol Head Neck Surg 2010;136(4):347–351

36. Yousem DM, Geckle RJ, Bilker WB, McKeown DA, Doty RL. Posttraumatic olfactory dysfunction: MR and clinical evaluation. AJNR Am J Neuroradiol 1996;17(6):1171–1179

37. Schechter PJ, Henkin RI. Abnormalities of taste and smell after head trauma. J Neurol Neurosurg Psychiatry 1974;37(7):802–810

38. Mott AE, Leopold DA. Disorders in taste and smell. Med Clin North Am 1991;75(6):1321–1353

39. Deems DA, Doty RL, Settle RG, et al. Smell and taste disorders, a study of 750 patients from the University of Pennsylvania Smell and Taste Center. Arch Otolaryngol Head Neck Surg 1991;117(5):519–528

40. Costanzo RM, Heywood P, Ward D, Young H. Neurosurgical application of clinical olfactory assessment. Ann N Y Acad Sci 1987;510:242–244

41. Duncan HJ, Seiden AM. Long-term follow-up of olfactory loss secondary to head trauma and upper respiratory tract infection. Arch Otolaryngol Head Neck Surg 1995;121(10):1183–1187

42. Rombaux P, Mouraux A, Bertrand B, Nicolas G, Duprez T, Hummel T. Retronasal and orthonasal olfactory function in relation to olfactory bulb volume in patients with posttraumatic loss of smell. Laryngoscope 2006;116(6):901–905

43. Dinardo L, Costanzo R. Post traumatic olfactory loss. In: Seiden AM, ed. Taste and Smell Disorders. New York: Thieme; 1997:79–87.

44. Smeets MA, Veldhuizen MG, Galle S, et al. Sense of smell disorder and health-related quality of life. Rehabil Psychol 2009;54(4):404–412

45. Miwa T, Furukawa M, Tsukatani T, Costanzo RM, DiNardo LJ, Reiter ER. Impact of olfactory impairment on quality of life and disability. Arch Otolaryngol Head Neck Surg 2001;127(5):497–503

46. Landis BN, Scheibe M, Weber C, et al. Chemosensory interaction: acquired olfactory impairment is associated with decreased taste function. J Neurol 2010;257(8):1303–1308

47. Hummel T, Sekinger B, Wolf SR, Pauli E, Kobal G. 'Sniffin' sticks': olfactory performance assessed by the combined testing of odor identification, odor discrimination and olfactory threshold. Chem Senses 1997;22(1):39–52

48. Lötsch J, Reichmann H, Hummel T. Different odor tests contribute differently to the evaluation of olfactory loss. Chem Senses 2008;33(1):17–21

49. Philpott CM, Rimal D, Tassone P, Prinsley PR, Premachandra DJ. A study of olfactory testing in patients with rhinological pathology in the ENT clinic. Rhinology 2008;46(1):34–39

50. Mrowinski D, Eichholz S, Scholz G. Objective test of smell with cognitive potentials. [Article in German] Laryngorhinootologie 2002;81(9):624–628

51. Rombaux P, Bertrand B, Keller T, Mouraux A. Clinical significance of olfactory event-related potentials

related to orthonasal and retronasal olfactory testing. Laryngoscope 2007;117(6):1096–1101

52. Rombaux P, Mouraux A, Bertrand B, Guerit JM, Hummel T. Assessment of olfactory and trigeminal function using chemosensory event-related potentials. Neurophysiol Clin 2006;36(2):53–62

53. Rombaux P, Mouraux A, Collet S, Eloy P, Bertrand B. Usefulness and feasibility of psychophysical and electrophysiological olfactory testing in the rhinology clinic. Rhinology 2009;47(1):28–35

54. Rombaux P, Mouraux A, Keller T, Hummel T. Trigeminal event-related potentials in patients with olfactory dysfunction. Rhinology 2008;46(3):170–174

55. Iannilli E, Gerber J, Frasnelli J, Hummel T. Intranasal trigeminal function in subjects with and without an intact sense of smell. Brain Res 2007; 1139:235–244

56. Rombaux P, Huart C, Collet S, Eloy P, Negoias S, Hummel T. Presence of olfactory event-related potentials predicts recovery in patients with olfactory loss following upper respiratory tract infection. Laryngoscope 2010;120(10):2115–2118

57. Blomqvist EH, Lundblad L, Bergstedt H, Stjärne P. Placebo-controlled, randomized, double-blind study evaluating the efficacy of fluticasone propionate nasal spray for the treatment of patients with hyposmia/anosmia. Acta Otolaryngol 2003; 123(7):862–868

58. Seo BS, Lee HJ, Mo JH, Lee CH, Rhee CS, Kim JW. Treatment of postviral olfactory loss with glucocorticoids, Ginkgo biloba, and mometasone nasal spray. Arch Otolaryngol Head Neck Surg 2009; 135(10):1000–1004

59. Seiden AM, Duncan HJ. The diagnosis of a conductive olfactory loss. Laryngoscope 2001;111(1):9–14

60. Heilmann S, Huettenbrink KB, Hummel T. Local and systemic administration of corticosteroids in the treatment of olfactory loss. Am J Rhinol 2004;18(1):29–33

61. Fukazawa K. A local steroid injection method for olfactory loss due to upper respiratory infection. Chem Senses 2005;30(Suppl 1):i212–i213

62. Henkin RI, Schecter PJ, Friedewald WT, Demets DL, Raff M. A double blind study of the effects of zinc sulfate on taste and smell dysfunction. Am J Med Sci 1976;272(3):285–299

63. Alexander TH, Davidson TM. Intranasal zinc and anosmia: the zinc-induced anosmia syndrome. Laryngoscope 2006;116(2):217–220

64. Viswaprakash N, Dennis JC, Globa L, et al. Enhancement of odorant-induced responses in olfactory receptor neurons by zinc nanoparticles. Chem Senses 2009;34(7):547–557

65. Stenner M, Vent J, Hüttenbrink KB, Hummel T, Damm M. Topical therapy in anosmia: relevance of steroid-responsiveness. Laryngoscope 2008; 118(9):1681–1686

66. Hummel T, Heilmann S, Hüttenbriuk KB. Lipoic acid in the treatment of smell dysfunction following viral infection of the upper respiratory tract. Laryngoscope 2002;112(11):2076–2080

67. Gudziol V, Hummel T. Effects of pentoxifylline on olfactory sensitivity: a postmarketing surveillance study. Arch Otolaryngol Head Neck Surg 2009;135(3):291–295

68. Henkin RI, Velicu I, Schmidt L. An open-label controlled trial of theophylline for treatment of patients with hyposmia. Am J Med Sci 2009; 337(6):396–406

69. Gudziol V, Pietsch J, Witt M, Hummel T. Theophylline induces changes in the electro-olfactogram of the mouse. Eur Arch Otorhinolaryngol 2010; 267(2):239–243

70. Panagiotopoulos G, Naxakis S, Papavasiliou A, Filipakis K, Papatheodorou G, Goumas P. Decreasing nasal mucus Ca++ improves hyposmia. Rhinology 2005;43(2):130–134

71. Zufall F, Leinders-Zufall T. The cellular and molecular basis of odor adaptation. Chem Senses 2000;25(4):473–481

72. Quint C, Temmel AF, Hummel T, Ehrenberger K. The quinoxaline derivative caroverine in the treatment of sensorineural smell disorders: a proof-of-concept study. Acta Otolaryngol 2002;122(8):877–881

73. Vent J, Wang DW, Damm M. Effects of traditional Chinese acupuncture in post-viral olfactory dysfunction. Otolaryngol Head Neck Surg 2010;142(4):505–509

74. Hummel T, Stuck BA. Treatment of olfactory disorders. [Article in German] HNO 2010;58(7):656–660

75. Hummel T, Rissom K, Reden J, Hähner A, Weidenbecher M, Hüttenbrink KB. Effects of olfactory training in patients with olfactory loss. Laryngoscope 2009;119(3):496–499

76. Jiang RS, Wu SH, Liang KL, Shiao JY, Hsin CH, Su MC. Steroid treatment of posttraumatic anosmia. Eur Arch Otorhinolaryngol 2010;267(10):1563–1567

77. Ikeda K, Sakurada T, Takasaka T, Okitsu T, Yoshida S. Anosmia following head trauma: preliminary study of steroid treatment. Tohoku J Exp Med 1995;177(4):343–351

78. Müller A, Landis BN, Platzbecker U, Holthoff V, Frasnelli J, Hummel T. Severe chemotherapy-induced parosmia. Am J Rhinol 2006;20(4):485–486

79. Fikentscher R, Rasinski C. Parosmias—definition and clinical picture. [Article in German] Laryngol Rhinol Otol (Stuttg.) 1986;65(12):663–665

80. Zilstorff K, Herbild O. Parosmia. Acta Otolaryngol Suppl 1979;360:40–41

81. Sarangi P, Aziz TZ. Post-traumatic parosmia treated by olfactory nerve section. Br J Neurosurg 1990; 4(4):358

82. Devere R, Calvert M. Food preparation. In: DeVere R, Calvert M, eds. Navigating Smell and Taste Disorders. New York: Demos Health/The American Academy of Neurology Publishers; 2011:81–149.

83. Seiden AM. Postviral olfactory loss. Otolaryngol Clin North Am 2004;37(6):1159–1166

84. Reden J, Mueller A, Mueller C, et al. Recovery of olfactory function following closed head injury or infections of the upper respiratory tract. Arch Otolaryngol Head Neck Surg 2006;132(3):265–269

85. Hummel T. Perspectives in olfactory loss following viral infections of the upper respiratory tract. Arch Otolaryngol Head Neck Surg 2000;126(6):802–803

86. Costanzo RM, Becker D. Smell and taste disorders in head injury and neurosurgery patients. In: Meiselman H, Rivlin R, eds. Clinical Measurement of Smell and Taste. New York: Macmillan Publishing Co; 1986:565–578

87. London B, Nabet B, Fisher AR, White B, Sammel MD, Doty RL. Predictors of prognosis in patients with olfactory disturbance. Ann Neurol 2008;63(2):159–166

88. Braak H, Braak E, Yilmazer D, de Vos RA, Jansen EN, Bohl J. Pattern of brain destruction in Parkinson's and Alzheimer's diseases. J Neural Transm 1996;103(4):455–490

9 Miscellaneous Causes of Olfactory Dysfunction

Philippe Rombaux

Introduction

Olfactory and gustatory disorders can be due to a wide variety of causes and can profoundly influence a patient's quality of life. This chapter covers toxicants, industrial agents, and therapeutic agents that cause olfactory dysfunction, idiopathic olfactory loss, congenital anosmia, endocrine diseases associated with olfactory dysfunction, postsurgical olfactory dysfunction, and tumor-related olfactory disorders. Miscellaneous causes of olfactory dysfunction, as defined in this chapter, account for less than 10% of cases.[1,2] A detailed history and examination is necessary to determine any lifestyle factors or toxicant or drug consumption that may be related to olfactory dysfunction. Counseling of the patient is mandatory to reduce toxicant exposure; change any implicated medications; give an accurate prognosis; or treat, as soon as possible, a tumor for which olfactory dysfunction is the sole and primary manifestation.

Diagnosis of olfactory dysfunction is often difficult, especially for toxicant and therapeutic agent exposure. The patient's history, including the delay between exposure and clinical manifestation, is the keystone of diagnosis. Moreover, the clinician must consider that combinations of causal factors may be present. This is especially true for a patient in whom a therapeutic agent is suspected to be the causative agent. It should also be stressed that in this category of miscellaneous causes of olfactory dysfunction, olfactory function needs to be objectively evaluated (see Chapter 6) because clinical findings may lead to legal action, changes in prescribed medications, changes in professional habit, or decisions concerning the surgical management of the patient.

Toxicants and Industrial Agents

Acute or chronic exposure to toxicants and industrial agents may have deleterious effects on olfactory function.

Although many reports in the literature suggest that a wide variety of toxicants may have a deleterious effect on the chemosensory function in general and on the olfaction in particular, specific information regarding the pathophysiology, the time–dose effect, and the potential of recovery is poor. The olfactory neuroepithelium is highly sensitive to the chemical or microbiological environment because it acts as an interface between the outside world in the upper airways and the inside world in the central nervous system. Many defense mechanisms exist at the olfactory neuroepithelial level to induce detoxification and rapid regeneration after chronic and repetitive or acute and brief exposure to irritants and toxins.

Exposure to toxic volatiles at levels sufficient to impair olfaction usually occurs by accident. The list of chemicals that is theoretically toxic to the olfactory system is extensive and reported cases are numerous even though toxicant exposure is thought to be responsible for less than 2% of cases of olfactory dysfunction (**Table 9.1**).[1,2] The degree of exposure, concentration, and intrinsic toxicity of the agent, as well as local conditions at the neuroepithelial level, may greatly influence the significance of the damage and its clinical manifestation.[3,4]

Chronic exposure to benzene (an industrial solvent used in the production of drugs, plastic, synthetic rubbers, and dyes), butyl acetate (a solvent used in the production of lacquers and synthetic fruit flavoring in foods), formaldehyde (a precursor of many chemical products used for resin and polymer formation), and paint solvent can cause varying degrees of olfactory dysfunction. Others compounds such as industrial dusts (cotton, silicone, cement, lead, coal, chromium, and nickel) and chemicals such as sulfuric acid, trichloroethylene and hydrogen have been also associated with olfactory dysfunction.

Chronic exposure to cadmium has been well reported in a large cohort of workers who handle electrical batteries containing cadmium and can lead to olfactory disorder. Chronic exposure to gases (carbon disulfide, carbon monoxide, sulfur dioxide) or to solvents (acetone, acetophenone, turpentine) can also induce smell disorders.[5–12]

Table 9.1 Major toxicants and industrial agents with the potential to induce olfactory disorder

Metallic compounds	Organic compounds
• Cadmium	• Acetaldehyde
• Dichromates	• Acetophenone
• Nickel	• Benzene
• Zinc	• Butyl acetate
• Alum	• Chlorometanes
• Arsenic	• Ethyl acetate
• Silver nitrate	• Trichloroethylene
• Copper arsenite	• Acetic acid
	• Formaldehyde
	• Trichloroethane
	• Chloroform
Metallurgical processes	**Dusts**
• Chromium	• Cement
• Nickel plating or refining	• Chemicals
• Lead smelting	• Hardwoods
• Magnet production	• Cotton
• Steel production	• Cyanides
• Zinc, copper, manganese, and tin fumes	• Wax
• Arsenic	• Potash
	• Silicon dioxide
Nonmetallic inorganic compounds	**Manufacturing processes**
• Ammonia	• Acids
• Carbon disulfide	• Asphalt
• Carbon monoxide	• Cutting oils
• Chlorine	• Fragrances
• Fluorides	• Lead paints
• Hydrogen	• Rubber vulcanization
• Nitric acid	• Spices
• Selenium dioxide	• Tobacco
	• Tanning

Pathophysiology focuses mainly on histological damage (replacement of the neuroepithelium by respiratory epithelium), decreased function in the Bowman gland, and direct toxicity to the olfactory receptor cell (by the molecule itself, or after enzymatic activation to the proximate toxicant). The health of the host is important and may influence the outcome of exposure of the olfactory epithelium to toxins. An upper respiratory infection, for example, may induce severe olfactory dysfunction if present at the same time as a toxic exposure that would not inflict severe damage if present alone.

Exposure of the olfactory neuroepithelium to a toxic agent stimulates defense mechanisms such as secretion of enzymes or proteins that protect the integrity of the neuroepithelium, or activation of the trigeminal reflex, which has a direct role in eliminating and reducing the risk of olfactory damage by inducing glandular secretions, sneezing, and watery discharge from the nasal mucosa and the eye. Protection of the olfactory neuroepithelium is achieved through structural recovery of olfactory tissue, an increase in metabolizing enzymes that facilitate olfactory receptor neuron (ORN) recovery, and an increase in metal chelating agents. Localization of membrane transporters and efflux mechanisms also protect the integrity of the neuroepithelium.

Epidemiological studies in workplaces known to be causative for olfactory dysfunction should be performed, along with animal studies to test compounds for potential olfactory toxicity. In the absence of such evidence, the precautionary principle should be applied to workers in whom toxicant-related olfactory dysfunction is suspected.[13]

Therapeutic Agents

> Therapeutic agents affect olfaction qualitatively more than quantitatively, and affect taste more often than olfaction. Drug-induced chemosensory dysfunction is often reversible.

Drug-induced olfactory dysfunction is often reversible and related to the duration of intake. In drug-related chemosensory dysfunction, taste is much more affected than smell[14,15] and qualitative disorders are more common than quantitative disorders.[16] Many different therapeutic agents may be responsible (**Table 9.2**), and documentation of the time course between medication intake and the development of clinical symptoms is essential. In clinical practice, it is sometimes difficult to differentiate between drug-induced chemosensory dysfunction and other conditions such as postinfectious olfactory loss. A comprehensive history is essential to aid the diagnosis. The condition for which the medication has been prescribed must be considered as a possible cause, as well as endocrine disorders, chronic renal failure, chronic hepatic dysfunction, severe infection, or diabetes.

Therapeutic agents can cause olfactory dysfunction at the periphery and at receptor level. Typically, the olfactory dysfunction is reversible once the medical treatment is discontinued (if possible). Recovery depends on many factors, such as age, sex, environmental status (e.g., tobacco intake, exposure to other toxicants), and sinonasal status (e.g., chronic rhinosinusitis, allergy). Therapeutic agents leading to a negative effect on olfactory perception may be distinguished as a class effect (e.g., quinolone antibiotics) or on an individual basis with single cases reported. Informing the pharmaceutical company of the potential association between a medication and a side effect on olfactory function is also mandatory.

Idiopathic Olfactory Disorder

> If no cause is found for the diagnosis, a patient is considered to have idiopathic olfactory loss. A preclinical state of neurodegenerative disease should not be forgotten.

Despite extensive work-up with psychophysical testing (uni- or bilateral), electrophysiological

Table 9.2 Therapeutic agents with well-demonstrated negative effects on olfactory function

Antibiotics • Aminoglycoside: rare • Penicillin: rare • Quinolone < 1% • Macrolides: rare (taste > smell) • Tetracycline: rare	**Cytostatics** • Cytarabine • Doxorubicin • Methotrexate • Vincristine
Topical intranasal drugs • Steroids: < 1% • Decongestants: 1–3% • Cocaine: 5–10%	**Antidepressants** • Amitriptyline • Clomipramine • Desipramine • Doxepin • Imipramine • Nortriptyline
Cardiovascular drugs • Calcium channel blockers • Antiarrhythmics • Lipid lowering agents	**Antipsychotics** • Clozapine • Trifluoperazine
Antithyroid agents • Carbimazole • Thiamazole	**Muscle relaxants** • Baclofen • Dantrolene
Antiparkinsonian drugs • Levodopa	

recording, structural magnetic resonance imaging (MRI), patient history, and endonasal endoscopic examination of the olfactory cleft, no explanation for olfactory symptoms is found in a significant number of patients. This is classified as idiopathic olfactory loss.

In a large cohort of patients, olfactory loss was classed as idiopathic in up to 18% of cases.[17] This must be a diagnosis of exclusion made after complete and extensive evaluation of the confirmed olfactory dysfunction. In patients with idiopathic olfactory loss, the olfactory bulb (OB) is smaller than in controls, which seems to suggest an involvement of the OB in its pathophysiology.[18] An unsuccessful oral corticosteroid trial should also serve as a diagnostic criterion.[19] Care must also be taken to remember that olfactory dysfunction may be a preclinical sign of neurodegenerative disorder (e.g., Alzheimer or Parkinson diseases). It is generally assumed that patients with idiopathic olfactory loss need to be re-examined after several months, with endonasal endoscopic examination, psychophysical testing, and even structural imaging, to rule out any developing disease such as neurodegenerative diseases.

Endocrine Disorders

> Various endocrine disorders may affect chemosensory function.

Many patients with endocrine disorders complain of olfactory dysfunction, but the pathophysiological mechanism is poorly understood.[20–22] This chemosensory dysfunction is often accompanied by other sensory (hearing, vision) or proprioceptive disorders. In general, endocrine disorder is associated with a decrease in olfactory function, although adrenocortical insufficiency (Addison disease) may lead to increased sensitivity to chemosensory stimuli. Turner syndrome (chromatin-negative gonadal dysgenesis), Cushing syndrome (excessive secretion of adrenal corticosteroids), hypothyroidism, and pseudohypoparathyroidism are also medical conditions where olfactory function is impaired. The mechanism seems to affect the neuroepithelial level, where endocrine dysfunction may alter transduction and sensorineural function. It is not clear if treatment of the endocrine disorder has a positive impact on olfactory

recovery, or if the prognosis of both conditions is linked.

Congenital Olfactory Disorder

> Absence or hypoplasia of the OB or abnormal depth of the olfactory sulcus may be related to a congenital olfactory disorder.

Olfactory dysfunction since birth or childhood may be classed as syndromic (genetic and complete) or nonsyndromic (isolated and incomplete). In complete and genetic dysfunction, the olfactory dysfunction is part of the general deficiency in the morphotype. In this field, Kalmann syndrome, Klinefelter syndrome, or CHARGE syndrome are well described.[23–30] Kalmann syndrome encompasses a hypogonadotrophic hypogonadism associated with severe olfactory dysfunction. Kalmann syndrome is an autosomal dominant condition with incomplete expressivity and with a morphotype including cryptorchidism, midline craniofacial abnormalities, tooth agenesis, deafness, and renal abnormalities. Its incidence is higher in men (1 in 10,000) than in women (1 in 50,000). This syndrome occurs far less often than isolated olfactory dysfunction, and the term isolated anosmia (IA) has been introduced to describe patients with an absence of any olfactory structure on MRI with no other endocrine, sensory, or renal disorders.

Congenital olfactory dysfunction is characterized by the absence of any olfactory perception since birth or childhood, and is typically related to aplasia or absence of the OB as revealed by MRI. Aplasia of the OB may be bilateral and symmetrical, more pronounced on one side, or unilateral. Absence of an OB is associated with decreased depth—or even complete absence—of the olfactory sulcus, and with absence of any olfactory tract.[28–30] In both syndromic and isolated congenital anosmia, three different variations have been reported: (1) hypoplasia of the OB with olfactory tracts present; (2) aplasia of the OB with olfactory tracts present; and (3) aplasia of both the OB and olfactory tracts (**Fig. 9.1**).

Time of diagnosis in children with nonsyndromic dysfunction is often around 8 to 14 years, when olfactory dysfunction is first reported by the patient. Absence of the OB on MRI examination is sometimes difficult to ascertain because of technical difficulties. Decreased olfactory depth, calculated in the plane posterior to the eyeball, is therefore an important feature that confirms the diagnosis of congenital absence of the OB. In a large cohort of patients, the minimal depth of olfactory sulcus associated with presence of the OB and olfactory tract, with a specificity of 1, was 8 mm. This means that, below this value, there is a high probability that the OB and olfactory tracts are absent.[31]

There is no treatment, medical or surgical, that improves olfactory function in congenitally affected patients. Counseling and discussion of coping strategies seem to be the best way to help these patients.

Tumoral Causes of Olfactory Disorder

(See **Table 9.3**)

Some head and neck tumors may present as an olfactory disorder or when exploring olfactory function, especially with unilateral dysfunction or when a significant discrepancy between the two nostrils is observed.

The diagnosis of a tumoral (benign or malignant) lesion with olfactory dysfunction as its primary and sole manifestation is very rare.

Extracranial (intranasal) tumoral lesions usually cause other clinical symptoms, such as nasal obstruction, and expresses unilateral symptoms: inverted papilloma, Schwannoma, angiofibroma, adenocarcinoma, esthesioneuroblastoma, and epidermoid carcinoma. Pathology of the olfactory cleft such as hamartoma adenomatoid or adenocarcinoma leads to homolateral olfactory dysfunction if explored with unilateral olfactory testing (**Figs. 9.2, 9.3 and 9.4**). Depending on the histological diagnosis, the age of the patient, the extent of the surgical procedure, or the proposed treatment, the evolution of the olfactory dysfunction may be variable.

Intracranial tumoral lesions may also impede olfactory function by compromising OB and olfactory tract function. Olfactory groove meningiomas, suprasellar ridge meningiomas, and pituitary growths extending above the diaphragm of the sella turcica may develop from the dura of the cribriform plate and surrounding tissue, and cause olfactory dysfunction (**Fig. 9.5**). Frontal or temporal lobe tumors or non-neoplastic space-filling lesions (e.g., aneurysm, hydrocephalus located in the area of the third ventricle) have also been reported with olfactory dysfunction.

Although olfactory evaluation is not the primary diagnostic tool in the clinical work-up of head and neck tumors, a unilateral disorder or an extensive side difference in olfactory function should arouse suspicion and lead to further evaluation using imaging techniques.[32,33]

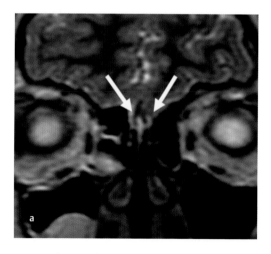 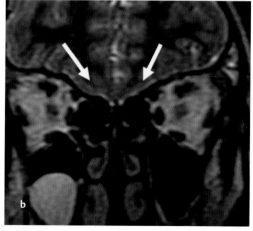

Fig. 9.1a, b Coronal magnetic resonance image (T2 sequence) of the anterior cranial base revealing no olfactory bulb structure (**a**, white arrows) and no olfactory sulcus (**b**, white arrows).

Table 9.3 Tumoral lesions associated with olfactory dysfunction

Tumor	Features
Extracranial	
Benign	
• Angiofibroma	• Pterygopalatine fossa, male, adolescent
• Inverted papilloma	• Ethmoid or maxillary, unilateral, male
• Schwannoma	• Very rare
• Adenomatoid hamartoma	• Olfactory cleft, old people
• Others (osteoma, etc.)	• Very rare
Malignant	
• Adenocarcinoma	• Olfactory cleft, woodworker
• Esthesioneuroblastoma	• From the olfactory neuroepithelium
• Epidermoid carcinoma	• Tobacco and alcohol consumption
• Others (carcinoma adenoid cystic, etc.)	
Intracranial	
Benign	
• Meningioma	• From the olfactory groove
• Pituitary tumors	• Extending outside the sella turcica
Malignant	
• Frontal or temporal tumors	• Olfactory dysfunction rare as a sole manifestation
Space-filling lesions	• Non-neoplastic (aneurysm, hydrocephalus)

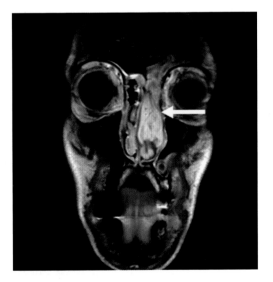

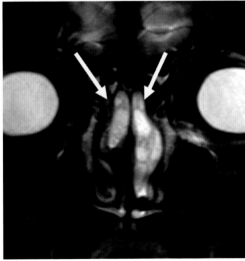

Fig. 9.2 Coronal magnetic resonance image (T1 sequence) of the paranasal sinuses showing a tumoral mass in the left olfactory cleft (white arrow): Schwannoma.

Fig. 9.3 Coronal magnetic resonance image (T2 sequence) of the paranasal sinuses showing a bilateral tumoral mass in the olfactory cleft (white arrows): adenomatoid hamartoma.

111

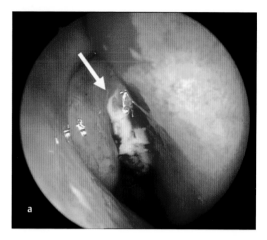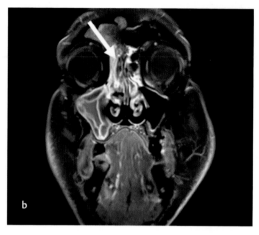

Fig. 9.4a, b Tumoral masses associated with olfactory loss.

a Endoscopic view (30°) of the right olfactory cleft showing a tumoral mass (white arrow) medial to the middle turbinate.

b Coronal magnetic resonance image (T1 sequence) of the paranasal sinuses showing a right tumoral mass in the olfactory cleft (white arrow): adenocarcinoma in woodworker.

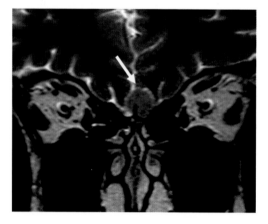

Fig. 9.5 Coronal magnetic resonance image (T2 sequence) of the anterior cranial base showing a tumoral mass (white arrow) in the olfactory groove: olfactory meningioma.

Complications of Surgery and Olfactory Dysfunction

> Even if nasal and sinus surgery have the primary goal of restoring olfactory function, some surgical procedures may be associated with a deterioration in chemosensory function.

Very rare case reports have been published where an olfactory dysfunction occurred during the course of surgery not associated with olfactory pathways. A variety of drugs given during a surgical procedure may impede olfaction after oral administration, systemic injection, or topical application. Halogenated volatile agents given during anesthesia may also induce an unpleasant smell perception during inhalational induction. Olfactory dysfunction is usually transient and a causal relationship between the anesthetic medication and the chemosensory dysfunction is often difficult to ascertain.[34–36]

After nasal surgery, olfactory function may be worse for several reasons: nasal packing; mucosal edema; olfactory neuroepithelial lesions; or scar tissue formation. Although very rare and time-limited, olfactory dysfunction after common nasal surgery (e.g., septoplasty, rhinoseptoplasty, turbinectomy, etc.) has been reported with variable prevalence (**Table 9.4**).[37–45]

Endoscopic endonasal surgery in the ethmoid sinuses and in the olfactory cleft may also induce severe olfactory dysfunction as a result of: metaplasia of the olfactory neuroepithelium; scar tissue formation in the olfactory cleft; superinfection with neurotoxin-producing bacteria; iatrogenic injury to the sinonasal mucosa, where olfactory receptor neurons are present; and iatrogenic injury to the olfactory cleft (e.g., cerebrospinal fluid leak, reconstruction of the anterior cranial base). This is especially true when extensive or radical surgery has been performed, inducing a complete atrophic rhinitis (**Fig. 9.6**).[46]

Table 9.4 Nasal surgery and olfactory function

Author	Operation	n	Improvement in olfactory function	Deterioration in olfactory function	Comment
Delank and Stoll 1998[38]	Sinus surgery	115		8%	
Pade and Hummel 2008[39]	Sinus surgery	206	23%	9%	
	Nasal surgery		16%	7%	
Damm et al 2003[40]	Septoplasty Partial turbinectomy	30		13%	Moderate decrease
Pfaar et al 2004[41]	Septoplasty	30		3%	Hyposmia
Dürr et al 2002[42]	Rhinoplasty	41		14%	
Briner et al 2003[43]	Septoplasty and sinus surgery	164		2.5–3%	Hyposmia

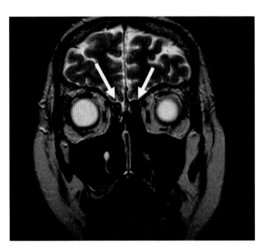

Fig. 9.6 Coronal magnetic resonance image (T2 sequence) of the paranasal sinuses showing a postoperative view after radical surgery (complete removal of inferior and middle turbinate, and ethmoid mucosa: white arrows) leading to atrophic rhinitis with olfactory disorder.

A classical approach to the anterior cranial fossa for skull base tumors is almost always associated with permanent postoperative olfactory dysfunction because olfactory structures are an obstacle to the approach. Alternative routes exist that better spare the olfactory apparatus, although these must not jeopardize the approach or the tumor removal.[45] Olfactory dysfunction can also be present after trans-sphenoidal hypophysectomy.[34]

The Olfactory Cleft Syndrome

> Congestion of the olfactory cleft without inflammation of the paranasal sinuses may have a negative impact on olfactory function and may be related to the so-called olfactory cleft syndrome.

Patients with obstructive inflammation of the olfactory clefts also have impaired olfactory function. This syndrome is considered as a new finding and is diagnosed when clear inflammatory obstruction of the olfactory cleft is demonstrated on imaging without any radiological sign of opacified sinuses (**Fig. 9.7**).[46] The obstruction corresponds to local inflammation of the mucosal tissue covering the olfactory cleft and may be secondary to a severe nasopharyngeal infection or to damage to the cleft region, leading to squamous metaplasia or fibrosis, with negative consequences on olfactory function. Association with hypertrophy of the middle turbinate (concha bullosa) and with obvious anatomical malformation has been underlined also. This diagnosis is radiological and endoscopic. Endonasal endoscopy typically detects bilateral and symmetrical congestion in the olfactory cleft with no extension to the more inferior part of the nasal fossa. Tentative treatment may be based on oral corticosteroid treatment (which is not really helpful for the vast majority of patients) or on concha bullosa reduction.

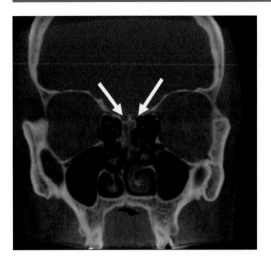

Fig. 9.7 Coronal computed tomography of the paranasal sinuses revealing a swelling of the mucosa in the olfactory cleft bilaterally (white arrows): olfactory cleft syndrome.

Conclusions

- Miscellaneous causes of olfactory dysfunction are numerous, and treatment needs to be adapted to each specific case. Eliminating the causative toxicant or drug seems the logical way to manage patients with toxicant- or drug-induced olfactory dysfunction.
- Endocrine-related disorders should receive appropriate treatment of the underlying disease, but olfactory recovery may not ensue.
- Idiopathic olfactory disorders should only be diagnosed if others causes have been ruled out. The possibility of developing neurodegenerative disease should be considered.
- Congenital olfactory disorders should be diagnosed by MRI techniques focusing on the OB and the olfactory sulcus, despite the fact that no treatment exists for these patients.
- Tumor-related olfactory dysfunction is rare as a sole and primary manifestation of the disease. MRI evaluation and appropriate surgical removal (aiming to spare the olfactory apparatus without jeopardizing tumor removal) should be proposed.
- Postsurgical complications leading to olfactory dysfunction may have multiple origins.
- The prevalence of these miscellaneous causes of olfactory dysfunction is very low. Amalgamating data from different cases at different smell and taste centers should add valuable information in this area.

References

1. Damm M, Temmel A, Welge-Lüssen A, et al. Olfactory dysfunctions. Epidemiology and therapy in Germany, Austria and Switzerland. [Article in German] HNO 2004;52(2):112–120
2. Deems DA, Doty RL, Settle RG, et al. Smell and taste disorders, a study of 750 patients from the University of Pennsylvania Smell and Taste Center. Arch Otolaryngol Head Neck Surg 1991;117(5):519–528
3. Watelet JB, Strolin-Benedetti M, Whomsley R. Defence mechanisms of olfactory neuro-epithelium: mucosa regeneration, metabolising enzymes and transporters. B-ENT 2009;5(Suppl 13):21–37
4. Hastings L, Evans JE. Olfactory primary neurons as a route of entry for toxic agents into the CNS. Neurotoxicology 1991;12(4):707–714
5. Yamagishi M, Hasegawa S, Nakano Y. Examination and classification of human olfactory mucosa in patients with clinical olfactory disturbances. Arch Otorhinolaryngol 1988;245(5):316–320
6. Reed CJ. Drug metabolism in the nasal cavity: relevance to toxicology. Drug Metab Rev 1993; 25(1–2):173–205
7. Mitchell AB, Parsons-Smith BG. Trichloroethylene neuropathy. BMJ 1969;1(5641):422–423
8. Bergman U, Ostergren A, Gustafson AL, Brittebo B. Differential effects of olfactory toxicants on olfactory regeneration. Arch Toxicol 2002;76(2): 104–112
9. Ling G, Gu J, Genter MB, Zhuo X, Ding X. Regulation of cytochrome P450 gene expression in the olfactory mucosa. Chem Biol Interact 2004; 147(3):247–258
10. Ding X, Dahl AR. Chapter 3: Olfactory mucosa: composition, enzymatic localization and metabolism. In: Doty RL, ed. Handbook of Olfaction and Gustation, 2nd ed. New York: Marcel Dekker; 2003: 51–73
11. Ahlström R, Berglund B, Berglund U, Lindvall T, Wennberg A. Impaired odor perception in tank cleaners. Scand J Work Environ Health 1986; 12(6):574–581
12. Schwartz BS, Doty RL, Monroe C, Frye R, Barker S. Olfactory function in chemical workers exposed to acrylate and methacrylate vapors. Am J Public Health 1989;79(5):613–618
13. Doty RL, Gregor T, Monroe C. Quantitative assessment of olfactory function in an industrial setting. J Occup Med 1986;28(6):457–460
14. Ackerman BH, Kasbekar N. Disturbances of taste and smell induced by drugs. Pharmacotherapy 1997; 17(3):482–496
15. Doty RL, Shah M, Bromley SM. Drug-induced taste disorders. Drug Saf 2008;31(3):199–215
16. Henkin RI. Drug-induced taste and smell disorders. Incidence, mechanisms and management related primarily to treatment of sensory receptor dysfunction. Drug Saf 1994;11(5):318–377
17. Temmel AF, Quint C, Schickinger-Fischer B, Klimek L, Stoller E, Hummel T. Characteristics of olfactory disorders in relation to major causes of olfactory loss. Arch Otolaryngol Head Neck Surg 2002;128(6):635–641

18. Rombaux Ph, Potier H, Markessis E, Duprez T, Hummel T. Olfactory bulb volume and depth of olfactory sulcus in patients with idiopathic olfactory loss. Eur Arch Otorhinolaryngol 2010;267(10):1551–1556

19. Heilmann S, Strehle G, Rosenheim K, Damm M, Hummel T. Clinical assessment of retronasal olfactory function. Arch Otolaryngol Head Neck Surg 2002;128(4):414–418

20. Henkin RI. Impairment of olfaction and of the tastes of sour and bitter in pseudohypoparathyroidism. J Clin Endocrinol Metab 1968;28(5):624–628

21. Doty RL, Fernandez AD, Levine MA, Moses A, McKeown DA. Olfactory dysfunction in type I pseudohypoparathyroidism: dissociation from Gs alpha protein deficiency. J Clin Endocrinol Metab 1997;82(1):247–250

22. Lewitt MS, Laing DG, Panhuber H, Corbett A, Carter JN. Sensory perception and hypothyroidism. Chem Senses 1989;14:537–546

23. Kallmann FJ, Schoenfeld WA, Barrera SE. The genetic aspects of primary eunuchoidism. Am J Ment Defic 1944;48:203–236

24. Pawlowitzki IH, Diekstall P, Schadel A, Miny P. Estimating frequency of Kallmann syndrome among hypogonadic and among anosmic patients. Am J Med Genet 1987;26(2):473–479

25. Assouline S, Shevell MI, Zatorre RJ, Jones-Gotman M, Schloss MD, Oudjhane K. Children who can't smell the coffee: isolated congenital anosmia. J Child Neurol 1998;13(4):168–172

26. Jafek BW, Gordon AS, Moran DT, Eller PM. Congenital anosmia. Ear Nose Throat J 1990;69(5):331–337

27. Leopold DA, Hornung DE, Schwob JE. Congenital lack of olfactory ability. Ann Otol Rhinol Laryngol 1992;101(3):229–236

28. Yousem DM, Geckle RJ, Bilker W, McKeown DA, Doty RL. MR evaluation of patients with congenital hyposmia or anosmia. AJR Am J Roentgenol 1996;166(2):439–443

29. Knorr JR, Ragland RL, Brown RS, Gelber N. Kallmann syndrome: MR findings. AJNR Am J Neuroradiol 1993;14(4):845–851

30. Yousem DM, Turner WJD, Li C, Snyder PJ, Doty RL. Kallmann syndrome: MR evaluation of olfactory system. AJNR Am J Neuroradiol 1993;14(4):839–843

31. Huart C, Meusel T, Gerber J, Duprez T, Rombaux P, Hummel T. The depth of the olfactory sulcus is an indicator of congenital anosmia. AJNR Am J Neuroradiol 2011;32(10):1911–1914

32. Elsberg CA. The localization of tumors of the frontal lobe of the brain by quantitative olfactory tests. Bull Neurol Inst NY. 1935;4:535–543

33. Welge-Lüssen A, Gudziol V, Wolfensberger M, Hummel T. Olfactory testing in clinical settings – is there additional benefit from unilateral testing? Rhinology 2010;48(2):156–159

34. Adelman BT. Altered taste and smell after anesthesia: cause and effect? Anesthesiology 1995;83(3):647–649

35. Zoanetti DC, Cyna AM. Distorting the perception of smell during gaseous induction. Paediatr Anaesth 2005;15(12):1148, author reply 1149

36. Fukumoto M, Arima H, Ito S, Takeuchi N, Nakano H. Distorted perception of smell by volatile agents facilitated inhalational induction of anesthesia. Paediatr Anaesth 2005;15(2):98–101

37. Kimmelman CP. The risk to olfaction from nasal surgery. Laryngoscope 1994;104(8 Pt 1):981–988

38. Delank KW, Stoll W. Olfactory function after functional endoscopic sinus surgery for chronic sinusitis. Rhinology 1998;36(1):15–19

39. Pade J, Hummel T. Olfactory function following nasal surgery. Laryngoscope 2008;118(7):1260–1264

40. Damm M, Eckel HE, Jungehülsing M, Hummel T. Olfactory changes at threshold and suprathreshold levels following septoplasty with partial inferior turbinectomy. Ann Otol Rhinol Laryngol 2003;112(1):91–97

41. Pfaar O, Hüttenbrink KB, Hummel T. Assessment of olfactory function after septoplasty: a longitudinal study. Rhinology 2004;42(4):195–199

42. Dürr J, Lindemann J, Keck T. Sense of smell before and after functional esthetic rhinoplasty. [Article in German] HNO 2002;50(7):626–629

43. Briner HR, Simmen D, Jones N. Impaired sense of smell in patients with nasal surgery. Clin Otolaryngol Allied Sci 2003;28(5):417–419

44. Huart C, Eloy P, Collet S, Rombaux P. Chemosensory function assessed with psychophysical testing and event-related potentials in patients with atrophic rhinitis. Eur Arch Otorhinolaryngol 2012;269(1):135–141

45. Feiz-Erfan I, Han PP, Spetzler RF, et al. Preserving olfactory function in anterior craniofacial surgery through cribriform plate osteotomy applied in selected patients. Neurosurgery 2005; 57(1, Suppl):86–93, discussion 86–93

46. Trotier D, Bensimon JL, Herman P, Tran Ba Huy P, Døving KB, Eloit C. Inflammatory obstruction of the olfactory clefts and olfactory loss in humans: a new syndrome? Chem Senses 2007;32(3):285–292

10 Chemosensory Function in Infants and Children

David G. Laing, Benoist Schaal

It is now established that chemosensory functions are behaviorally and cognitively significant in human neonates, infants, and children. This chapter aims to summarize current knowledge on the development of nasal and oral chemoreception, and corresponding behavioral functions. Further, it will discuss different methods available to assess olfactory and taste capabilities in children both qualitatively and quantitatively.

Development of Chemosensory Functionality

The Fetus and Prematurely Born Infant

Nasal Chemoreception

The strongest evidence for human prenatal olfactory function comes from studies on newborns in which the odor of amniotic fluid,[1] or of flavor compounds (e.g., anise, alcohol, carrot) transferred into it, induce appetitive responses in the newborn.[2,3] Thus, from late gestation, the human fetus is able to detect, selectively encode, and retain some odor information in the womb. Near-term fetuses may be as competent as neonates. Sarnat,[4] however, found that the proportion of premature newborns detecting mint odor at birth (assessed by sucking or arousal responses) was related to gestational age. While most infants born between 29 and 36 weeks' gestation responded, less predictable reactions arose before week 29. After gestational week 32, infants born prematurely responded to the mint odor equally to infants born at term. Near-infrared spectroscopy also showed that preterm infants aged 33.7 gestational weeks (tested 12.5 days post birth) evince differential cortical hemodynamic variations when exposed to the odor of colostrum or vanilla or to trigeminal stimuli carried in disinfectants or detergents: after 10 seconds of stimulation, an increase or decrease, respectively, was noted in oxygenated hemoglobin over the parietal region.[5]

Oral Chemoreception

Taste buds of all types are evident as early as gestational week 10, and by the end of gestational month 4 receptor cells become accessible to potential stimuli through open taste pores. Human fetal responses to sapid agents infused in utero remain equivocal, but functional taste has been established in infants born preterm within gestational months 6 to 9. Sweet, bitter, or acid tastants elicit responses indicating that, from early gestational month 6, taste buds are connected with the central systems controlling behavioral and autonomic (salivation) responses. Sweet solutions lead to mouthing/sucking and positive hedonic responses (sucking, calming, facial expression indicating acceptance) in preterm infants, whereas bitter, acid, and salty stimuli tend to inhibit these responses or do not affect them (e.g., ref. 6).

The Newborn[*]

Nasal Chemoreception

When tested within 12 hours after birth and before any postnatal ingestion, odorants chosen to be pleasant or unpleasant to adults (banana, vanilla, and milky odorants versus fishy and rotten odorants, respectively) elicited typical facial responses.[7] When photographs of these responses were evaluated by an adult panel for their hedonic meaning, the odors considered pleasant induced expressions of acceptance (relaxed face, rising mouth corners, licking, sucking), while unpleasant odors provoked rejection expressions (lowering mouth corners, lip/tongue protrusion, gaping) (**Fig. 10.1**). As one anencephalic newborn reacted with similar facial expressions to odors as normal infants, an "innate" brainstem mechanism controlling hedonic facial reactivity was proposed, and termed the olfactofacial reflex.[7] However, it was later shown that prenatal experience with odorants can strongly bias such neonatal responses,[3] casting doubt on the innate nature of the "reflex".

---

[*] The human neonatal period is generally considered as extending from birth to the first month.

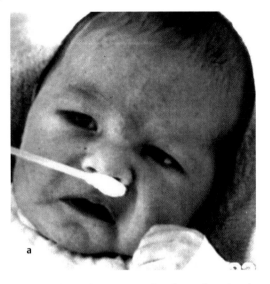 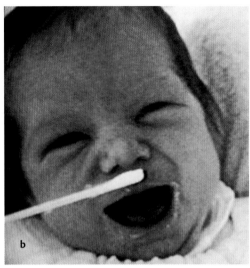

Fig. 10.1a, b Facial expressions of newborn infants (aged 2–3 days) during 10-second exposure to negative and positive odorants on Q-tips. (From Soussignan et al.[15])

a Butyric acid 0.125%.

b Cow-based formula milk.

Oral Chemoreception

Taste stimuli are well discriminated by term-born newborns. Facial and oral movements expressing acceptance (sucking, relaxed and "smiley" face, eye opening, hand–mouth contact) are elicited by water solutions of sweet tastants (sucrose, lactose, or saccharin), or by monosodium glutamate (savory) administered in a soup. In contrast, facial–oral responses expressing avoidance (grimaces, crying, gaping, eye closure) occur with acid and bitter tastants, while salty solutions remain hedonically ambiguous during the first postnatal months.[7] Reactivity measured by comparing differential ingestion from bottles containing various taste solutions against a reference bottle (generally water) provided less convincing data, probably because the sucking drive over-rides taste regulation of intake at this early age. While the acceptance for sweet solutions remained, infants consumed salt and bitter (urea) solutions as much as water, suggesting indifference to these latter tastants, while sour tastes were generally rejected.[8] Taste can regulate infants' activation states by inhibiting crying and facilitating calmness. The oral administration of sucrose activates mouthing/licking/sucking motions. This sweetness–calming link appears to fade out after 2 months of age, however.

Infants and Children

Nasal Chemoreception

Owing to difficulties in compliance and in designing tests for preverbal children, our understanding of nasal chemosensation remains scanty between the ages of 1 month and 3 years. However, there is no a priori reason why nasal chemosensation should not function well over this period:

- Below 3 years of age, reactivity to odors is attested by infants' selective responsiveness to foods and persons[9]; between 3 and 4 years, rare studies indicate good odor detection abilities; and by age 5 children's responses become accessible to more systematic psychophysical testing (see pp. 58–75).
- The best evidence for infants' and children's olfactory responsiveness comes from studies on preferences and aversions, which suggest a generally greater tolerance to unpleasant odors before 5 years of age, and converging hedonic responses in children and adults.[10] Early stability in categorizing odors as pleasant or unpleasant occurs, although considerable interindividual differences exist because of exposure and learning effects.
- Sensitivity to trigeminal agents in infants and children under 5 years of age has not been clearly established.

- Puberty is a period of change in sensitivity and hedonic rating for certain odorant qualities in or resembling body odors (e.g., steroids, musks); thus, boys become increasingly insensitive to androstenone with advancing puberty, while girls become more sensitive to it.[11] However, this pubertal variation in olfactory sensitivity and preferences does not seem to affect food odorants.[12]

Oral Chemoreception

The sense of taste continues to mature until at least 8 years of age, and possibly into adolescence. Measurement of taste detection thresholds indicate that 8-year-old females, but not males, have similar detection thresholds to adults, and 6- to 10-year-olds require larger differences between the concentrations of a tastant to perceive a difference.[13] In addition, 8-year-olds cannot perceive tastes in mixtures similarly to adults, and fail to detect both tastes in some two-component mixtures. Adults and children also differ in their taste preferences (e.g., higher levels of sourness are preferred by many children of this age, while 9- to 15-year-olds prefer higher salt concentrations than adults). These behavioral differences are accompanied by anatomical changes in 8-year-olds, with greater numbers of fungiform papillae per unit area occurring on the anterior tongue than in adults, which is reflected in higher taste sensitivity in localized areas of the tongue. Nevertheless, 8-year-olds and adults have similar response functions for suprathreshold sweet stimuli.

Importance of Chemoreception in Infancy and Childhood

The Range of Organismic Responses Influenced by Chemosensation

In general, responses elicited by odorants, tastants, or irritants appear dichotomous, with opposite trends in arousal and related attention, directional actions, information intake (sniffing and lingual actions), and lastly preferential choices and ingestion.

Arousal

Odors and tastes can markedly affect an infant's activation state. Thus, between 2 and 10 days of age, upset infants become less agitated when exposed to the breast odor of a lactating mother, which can also counteract the hyperarousal elicited by acute pain. Attenuation of agitation is even more pronounced when the odors originate from the infant's own mother.[9]

Directional Responses

Head orientation is a much used index of olfactory discrimination in infants. A two-choice test was developed that recorded supine newborns' head-turning responses to two odor stimuli, hanging on each side of their faces.[14] It demonstrated that 6-day-old infants spent more time turned toward their mother's breast odor rather than to another mother's breast odor. Infants were later shown to orient more insistently to the odor of milk from an unfamiliar woman rather than toward an unfamiliar odor of similar intensity.[9] Odors can also motivate infants to crawl toward a distant odor source.

Stimulus Sampling Responses

Volitional sniffing remains poor in infants below 2 years of age, but their respiratory pattern is nevertheless affected by the hedonic nature of an odor. For example, newborns show accelerated and decreased respiratory rates, respectively, to vanilla and butyric acid.[15] Maternal odor of very low intensity can also elicit specific patterns of respiration in newborns.[16] Thus, infants tend to adjust their nasal airflow depending on whether it carries a pleasant/familiar or unpleasant/unfamiliar odorant. Maternal odors also stimulate oral (chewing) and lingual (licking, sucking) motions that favor stimulation by taste. Four-day-olds display increased oral responses to the odor of their mother's milk than the odor of another mother's milk, or when they perceive their amniotic fluid odor. Oral movements do, therefore, express an individual's motivation to grasp the offered stimulus orally. In addition to the effects of odorants administered orthonasally, infants detect retronasal odorants during feeds, and modulate their ingestive decisions accordingly.[17]

Physiological Interactions

Odorants and tastants affect various responses controlled by the autonomic nervous system (i.e., heart and respiration rates, endocrine release).[15] Conversely, the metabolic state influences infantile responses to odors. When 3-day-old, bottle-fed infants are exposed to the odor of their usual formula milk 1 hour before and 1 hour after a feed, they respond more negatively to it during the postprandial than during the preprandial stage.[18] This fluctuation in hedonic responsiveness of infants resembles the phenomenon of negative alliesthesia* described in adults, and is an important factor of variation to consider in the testing of olfactory or taste abilities.

Everyday Adaptive Functions of Olfaction and Taste

The processes that have been most investigated are perceptual (i.e., detection, discrimination, recognition), affective (i.e., preferences, mood, attitudes), and cognitive (i.e., attention, learning, categorization, memory, semantics, lexicalization) in nature. With some obvious conceptual or linguistic limitations as a function of age, these processes are competent from earliest development to help individuals to make sense of the world. Infantile chemosensory abilities are fine-tuned by sensory experience received in the womb or in contact with the mother, and in confrontation with the ever-expanding variety in food and environment. Infants can sense flavors associated with milk and the mother's breast and recall them in tests more than a year later.[19] Olfaction is thus in a position to trace "continuity cues" to deal adaptively with the ever-changing environment, especially during episodes of instability in self-regulation (separation, stress) or periods of social or food transitions (birth, weaning, puberty, social networking). When such "odor bridges" are provided to the infant or child, adaptive responses generally ensue at individual or interactional levels. In contrast, when such olfactory continuity is ignored by caretaking routines, or disrupted by

pathological causes or iatrogenic interventions, maladaptive consequences can occur. For example, applying novel odorants to the breasts triggers distress in newborns, while smearing the breasts with their amniotic fluid facilitates initial latching responses. In older infants undergoing transition to postlacteal food, the simple technique of introducing maternal milk in a novel food facilitates its acceptance.

Chemosensation also appears to promote early perceptual unitization with inputs from other sense modalities. Thus, olfaction and taste become part of the developmental springboard that engages the multisensory processing of persons, the establishment of attachments, and the learning of the environment at large. In conclusion, it appears that odor, taste, and flavor cues are attended, processed, and recalled from earliest infancy, and that such early memories contribute to current and subsequent adaptive social and feeding responses. The following sections present different ways to characterize the performance of early nasal and oral chemosensations.

> Infantile chemosensory abilities are fine-tuned by sensory experience received in the womb or in contact with the mother, and by an ever-expanding variety in food and in the environment.

Evaluation of Chemosensory Functions in Newborns and Infants

Although olfaction and taste have been abundantly studied for functionality in early development, they have rarely been a topic of systematic psychophysical screening before the age of 3 years. Such investigations are dependent on the accessibility of pediatric populations, and more data are available for easily reachable newborns than for infants aged between 2 weeks and 3 years. Thus, efforts should be made to develop psychophysical testing adapted over this early age range.

Few such studies have been attempted in newborn olfaction. Three[4,20,21] used peppermint and indicated that nearly all term-born infants (cumulated $n = 278$) responded by oral, facial, segmental, or general motions. However, infants

---

* Alliesthesia defines the change in the level of pleasure associated with sensory stimulation. Negative alimentary alliesthesia denotes the decrease in pleasure of food-related stimuli after a meal.

born prematurely or with birth complications (asphyxia) or malformations responded at lower rates or not at all. In another assessment of neonatal olfaction,[22] the odorants phenylethyl alcohol, cyclotene, isovaleric acid, undecalactone, and skatole were delivered orthonasally to infants while their heart rate, respiration, and motor activity was recorded. Term-born neonates responded at a rate similar to adults; premature infants had lower detection performance. Finally, a few studies have measured brain responses to odors, with mixed success. Although the odors of coffee, citral, vanillin, and pyridine did not cause significant alterations in the electroencephalography (EEG) before postnatal day 6, reliable variations were seen after day 6.[23] EEG in 3- to 4-month-olds also reveals inconsistent results.[24,25] Such variability in cerebral response might be attributed to recording conditions (awake versus sleeping states) and choice of odorants.

An objective clinical test of taste dysfunction in neonates and children aged up to 4 years has not been carried out. However, measures of ingestion of water versus a tastant (volume consumed, sucking rates, facial expressions) can provide a qualitative indication of taste function and have the potential to be developed into a practical measure of taste.

> Olfaction and taste have rarely been a topic of systematic psychophysical screening before the age of 3 years.

Measurement of Chemosensory Functions in School-age Children

The greatest limitation to determining chemosensory function in children is their cognitive ability to understand the requirements of the test and their ability to maintain attention during the task. Clinical tests for children should (1) require minimal or no training for a child to be able to complete the test successfully; (2) have a low withdrawal rate; (3) be reliable; (4) be suitable for use at the bedside, outpatient clinic, school, or home; and (5) produce data that allow classification of children of different ages as normative, hyposmic/hypogeusic, or anosmic/ageusic.

Olfactory Function

> By 5 years of age, children are familiar with many smells, and this provides the basis of highly reliable smell tests.

Sydney Children's Hospital Odor Identification Test

The Sydney Children's Hospital Odor Identification Test (SCHOT) was specifically developed for the clinical measurement of olfactory function in school-age children. SCHOT involves the identification of 16 odors that are highly familiar to Australian children and has a test–retest reliability of $r = 0.98$.[26] The test requires a child to sniff an odorant contained in a white opaque flip-top squeeze bottle marked with a three-digit code number, and indicate which of three labeled photographs best represents the odor. The 16 sets of photographs (one set for each odor) are contained in a booklet. The odorants represent floral, orange, strawberry, fish, chocolate, baby powder, paint, cut grass, sour, minty, onion, Vicks VapoRub, spicy, Dettol, cheese, and petrol (**Fig. 10.2**).

The test has not been used with other cultures and a few of the odorants may need to be replaced by odors that are more familiar to a particular culture. Advantages of this test are as follows: only one practice trial is required to familiarize a

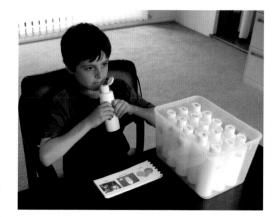

Fig. 10.2 Child sniffing 1 of 16 odor containers. A booklet of 16 sets of three photographs representing each odor and two distraction odors is provided. The child chooses the photograph that best represents the odor the child has perceived.

child with the test; it is rare for a child to refuse or not complete the test; it is completed within 5 minutes; and there are sufficient odors to provide a range of scores to enable ready classification of normosmics, hyposmics, and anosmics. To date, normative data have been obtained for 642 children and indicate that the prevalence of olfactory dysfunction in children aged 5 to 12 years is low at 0.38%. The test has been used at the bedside of patients, in outpatient clinics, and at schools. Regarding the definition of normality in this test, the following two criteria have been found to produce similar outcomes: (1) The first commonly applied clinical criterion defines normality as the score obtained by 90% of a population group; and (2) the second defines normality as two standard deviations below the mean score of a population group. These criteria indicate that a child has normal olfactory function if they correctly identify 13 out of 16 of the odorants, hyposmia if the score is 8 to 12 out of 16, and anosmia if the score is < 8 out of 16. Scores of 11 out of 16 and 12 out of 16 indicate normal function for 5- and 6-year-olds, respectively. Two of the odorants, namely, Vicks VapoRub (methyl salicylate) and sour (acetic acid), are also trigeminal nerve stimulants and provide an indication of function in this nerve. The test has been used to assess olfactory function in children with otitis media,[26] chronic renal disease,[27] cystic fibrosis,[28] nasopharyngeal carcinomas, and bone marrow transplants (unpublished studies at Sydney Children's Hospital).

"Sniffin' Sticks" (Threshold, Discrimination, and Identification Test)

This test is described in Chapter 6. Recently, it was used with 230 children aged 4 to 15 years and was found to be suitable for use with children aged 7 years and above.[29] Normative data were obtained for 102 7- to 9-year-olds and 73 10- to 15-year-olds. The failure of 4- to 6-year-olds to identify the odorants was a result of issues of familiarity with the odorants used (identification task) and attending and understanding the test procedures (discrimination and threshold tasks), with 33% failing to complete the threshold test. Also, three odors (turpentine, anise, and cloves) were unfamiliar to many of the children and need to be replaced to provide a more appropriate set of odorants in the identification test. The main disadvantage of

the test is that it requires 30 minutes to complete, making it less suitable for use with patients experiencing chronic pain or nausea, or when large groups of children are screened for olfactory dysfunction in schools where limited time is allowed away from classroom activities.

Other olfactory tests described for use with children include the San Diego Odor Identification test (SDOIT),[30] Sniff Magnitude test (SMT),[31] Alcohol Sniff test (AST),[32] and Match-to-Sample Odor Identification test (MTST).[33] Except for MTST in a study of 825 healthy children, none has been used with significant numbers of children and the AST and SMT tests have been limited to one odorant at a single concentration. Accordingly, they cannot indicate, for example, whether a child who is hyposmic is also dysosmic. The main limitation of the SDOIT and the MTST is that the use of only eight and five odorants, respectively, provides a very narrow range of scores on which to classify a child as normosmic, hyposmic, or anosmic. No reports on the use of the MTST have appeared since 1995.

Retronasal Function

A simple but reliable test of retronasal function in children aged 7 years and above, termed the Candy Smell Test (CST), was reported recently.[29] The test was not suitable for the 4- to 6-year-olds who participated. In this test, subjects placed candy on their tongues and chewed until they had selected one of four possible odor choices, as in the "Sniffin' Sticks" test. A minor modification was that children were presented with pictures of the object odors in addition to the usual words. Reliability for children aged 4 to 15 years was $r = 0.71$, which compared favorably with that for adults of $r = 0.84$. Comparison with data from the "Sniffin' Sticks" test allowed classification of participants. Thus, using a threshold, discrimination, and identification test (TDI) value of 30.3 as the cut-off for normosmics gave a score of 16 out of 23 for the CST. A CST score of 16 correctly classified 83% subjects with TDI scores below 30.3, while a CST score of 17 correctly classified 88% of subjects with TDI scores > 30.3 (i.e., normosmics). However, as indicated by the authors, the test needs refining regarding choice of odorants, as adults had low identification scores (< 80%) for six odors, and children < 16 years old had low scores for eight odors. This test should not be used in children with fructosemia.

Finally, data from the CST and "Sniffin' Sticks" tests that included all age groups tested (other than 4- to 6-year-olds) showed a significant correlation of $r = 0.84$. Importantly, the CST could be used as a test of olfaction as it provided a similar classification of adults to the "Sniffin' Sticks" test.

Qualitative Assessment of Olfaction in Everyday Life

The Children's Olfactory Behaviors in Everyday Life questionnaire was developed to assess attention to, and reliance on, odors in real-life situations, and to evaluate individual variations.[34] It consists of 16 items prompting self-reports of active seeking of, awareness of, and affective reactivity to odors imagined in connection with food, people, and the environment (**Table 10.1**). The questionnaire has been used with 215 children aged 6 to 10 years. It revealed that girls were significantly more olfaction-oriented than boys in their everyday life. An increasing ability of children to describe the odor facets of their perceptual world was found between

Table 10.1 The Children's Olfactory Behavior in Everyday Life questionnaire, a qualitative tool used from 6 years of age. It consists of 16 items in a given order on food, social relations, and the general environment. For full details and the scoring method, see ref. 34

1. Odor in food dislikes	Are there some foods/drinks that you hate (yes/no)? Which ones (up to six)? For which reasons (for each cited food)?
2. Response to unknown food	Imagine your parents present you with a dish you do not know: will you do something before putting it in your mouth (yes/no)? What do you do? Will you smell it (yes/no)?
3. Senses in nature	When you walk in nature, what do you prefer (rank from 1 to 4: touching, smelling, watching, listening)?
4. Yesterday odors (memory)	Do you remember odors you smelled yesterday (food odors not acceptable)? Which ones?
5. Odors sought when sad	Are there odors you like smelling when you feel sad? Which ones?
6. Beloved odorous objects	Are there things you treasure just because they smell very good? Which ones?
7. Outside odors	Imagine there were no odors outside anymore: would you not care/would it bother you/would it suit you?
8. Smelling school tools	Do you happen to smell your school things (never/sometimes/often)? Which ones?
9. Odor in cars	In your parents' car, does it smell of something or nothing? Do you love/like/not care/not like this odor/feel ill?
10. Odor of bathroom objects	Please list objects of your bathroom (up to eight). Which ones smell of something?
11. Family odors	Do you find that your parents/siblings smell of something? Imagine they would not smell of anything anymore: would you not care/would it bother you/would it suit you—a little/a lot? Why?
12. People's natural odor	Do you find that people smell of something, even without perfume or deodorant (no/yes some people/yes everyone)?
13. Smelling clothes	Do you happen to smell your clothes (never/sometimes/often)? Why?
14. Smelling self-odor	Do you happen to smell parts of your body (never/sometimes/often)? Which parts? Why?
15. Tobacco smell	Imagine someone is smoking next to you. Do you love/like/not care/not like/hate this odor?
16. Guessing food odor	When you smell a food odor, do you try to guess for fun what it is (never/sometimes/often)?

6 and 10 years, partly due to their improving cognitive skills and olfactory experiences.

Nasal Trigeminal Function

Trigeminal sensitivity can be assessed using the lateralization task described in Chapter 12, where a child is requested to identify the side of the nose to which an odorous stimulus was presented. Only one detailed measure of nasal trigeminal function in children has been reported.[35] This involved 262 children and 86 adults, and indicated that the method can be used by 5-year-olds, with little change in performance from 7 years of age. Although the phenomenon of lateralization appears to be an excellent working tool for determining nasal trigeminal function, its reliability has yet to be demonstrated.

Gustatory Function

> Loss of one or more taste qualities is more common than not being able to perceive any taste. Complete loss of all qualities is rare and is due to the tongue, palate, and throat being innervated by several taste nerves.

Whole-mouth Test

The Sydney Children's Hospital Gustatory Test (SCHGT) is the only clinical taste test that has been specifically developed for use in children.[27,28,36] The test is a three-choice task that requires the identification of 25 samples of sweet (sucrose), sour (citric acid), salt (sodium chloride), and bitter (quinine hydrochloride) tastes and water. Each tastant is presented at five concentrations that range from weak but identifiable for a healthy 5-year-old, to very strong. Children are required to identify each sample using a set of three photographs labeled with appropriate words, by choosing the photo that best represents the taste (**Fig. 10.3**). Different sets are used with each sample, and each set contains a photograph of a glass of water. Water is always given as one of the choices to provide an appropriate choice if a child cannot perceive a taste. Thus, a child who chooses water consistently instead of a specific taste can be classified as hypogeusic. One who consistently chooses a taste other than the correct one is classified as dysgeusic. The stimuli

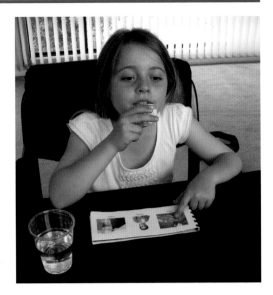

Fig. 10.3 Child sipping a tastant and pointing to the photograph that best represents the taste she has perceived.

are presented in a random order with an intertrial interval of 30 seconds, during which time children rinse their mouths with water. Mean identification scores for healthy children for each of the tastants and water have exceeded 90% in three clinical studies with children,[27,28,36] and comparison of the overall identification scores over two test days indicated a reliability of $r = 0.52$. However, classification of a child as having a taste disorder is not based on the overall identification score but on the identification of at least three of the five concentrations of a taste quality. Loss of one or more taste qualities appears to be much more common than not being able to perceive any taste. Indeed, complete loss of taste for all qualities is rare, and perception of at least some tastes is owing, in part, to the tongue, palate, and throat being innervated by several taste nerves. For example, damage to the chorda tympani in the middle ear by otitis media pathogens[37] is not accompanied by damage to the glossopharyngeal nerve, which is the other main nerve innervating the tongue. Prevalence of taste dysfunction appears to be high, reported at 12 and 7.9% for 8- to 12-year-old Australian Aboriginal and non-Aboriginal children, respectively.[36] Other tests have been used to assess taste function in child patients, but none have been developed specifically for use in children, or had their reliability established.

Regional Taste Function

Clinical measurement of disorders within taste-sensitive parts of the mouth, including the tongue and palate, has rarely been reported in children. The only report concerning regional measurements in children involved a taste identification task with 5- to 7-year-olds, where moderate strength aqueous solutions were delivered to four regions of the tongue.[38] The test was a modified version of the clinical test used with adults[39] and used the same tastants at the following concentrations: sweet, 1 M; sour, 0.0032 M; salty, 1 M; and bitter, 0.001 M. Modification of the test was necessary because the adult test requires participants to use a rating scale to estimate the strength of tastants, and children under ~8 years of age cannot do this without substantial training. Accordingly, a much easier identification task was adopted. The four regions examined were two regions on each side of the dorsal tongue, namely, the tip of the tongue and laterally just forward of the most anterior circumvallate papilla. Stimuli were delivered using cotton buds. To be consistent in the size of the area stimulated, the cotton bud was dipped in a tastant solution and then rolled ~1 cm toward the posterior tongue at the chosen region. To achieve this, children were asked to protrude their tongues as far as was comfortable until they had identified the tastant in a region. It was explained that withdrawal of the tongue would spread the solution over much of the tongue and the test would have to be repeated. Subjects indicated the identity of a tastant by pointing to one of three photographs. The sets of photographs were the same as those used in the whole-mouth test. The order of presenting the stimuli was randomized across subjects and across the four tongue regions, to result in 20 presentations during the test. To familiarize a child with the tastants and the general identification procedure, a child sampled each tastant from a small cup and identified it from sets of the photographs. There was an intertrial interval of 30 seconds, during which the child rinsed his or her mouth with water. The data, based on 212 children, indicate that 90% of 5-, 6-, and 7-year-olds can be expected to identify at least three of the five tastes at each of the four regions, which is similar to the results achieved by 52 adults.[38] More recently, this test was used with 218 9- to 12-year-old Australian Aboriginals to assess the effects of otitis media on regions of the tongue that coincided with the side(s) and ear

that had been shown to exhibit hearing loss (Armstrong and Laing, in preparation).

Electrogustometry

Electrogustometric measurement (see Chapter 14) of detection thresholds has been used to assess taste function in 160 children aged 4 to 18 years who had undergone otological surgery.[40] Taste dysfunction was found in patients who had experienced tympanoplasty (27%), mastoidectomy (30%), or cochlear implantation (26% unilateral; 5% bilateral). Interestingly, 9% of controls exhibited taste dysfunction, which is similar to the prevalence in children reported recently using the SCHGT.[36] A limitation of electrogustometry is that it does not indicate the nature of the taste loss. For example, it cannot indicate whether taste loss is confined to one or more qualities, or the extent of such a loss.

Summary

This chapter summarizes the functional development of the human chemical senses and describes methods for measuring function at different ages. Cognitive abilities limit the use of psychophysical tests until ~6 to 7 years of age, and only qualitative tests have been used in nonclinical assessments of olfactory function in newborns and infants. As yet, no test used with children has become a "gold standard" for assessing the chemical senses, although reliable olfactory and gustatory tests have been reported for older children. The most glaring shortcoming is the absence of objective clinical tests of smell and taste for newborns and children < 6 years of age.

References

1. Schaal B, Marlier L, Soussignan R. Olfactory function in the human fetus: evidence from selective neonatal responsiveness to the odor of amniotic fluid. Behav Neurosci 1998;112(6):1438–1449
2. Mennella JA, Jagnow CP, Beauchamp GK. Prenatal and postnatal flavor learning by human infants. Pediatrics 2001;107(6):E88
3. Schaal B, Marlier L, Soussignan R. Human foetuses learn odours from their pregnant mother's diet. Chem Senses 2000;25(6):729–737
4. Sarnat HB. Olfactory reflexes in the newborn infant. J Pediatr 1978;92(4):624–626
5. Bartocci M, Winberg J, Papendieck G, Mustica T, Serra G, Lagercrantz H. Cerebral hemodynamic response to unpleasant odors in the preterm

newborn measured by near-infrared spectroscopy. Pediatr Res 2001;50(3):324–330

6. Tatzer E, Schubert MT, Timischl W, Simbruner G. Discrimination of taste and preference for sweet in premature babies. Early Hum Dev 1985;12(1): 23–30

7. Steiner JE. Human facial expressions in response to taste and smell stimulations. Adv Child Dev Behav 1979;13:257–295

8. Desor JA, Maller O, Andrews K. Ingestive responses of human newborns to salty, sour, and bitter stimuli. J Comp Physiol Psychol 1975;89(8):966–970

9. Schaal B. Olfaction in infants and children: developmental and functional perspectives. Chem Senses 1988;13:145–190

10. Schmidt HJ, Beauchamp GK. Adult-like odor preferences and aversions in three-year-old children. Child Dev 1988;59(4):1136–1143

11. Dorries KM, Schmidt HJ, Beauchamp GK, Wysocki CJ. Changes in sensitivity to the odor of androstenone during adolescence. Dev Psychobiol 1989; 22(5):423–435

12. Laing DG, Clark PJ. Puberty and olfactory preferences of males. Physiol Behav 1983;30(4):591–597

13. Kimmel SA, Sigman-Grant M, Guinard JX. Sensory testing with young children. Food Technol 1994; 94:92–99

14. Macfarlane AJ. Olfaction in the development of social preferences in the human neonate. Ciba Found Symp 1975;33(33):103–117

15. Soussignan R, Schaal B, Marlier L, Jiang T. Facial and autonomic responses to biological and artificial olfactory stimuli in human neonates: re-examining early hedonic discrimination of odors. Physiol Behav 1997;62(4):745–758

16. Doucet S, Soussignan R, Sagot P, Schaal B. The secretion of areolar (Montgomery's) glands from lactating women elicits selective, unconditional responses in neonates. PLoS ONE 2009;4(10):e7579

17. Mennella JA, Beauchamp GK. Maternal diet alters the sensory qualities of human milk and the nursling's behavior. Pediatrics 1991;88(4):737–744

18. Soussignan R, Schaal B, Marlier L. Olfactory alliesthesia in human neonates: prandial state and stimulus familiarity modulate facial and autonomic responses to milk odors. Dev Psychobiol 1999;35(1):3–14

19. Delaunay-El Allam M, Soussignan R, Patris B, Marlier L, Schaal B. Long-lasting memory for an odor acquired at the mother's breast. Dev Sci 2010; 13(6):849–863

20. Datta T, Prasad SS, George S. Response to olfactory stimulation in normal newborn infants. Indian Pediatr 1982;19(7):591–595

21. Gauthaman G, Jayachandran L, Prabhakar K. Olfactory reflexes in newborn infants. Indian J Pediatr 1984;51(4):397–399

22. Shimada M, Takahashi S, Imura S, Baba K. Olfaction in neonates. Chem Senses 1987;12:518

23. Fusari C, Pardelli L. Electroencephalographic olfactometry in infants. [Article in Italian] Boll Mal Orecch Gola Naso 1962;80:719–734

24. Kendal-Reed M, Van Toller S. Brain electrical activity mapping: an exploratory study of infant response to odours. Chem Senses 1992;17:765–777

25. Yasumatsu K, Uchida S, Sugano H, Suzuki T. The effect of the odour of mother's milk and orange on the spectral power of EEG in infants. [Article in Japanese] J UOEH 1994;16(1):71–83

26. Armstrong JE, Laing DG, Wilkes FJ, Laing ON. Olfactory function in Australian Aboriginal children and chronic otitis media. Chem Senses 2008;33(6):503–507

27. Armstrong JE, Laing DG, Wilkes FJ, Kainer G. Smell and taste function in children with chronic kidney disease. Pediatr Nephrol 2010;25(8):1497–1504

28. Laing DG, Armstrong JE, Aitken M, et al. Chemosensory function and food preferences of children with cystic fibrosis. Pediatr Pulmonol 2010;45(8):807–815

29. Renner B, Mueller CA, Dreier J, Faulhaber S, Rascher W, Kobal G. The Candy Smell Test: a new test for retronasal olfactory performance. Laryngoscope 2009;119(3):487–495

30. Sandford AA, Davidson TM, Herrera N, et al. Olfactory dysfunction: a sequela of pediatric blunt head trauma. Int J Pediatr Otorhinolaryngol 2006;70(6):1015–1025

31. Frank RA, Dulay MF, Niergarth KA, Gesteland RC. A comparison of the Sniff Magnitude test and the University of Pennsylvania Smell Identification Test in children and nonnative English speakers. Physiol Behav 2004;81(3):475–480

32. Davidson TM, Freed C, Healy MP, Murphy C. Rapid clinical evaluation of anosmia in children: the Alcohol Sniff Test. Ann N Y Acad Sci 1998;855:787–792

33. Richman RA, Wallace K, Sheehe PR. Assessment of an abbreviated odorant identification task for children: a rapid screening device for schools and clinics. Acta Paediatr 1995;84(4):434–437

34. Ferdenzi C, Coureaud G, Camos V, Schaal B. Human awareness and uses of odor cues in everyday life: Results from a questionnaire study in children. Int J Behav Dev 2008;32:422–431

35. Hummel T, Roudnitzky N, Kempter W, Laing DG. Intranasal trigeminal function in children. Dev Med Child Neurol 2007;49(11):849–853

36. Laing DG, Wilkes FJ, Underwood N, Tran L. Taste disorders in Australian Aboriginal and non-Aboriginal children. Acta Paediatr 2011;100(9):1267–1271

37. Gedikli O, Doğru H, Aydin G, Tüz M, Uygur K, Sari A. Histopathological changes of chorda tympani in chronic otitis media. Laryngoscope 2001;111(4 Pt 1):724–727

38. Laing DG, Segovia C, Fark T, et al. Tests for screening olfactory and gustatory function in school-age children. Otolaryngol Head Neck Surg 2008; 139(1):74–82

39. Bartoshuk LM. Clinical evaluation of the sense of taste. Ear Nose Throat J 1989;68(4):331–337

40. Leung RM, Ramsden J, Gordon K, Allemang B, Harrison BJ, Papsin BC. Electrogustometric assessment of taste after otologic surgery in children. Laryngoscope 2009;119(10):2061–2065

11 Neurological Diseases and Olfactory Disorders

Antje Haehner, John E. Duda

Impairment of olfaction is a characteristic feature of many neurological diseases. This chapter summarizes the available information about olfactory function in neurodegenerative and other neurological conditions, and describes the advantageous use of olfactory testing in the diagnosis of several disorders, including Parkinson disease (PD) and Alzheimer dementia.

Olfactory Loss in Neurodegenerative Disorders

Neurodegenerative disorders are characterized by a progressive loss of structure or function of neurons. Impaired olfaction has been associated with a variety of age-related neurodegenerative conditions that impair cognitive and motor function, including PD,[1-5] Alzheimer disease (AD),[6] Huntington disease,[7] and motor neuron disease.[8] Smell loss may therefore be considered an important contribution to the diagnosis of these diseases, and physicians should be familiar with this attendant symptom.

Parkinsonian Syndromes

Prevalence of Olfactory Loss in Parkinson Disease

The association between olfactory dysfunction and PD was noted more than 30 years ago.[9] Virtually all studies performed since then have shown olfactory disturbances in patients with PD. The reported prevalence of olfactory dysfunction in PD, however, ranges from 45 and 49% in the pioneering studies of Ansari and Johnson[9] and Ward et al,[2] respectively, up to 74% in the work of Hawkes et al,[3] or as high as 90% in a study published by Doty et al.[1] In a recent multicenter study[10] using a comprehensive testing method in a large sample of patients with PD ($n = 400$) from three independent populations, the prevalence of olfactory dysfunction in people with PD was greater than previously reported. More than 96% of patients with PD were found to present with significant olfactory

dysfunction compared with young, normosmic patients. When using age-dependent normative criteria, 74.5% of this study population was diagnosed with olfactory loss (**Fig. 11.1**). Furthermore, of the patients with PD with smell loss, more than 80% were functionally anosmic or severely hyposmic regardless of the olfactory test being used for diagnosis. These data also confirmed numerous previous studies regarding a lack of correlation between olfactory loss and both duration of disease[1,3,11] and the clinical severity of PD, as measured by means of the Hoehn and Yahr scale and the Unified Parkinson Disease Rating Scale (compare with ref. 12)—although some studies found a correlation between the severity of PD and certain measures of olfactory function (namely latencies of olfactory event-related potentials[13] or results from an odor discrimination task).[14] However, this inability to demonstrate a relationship between disease duration and olfactory loss may be partially owing to a "basement effect" of olfactory dysfunction in patients with PD with moderate-to-severe disease, and if only patients with early PD are assessed it might be possible to demonstrate a worsening function with disease duration. With regard to olfactory function, no major differences were found among subtypes of PD (tremor-dominant PD, akinetic-rigid PD, or mixed-type PD). While this confirms previous observations in small sample sizes,[15,16] the present findings are in contrast to reports by Stern and colleagues,[11] who reported significantly better odor identification scores in patients with tremor-predominant PD ($n = 40$) than in patients with postural instability-gait disorder–predominant PD ($n = 23$). While differences among studies may be due to the type of olfactory test used, sample size, normative data, and age distribution (which varied among these investigations), available data allow the conclusion that olfactory dysfunction is a highly reliable symptom of the disease. This concurs with the results of a case–control study of 90 patients with PD and healthy controls by Bohnen et al,[17] who found that the accuracy of smell testing in PD diagnosis outweighs the accuracy of motor test batteries and nonmotor tests of depression, and anxiety.

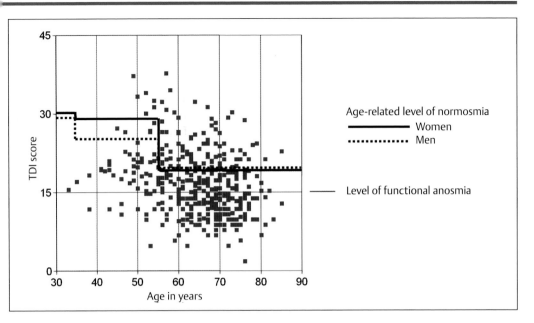

Fig. 11.1 Olfactory function of 400 patients with PD. Results are shown as a composite TDI score (sum of odor threshold, odor discrimination, and odor identification score) adjusted to age-related norms. (From Haehner et al.[10])

Olfactory Dysfunction in Early Parkison Disease Diagnosis

Patients with PD frequently report a reduction in their sense of smell that occurs a few years prior to the onset of motor symptoms. Support for the existence of a prodromal phase of PD, including a long premotor phase, comes from imaging, neuropathology, and various clinical or epidemiological surveys. The best evidence for a long premotor phase is derived from large prospective studies examining olfaction, constipation, rapid eye movement (REM) sleep behavior disorder, and depression.[18-20] Estimates for the duration of the prodrome range from 2 to 50 years depending on the symptom, duration of follow-up, accuracy of diagnosis, and individual variation.

However, patients' lack of awareness of smell deficits may account for the inconsistent results described in retrospective surveys. In two small studies,[21,22] upon questioning prior to olfactory testing, 24 and 39% of respondents indicated an awareness of decreased olfactory function which actually preceded their diagnosis of PD. Several studies could show evidence of olfactory dysfunction in untreated, newly diagnosed patients.[1] A plethora of evidence from recent studies supports the view that deficits in the sense of smell

may precede clinical motor symptoms by years. A study by Ponsen et al[23] of 361 asymptomatic relatives of patients with PD selected 40 relatives with the lowest olfactory performance. Within 2 years of follow-up, 10% of these first-degree relatives of patients with PD with significant olfactory loss developed clinical PD. In a follow-up study 5 years from baseline testing, five relatives had developed clinical PD as defined by the United Kingdom Parkinson's Disease Society Brain Bank Diagnostic Criteria for Parkinson's Disease. Initial clinical (motor) symptoms appeared 9 to 52 months (median 15 months) after baseline testing. Poorer performance on each of three olfactory processing tasks was associated with an increased risk of developing PD within 5 years.

In 2007, Haehner et al[24] published data on a clinical follow-up of 30 patients diagnosed with idiopathic olfactory loss. Four years from baseline, 7% (n = 2) of the individuals with idiopathic olfactory loss who were available for follow-up examination (n = 24) had newly developed clinical PD symptoms. Altogether, 13% (n = 4) of the patients presented with PD-relevant abnormalities of the motor system. The results indicated that unexplained olfactory loss may be associated with an increased risk of developing PD-relevant motor symptoms.

By contrast, authors of a twin study[25] concluded that smell identification ability may not be a sensitive indicator of future PD, even in a theoretically at-risk population. This was based on the fact that patients who subsequently developed PD had no evidence of significant smell loss when they were initially tested. However, as pointed out by the authors themselves, the reason for this negative finding might lie in the very long delay of 7 years between baseline assessment and follow-up visit. The initial test may have been too early for their subjects to have developed signs of smell dysfunction.

This is in accordance with the results of a large longitudinal study by Ross and colleagues.[26] They assessed olfactory function in 2,267 elderly men in the Honolulu Heart Program and found an association between smell loss and future development of PD. They came to the conclusion that impaired olfaction can predate PD by at least 4 years and may be a useful screening tool to detect those at high risk for development of PD in later life. However, this relationship appears to weaken beyond the 4-year period.

Along with quantitative smell loss, idiopathic phantosmia has also been proposed to herald PD. Several case reports show that some patients have experienced phantosmia very early in the course of the disease.[27,28] According to a recent study by Landis et al,[29] however, idiopathic phantosmia as an early sign of PD probably remains a rather exceptional presentation and the overwhelming majority of people with idiopathic phantosmia will not develop PD.

Recent data on olfactory loss as an early PD symptom are compatible with predictions made on the basis of neuropathological investigations. Braak et al[30] (**Fig. 11.2**) describe involvement of olfactory pathways and lower brainstem regions before nigrostriatal pathways are affected, which might cause early nonmotor symptoms. Documented pathological alterations in the olfactory bulb (OB) include neuronal loss and the accumulation of Lewy bodies and Lewy neurites within the intrabulbar portions of the anterior olfactory nucleus (**Fig. 11.3**). Other layers of the OB also exhibit accumulation of Lewy bodies and Lewy neurites to a lesser degree. Indeed, it has been suggested that the olfactory system is an ideal location to try to better understand the pathophysiology of Lewy neurodegeneration.[31] In another attempt

to understand the etiology of olfactory dysfunction in PD, Huisman et al[32] found an increase of periglomerular dopaminergic neurons in the OB in patients with PD (**Fig. 11.3**). They interpreted their finding within the context of a possible compensatory mechanism in response to the loss of dopaminergic neurons in the basal ganglia. This concurs with their observation that dopaminergic neurogenesis in the glomerular layer tripled after nigrostriatal lesioning and, consistent with this finding, the total number of tyrosine hydroxylase positive cells increased.[33] However, results of a follow-up study[34] indicated a gender-related change, namely that the number of dopaminergic cells in the OB of both male and female patients with PD equals that of healthy males of the same age group. The authors therefore concluded that the hyposmia in patients with PD cannot simply be ascribed to dopamine in the OB. In another attempt to explain the mechanism of olfactory dysfunction in PD, Sobel and colleagues demonstrated a deficit in the magnitude of sniffing in patients with PD and reported small improvements in odor identification performance with forced vigorous sniffing.[35]

Several prospective studies currently underway will help to determine if olfactory loss may become a useful biomarker of PD development within populations at risk for PD. For instance, the current Parkinson-associated risk syndrome study,[36] which is examining the use of olfactory dysfunction and dopaminergic functional imaging as predictors of risk in first-degree relatives of patients with PD, will advance our understanding of early PD presentation.

Olfactory Dysfunction in the Differential Diagnosis of Parkinsonian Syndromes

Numerous studies suggest that olfactory disturbances in PD may have diagnostic utility for the differentiation of PD from other movement disorders. Wenning et al[37] presented data suggesting that olfactory function is differentially impaired in distinct parkinsonian syndromes. They reported a preserved or mildly impaired olfactory function to be more likely in atypical parkinsonism such as multiple system atrophy (MSA), progressive supranuclear palsy (PSP), or corticobasal degeneration (CBD), whereas pronounced olfactory loss appeared to suggest PD. In a study on 50 patients with parkinsonian syndromes, Müller et al[21] also found evidence for olfactory loss in MSA, but little or no olfactory loss in (the few investigated) patients with PSP and CBD. With regard to the differentiation between MSA and PD, a combined odor thresholds, odor discrimination, and odor identification (TDI) score cut-off of 19.5 had a sensitivity of 78% and a specificity of 100%. When the TDI score cut-off was increased to 24.8, sensitivity in this sample was 100% while specificity fell to 63%. This moderate specificity seems to be the limiting parameter for diagnostic purposes. A recent American Academy of Neurology practice parameter on the diagnosis and prognosis of PD concluded that olfactory testing "should be considered" to differentiate PD from PSP and CBD but not from MSA.[38] Furthermore, Liberini et al[39] reported a significant olfactory impairment in Lewy body disease (LBD), which does not allow differentiation from PD. In a sample of 116 patients with mild LBD, mild AD, and mild cognitive impairment and controls, Williams et al[40] describe even more marked olfactory impairment in patients with mild dementia with Lewy bodies than in those with mild AD. This lends significance to the role of Lewy body pathology in olfactory dysfunction, which would be in line with the observation that patients with nondegenerative causes of parkinsonism, such as vascular parkinsonism,[41] present with preserved smell function. There is also evidence for less olfactory disturbance in familial parkinsonism. In PARK2 PD, the olfactory sense is relatively well preserved, whereas PARK1 PD subjects are hyposmic (**Table 11.1**; reviewed in ref. 4). Two studies examined olfactory dysfunction in autosomal recessive PARK6 PD and found impaired olfactory function in symptomatic homozygotes as well as asymptomatic heterozygotes.[42,43] Recent data[44] suggest that patients with PARK8 PD present with impaired olfactory identification while asymptomatic carriers show normal olfactory performance, although the studies have included relatively few subjects (reviewed in ref. 45).

Results from studies of secondary parkinsonism also indicate a relationship between parkinsonian symptoms and olfactory dysfunction. Krüger et al[46] found an association between medication-induced parkinsonism and olfactory dysfunction in patients with psychotic depression treated with dopamine D2 receptor–blocking neuroleptic drugs. Here, the severity of motor symptoms positively correlated with the degree of olfactory dysfunction, which might indicate patients with latent basal ganglia dysfunction of neurodegenerative etiology. Similar to the results seen in drug-induced parkinsonism, a recent study of patients with Wilson disease revealed that those with neurological symptoms showed significant olfactory dysfunction compared with those with hepatic symptoms.[47] Individuals who were more severely neurologically affected also presented with more pronounced olfactory deficits. Based on these observations, olfactory testing should not be considered to differentiate PD from these specific conditions by itself. However, olfactory testing can inform the differential diagnosis of parkinsonism in the same way that many other examinations, including deep tendon reflex, extraocular movement, and cerebellar function assessments, cannot distinguish parkinsonian disorders in isolation, but can be helpful in the context of a complete history and physical examination. In particular, olfactory dysfunction assessment can be important in cases where patients present with parkinsonian features but preserved olfaction, when it appears to be valid to question a diagnosis of PD.

Conclusions

Recent data suggest that inexpensive olfactory probes improve the diagnostic process in patients with PD. In contrast to imaging procedures, olfactory testing is quick and easy to perform. Validated tests can be used as reliable diagnostic tools even in nonspecialized centers. Deeb et al[22] found that a basic smell test is as sensitive as a dopamine transporter scan (DaTSCAN). According to this study, the sensitivities of the University of Pennsylvania Smell Identification Test and DaTSCAN are high at 86% and 92%, respectively. Although DaTSCAN is superior for "localization," a smell test is considerably cheaper, and neither is disease specific. In a recent biopsy study,[48] it was shown that subjects with PD did not present specific histomorphological abnormalities of the olfactory mucosa compared with younger hyposmic controls. Consequently, structured and validated tests of olfactory function should be considered in the diagnosis of early PD and in differentiating PD from other secondary and atypical forms of parkinsonism.

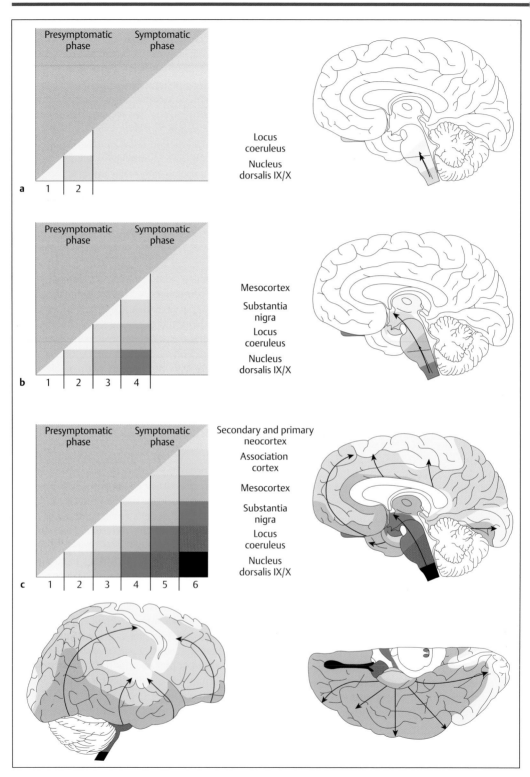

Fig. 11.2a–c

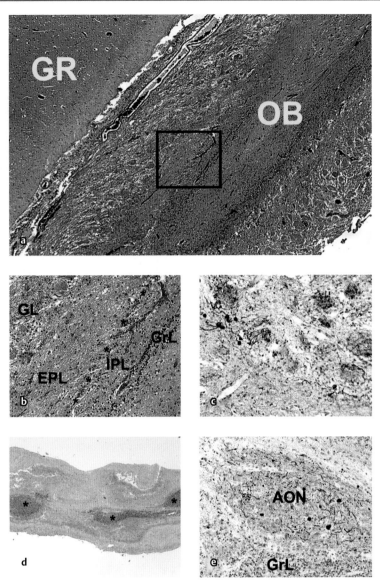

Fig. 11.3a–e Olfactory bulb anatomy and pathology.

a The human olfactory bulb (OB) rests on the inferior surface of the frontal lobes, adjacent to the gyrus rectus (GR).

b The olfactory bulb consists of six layers (enlarged view representative of boxed portion of **a**), which are not always well preserved in the elderly. These include the olfactory nerve layer, where axons of olfactory receptor neurons traverse the bulb en route to odorant-specific glomeruli in the glomerular level (GL), where they synapse with dendrites of mitral and tufted neurons; the external plexiform layer (EPL); the mitral cell layer (asterisks); the internal plexiform layer (IPL); and the granular layer (GrL).

c Tyrosine hydroxylase immunostaining of the olfactory bulb reveals dopaminergic periglomerular neurons (cell bodies surrounding glomeruli and processes within glomeruli) that modulate transmission between olfactory receptor neurons and mitral and tufted neurons.

d In Parkinson disease, Lewy bodies and Lewy neurites (identified by α-synuclein immunostaining) are concentrated within the anterior olfactory nucleus (asterisks).

e At higher power magnification, the anterior olfactory nucleus (AON) in Parkinson disease is characterized by neuronal loss and accumulation of Lewy bodies (round inclusions within cells) and Lewy neurites (curvilinear inclusions within cell processes).

◁ **Fig. 11.2a–c** Six stages of brain pathology in Parkinson disease. Whereas first lesions appear in stage one in the olfactory bulb, anterior olfactory nucleus, and dorsal nucleus of the vagus nerve (**a**), lesions in the substantia nigra are not present before stage three (**b**). At stage four the presymptomatic phase yields to the symptomatic phase of the disorder. Eventually, associate areas of the neocortex presymptomatic phase become involved (**c**). (From Hummel T, Welge-Lüssen A. Riech- und Schmeckstorungen: Physiologie, Pathophysiologie und Therapeutische Ansatze. Stuttgart: Thieme; 2009.)

Table 11.1 Relative degree of olfactory dysfunction in neurological disorders

Disease	Relative olfactory dysfunction
Parkinson disease, Alzheimer dementia, Lewy body dementia, PARK1 Parkinson disease, PARK8 Parkinson disease	Severe
Multiple system atrophy, Huntington disease, Multiple sclerosis, PARK6 Parkinson disease	Moderate
Motor neuron disease, Friedreich ataxia, spinocerebellar ataxia type 2, progressive supranuclear palsy	Mild
Corticobasal degeneration, spinocerebellar ataxia type 3, PARK2 Parkinson disease, essential tremor, restless legs syndrome	Slight to normal

> Impairment of olfaction is a characteristic and early feature of PD. Recent data indicate that >95% of patients with PD develop significant olfactory loss. Deficits in the sense of smell may precede clinical motor symptoms by years and can be used to assess the risk for developing PD in otherwise asymptomatic individuals. Numerous studies suggest that olfactory disturbances in PD may have diagnostic utility for the differentiation of PD from other movement disorders.

Alzheimer Dementia

Similar olfactory deficits have been shown in AD as in PD. In a meta-analysis,[6] defects in olfactory function in patients with AD and PD were relatively uniform, although there was a trend toward better performance in patients with AD on threshold tests than on odor identification tests. Therefore, no measure can distinguish the two conditions. As in PD, olfactory impairment is an early feature of AD. Postmortem studies have demonstrated that olfactory and transentorhinal regions are the earliest to be affected in the course of the disease.[49] Impaired olfaction in AD may be due to the deposition of amyloid plaques and neurofibrillary tangles in the OB and the entorhinal cortex, a structure which is also mainly involved in cognitive processing. In contrast to PD, a correlation between dementia severity and anosmia can be seen in AD. Furthermore, it has been found that the volume of the OB significantly correlates with global cognitive performance in AD patients. OB atrophy appears very early in the course of the disease,[50] which may contribute to early diagnosis. This is contrary to the findings of a small study of OBs in

patients with PD,[51] which demonstrated little or no difference in bulb size between patients with PD and healthy controls.

Patients with mild cognitive impairment who are considered at risk for developing AD demonstrate significant olfactory impairment compared with controls.[52] This association between smell loss and later conversion to dementia also applies to healthy elderly people. In a longitudinal study of 471 cognitively normal elderly people by Wilson et al,[53] olfactory dysfunction was a strong predictor of postmortem AD pathology.

In addition to LBD, which was discussed previously, other forms of dementia, including frontotemporal dementia, have been associated with varying degrees of olfactory dysfunction.[54]

> As in PD, olfactory impairment is an early feature of AD and can be observed in patients with mild cognitive impairment. Other forms of dementia have also been associated with olfactory dysfunction.

Huntington Disease

Patients with Huntington disease present with moderate hyposmia affecting olfactory detection threshold, odor discrimination, and odor identification.[7] Subsequent studies using discrimination and identification tests have not shown abnormalities in presymptomatic relatives of unknown genotype (e.g., ref. 55), implying that olfactory abnormalities do not occur before the onset of cognitive or motor symptoms. This is in contrast to the results of Larsson et al,[56] who reported impairment of odor discrimination, but not other olfactory assessments, in at-risk persons.

Other Neurodegenerative Diseases

Olfactory function has been assessed in patients with cerebellar ataxia due to Friedreich ataxia and spinocerebellar ataxias (SCA) type 2 and 3. Patients with SCA2 present with slight olfactory abnormality involving olfactory detection threshold, odor discrimination, and odor identification.[57] Patients with SCA3, however, have normal smell function,[58] which might have diagnostic utility, as they can present with parkinsonian features. In Friedreich ataxia, slight olfactory dysfunction was observed.[59]

Mild olfactory impairment has also been demonstrated in motor neuron disease. However, study results vary considerably,[60,61] possibly because of the fact that mainly patients with bulbar dysfunction are affected. Similar to olfactory dysfunction in PD, there is probably a small effect from reduced sniffing.[35]

> Olfactory dysfunction has also been demonstrated in some forms of inherited ataxia and motor neuron disease.

Therapy of Smell Loss

To date, no therapeutic interventions for olfactory loss in neurodegenerative disorders are available. Several studies indicate that pharmacological treatment of PD, including levodopa and the dopamine agonist apomorphine, fails to restore olfactory function in patients with PD.[1] However, recent experiments indicate that deep-brain stimulation of the subthalamic nucleus in patients with PD may improve odor discrimination, but not odor detection thresholds.[62] In addition, it is possible that improvement of olfactory function may be achieved with improvements in sniffing, which has been shown to be dysfunctional in patients with PD and motor neuron disease. Despite the lack of therapeutic options, patients should be advised of potential risks of smell loss, including inability to smell smoke, natural gas, and spoiled food products, and offered follow-up examinations of their sense of smell. In addition, regardless of the presence of neurological disease, other common causes of olfactory impairment should always be considered.

> Although there are no proven treatments for olfactory dysfunction in most neurological diseases, it is important to counsel patients with olfactory dysfunction about the possible risks that this impairment poses to their wellbeing.

Our experience suggests that it takes little time to follow up patients with a diagnosis of idiopathic smell loss neurologically as an essential part of their regularly scheduled visit to the smell and taste Clinic. In addition, elderly patients with idiopathic smell loss should be considered for referral to a neurologist as they have an increased risk of developing PD or AD. Such a comprehensive, multidisciplinary approach might enable the physician to detect slight motor or cognitive abnormalities in an at-risk population as early as possible. This may give rise to clinical studies that allow administration of neuroprotective substances in individuals with unexplained smell loss. Therapeutic studies with neuroprotective agents in patients with hyposmia and PD are currently underway and may help us to evolve preventive strategies for neurodegenerative diseases in the future.

> **Case Report: Unexplained Smell Loss**
>
> A 63-year-old man was referred because of severe olfactory dysfunction holding him back from his passion to cook. Four years earlier, he had noticed unpleasant olfactory sensations for the first time. During the following months, these sensations became less troublesome in terms of intensity and unpleasantness. Finally, the unpleasant sensations disappeared. He noticed, however, that his sense of smell deteriorated gradually.
>
> Psychiatric, neurological, and ear, nose, and throat examinations were normal. Detailed chemosensory testing revealed functional anosmia. In addition, the patient's history showed elements of phantosmia: they were not triggered by odors, they were difficult to explain verbally, and odors were unfamiliar to the patient. Taste was normal. The diagnosis of "idiopathic" olfactory loss was based on (1) negative magnetic resonance imaging and computed tomography;
>
> continued ▷

◁ continued

(2) no history of an association between olfactory loss and head trauma or infections of the upper respiratory tract; (3) gradual onset of olfactory loss over months or years; (4) absence of signs of sinonasal disease on detailed nasal endoscopy; (5) lack of response to short-term systemic treatment with corticosteroids; (6) no complaint of Parkinson-like motor symptoms or history of neurological disorders; and (7) no history of exposure to toxins or drugs potentially leading to olfactory disturbances.

At a follow-up visit to the clinic 12 months later, the patient reported left shoulder pain and subtle slowness of movement. His sense of smell had not improved. Neurological examination revealed reduced left-sided arm-swing and slight bradykinesia of the left hand that improved markedly following a positive test with levodopa 200 mg. Consequently, the patient was suspected of suffering from Parkinson disease. The diagnosis was confirmed by 18-fluoro-dihydroxyphenylalanine positron emission tomography, which showed decreased levels of the neurotransmitter dopamine in the basal ganglia.

Conclusion

We report a case of idiopathic phantosmia and anosmia with eventual manifestation of Parkinson disease. This case illustrates the significance of neurological examination in patients with idiopathic olfactory loss. Unexplained smell loss should be considered a first sign of neurodegenerative disorders.

Non-neurodegenerative Disorders

Multiple Sclerosis

The data on the prevalence of olfactory impairment in multiple sclerosis (MS) vary between 15 and 45%, although smell changes are rarely reported by patients with MS. Correlations have been demonstrated between plaque activity within olfactory-related central brain regions (e.g., the inferior frontal and temporal lobes) and the olfactory deficit (**Fig. 11.4**).[63] Recent studies report

that the frequency of olfactory impairment is higher in patients with secondary progressive MS than in those with relapsing–remitting or primary progressive courses. The observed association between decreased odor identification ability and symptoms of anxiety and depression in patients with MS suggests that mood and anxiety disorders should be considered in assessing olfaction in patients with MS.[64] There are a few anecdotal case reports on olfactory impairment as an early feature of MS even before optical neuritis occurs.

In patients with MS, smell loss has been correlated with the lesion load in brain regions involved in olfaction.

Epilepsy

It is generally accepted that temporal lobe epilepsy (TLE) may cause a brief olfactory aura prior to seizures. Olfactory assessment revealed that patients with TLE do not show abnormalities of odor thresholds compared with healthy controls.[65] They do, however, show impairment of higher level olfactory functions such as odor identification and discrimination.[65,66] Furthermore, latencies of chemosensory evoked potentials in these patients are prolonged.[67]

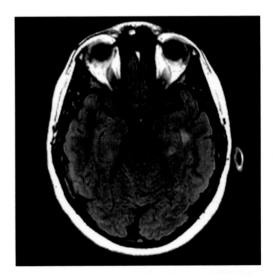

Fig. 11.4 Fluid-attenuated inversion–recovery sequence in a 29-year-old patient with temporal multiple sclerosis lesions and concomitant hyposmia. (Figure courtesy of Dr. Hagen Kitzler.)

Migraine

Similar to an epileptic aura, migraine aura may present with olfactory hallucinations, but these are much less common than visual auras. Migraine patients often report intolerance to odors in terms of hypersensitivity.[68] This applies during migraine attacks as well as in the time in between attacks. Consequently, odors may trigger attacks.[69] Some patients experience osmophobia during attacks, which might be important in distinguishing migraine from tension headache.

Meningioma

Meningiomas can present with olfactory disturbances. Unilateral or bilateral olfactory dysfunction is thought to be a very early symptom of olfactory groove meningioma. According to a study by Welge-Luessen et al,[70] however, olfactory testing seems to be of little help in detecting olfactory meningioma, as few patients complain of olfactory dysfunction. The likelihood of normal postoperative olfactory function contralateral to the tumor was high when the tumor was less than 3 cm in diameter and preoperative normosmia had been established. Further, preservation of olfactory function ipsilateral to the tumor seems to be extremely difficult, irrespective of tumor size or surgical approach.

Ischemic Lesions

Olfactory dysfunctions have been infrequently reported in patients following stroke.[71] Systematic studies of patients with cerebral ischemia have not been performed to date. Mainland et al[72] examined olfactory function in patients with unilateral cerebellar lesions due to ischemia or tumors. Testing revealed that patients had a contralesional impairment in olfactory function. Findings of this study strongly implicate an olfactocerebellar pathway in odor identification and detection that functionally connects each nostril primarily to the contralateral cerebellum.

Psychiatric Diseases

Compared with healthy controls, the prevalence of olfactory dysfunction is higher in patients with accompanying schizophrenia or acute depression.

Patients with acute major depressive disorder show significantly lower olfactory sensitivity,[73] but there is no difference in olfactory performance after successful therapy with antidepressants. Patients with acute major depressive disorder also present with smaller OB volumes than healthy controls, and a significant negative correlation between OB volume and depression score.[74] In schizophrenia, impairment of olfactory sensitivity, identification, and discrimination abilities were observed in patients and first-degree relatives,[74] suggesting a genetic vulnerability for chemosensory deficits.

> In addition to neurological diseases, several psychiatric conditions have been associated with olfactory dysfunction, including schizophrenia and acute depression.

References

1. Doty RL, Deems DA, Stellar S. Olfactory dysfunction in parkinsonism: a general deficit unrelated to neurologic signs, disease stage, or disease duration. Neurology 1988;38(8):1237–1244
2. Ward CD, Hess WA, Calne DB. Olfactory impairment in Parkinson's disease. Neurology 1983; 33(7):943–946
3. Hawkes CH, Shephard BC, Daniel SE. Olfactory dysfunction in Parkinson's disease. J Neurol Neurosurg Psychiatry 1997;62(5):436–446
4. Kranick SM, Duda JE. Olfactory dysfunction in Parkinson's disease. Neurosignals 2008;16(1):35–40
5. Morley JF, Duda JE. Olfaction as a biomarker in Parkinson's disease. Biomark Med 2010;4(5):661–670
6. Mesholam RI, Moberg PJ, Mahr RN, Doty RL. Olfaction in neurodegenerative disease: a meta-analysis of olfactory functioning in Alzheimer's and Parkinson's diseases. Arch Neurol 1998;55(1):84–90
7. Nordin S, Paulsen JS, Murphy C. Sensory- and memory-mediated olfactory dysfunction in Huntington's disease. J Int Neuropsychol Soc 1995; 1(3):281–290
8. Hawkes CH, Shephard BC, Geddes JF, Body GD, Martin JE. Olfactory disorder in motor neuron disease. Exp Neurol 1998;150(2):248–253
9. Ansari KA, Johnson A. Olfactory function in patients with Parkinson's disease. J Chronic Dis 1975;28(9):493–497
10. Haehner A, Boesveldt S, Berendse HW, et al. Prevalence of smell loss in Parkinson's disease—a multicenter study. Parkinsonism Relat Disord 2009; 15(7):490–494
11. Stern MB, Doty RL, Dotti M, et al. Olfactory function in Parkinson's disease subtypes. Neurology 1994;44(2):266–268

12. Ramaker C, Marinus J, Stiggelbout AM, Van Hilten BJ. Systematic evaluation of rating scales for impairment and disability in Parkinson's disease. Mov Disord 2002;17(5):867–876

13. Hummel T. Olfactory evoked potentials as a tool to measure progression of Parkinson's disease. In: Chase T, Bedard P, eds. Focus on Medicine Vol. 14—New Developments in the Drug Therapy of Parkinson's Disease. Oxford, UK: Blackwell Science; 1999:47–53.

14. Tissingh G, Berendse HW, Bergmans P, et al. Loss of olfaction in de novo and treated Parkinson's disease: possible implications for early diagnosis. Mov Disord 2001;16(1):41–46

15. Müller A, Müngersdorf M, Reichmann H, Strehle G, Hummel T. Olfactory function in Parkinsonian syndromes. J Clin Neurosci 2002;9(5):521–524

16. Ondo WG, Lai D. Olfaction testing in patients with tremor-dominant Parkinson's disease: is this a distinct condition? Mov Disord 2005;20(4):471–475

17. Bohnen NI, Studenski SA, Constantine GM, Moore RY. Diagnostic performance of clinical motor and non-motor tests of Parkinson disease: a matched case-control study. Eur J Neurol 2008;15(7):685–691

18. Hawkes CH, Del Tredici K, Braak H. A timeline for Parkinson's disease. Parkinsonism Relat Disord 2010;16(2):79–84

19. Leentjens AF, Van den Akker M, Metsemakers JF, Lousberg R, Verhey FR. Higher incidence of depression preceding the onset of Parkinson's disease: a register study. Mov Disord 2003;18(4):414–418

20. Postuma RB, Gagnon JF, Vendette M, Fantini ML, Massicotte-Marquez J, Montplaisir J. Quantifying the risk of neurodegenerative disease in idiopathic REM sleep behavior disorder. Neurology 2009;72(15):1296–1300

21. Müller A, Reichmann H, Livermore A, Hummel T. Olfactory function in idiopathic Parkinson's disease (IPD): results from cross-sectional studies in IPD patients and long-term follow-up of de-novo IPD patients. J Neural Transm 2002;109(5–6):805–811

22. Deeb J, Shah M, Muhammed N, et al. A basic smell test is as sensitive as a dopamine transporter scan: comparison of olfaction, taste and DaTSCAN in the diagnosis of Parkinson's disease. QJM 2010;103(12):941–952

23. Ponsen MM, Stoffers D, Booij J, van Eck-Smit BL, Wolters ECh, Berendse HW. Idiopathic hyposmia as a preclinical sign of Parkinson's disease. Ann Neurol 2004;56(2):173–181

24. Haehner A, Hummel T, Hummel C, Sommer U, Junghanns S, Reichmann H. Olfactory loss may be a first sign of idiopathic Parkinson's disease. Mov Disord 2007;22(6):839–842

25. Marras C, Goldman S, Smith A, et al. Smell identification ability in twin pairs discordant for Parkinson's disease. Mov Disord 2005;20(6):687–693

26. Ross GW, Petrovitch H, Abbott RD, et al. Association of olfactory dysfunction with risk for future Parkinson's disease. Ann Neurol 2008;63(2):167–173

27. Landis BN, Burkhard PR. Phantosmias and Parkinson disease. Arch Neurol 2008;65(9):1237–1239

28. Hirsch AR. Parkinsonism: the hyposmia and phantosmia connection. Arch Neurol 2009;66(4):538–539, author reply 539

29. Landis BN, Reden J, Haehner A. Idiopathic phantosmia: outcome and clinical significance. ORL J Otorhinolaryngol Relat Spec 2010;72(5):252–255

30. Braak H, Del Tredici K, Rüb U, de Vos RA, Jansen Steur EN, Braak E. Staging of brain pathology related to sporadic Parkinson's disease. Neurobiol Aging 2003;24(2):197–211

31. Duda JE. Olfactory system pathology as a model of Lewy neurodegenerative disease. J Neurol Sci 2010;289(1–2):49–54

32. Huisman E, Uylings HB, Hoogland PV. A 100% increase of dopaminergic cells in the olfactory bulb may explain hyposmia in Parkinson's disease. Mov Disord 2004;19(6):687–692

33. Winner B, Geyer M, Couillard-Despres S, et al. Striatal deafferentation increases dopaminergic neurogenesis in the adult olfactory bulb. Exp Neurol 2006;197(1):113–121

34. Huisman E, Uylings HB, Hoogland PV. Gender-related changes in increase of dopaminergic neurons in the olfactory bulb of Parkinson's disease patients. Mov Disord 2008;23(10):1407–1413

35. Sobel N, Thomason ME, Stappen I, et al. An impairment in sniffing contributes to the olfactory impairment in Parkinson's disease. Proc Natl Acad Sci U S A 2001;98(7):4154–4159

36. Stern MB, Siderowf A. Parkinson's at risk syndrome: can Parkinson's disease be predicted? Mov Disord 2010;25(Suppl 1):S89–S93

37. Wenning GK, Shephard B, Hawkes C, Petruckevitch A, Lees A, Quinn N. Olfactory function in atypical parkinsonian syndromes. Acta Neurol Scand 1995;91(4):247–250

38. McKinnon JH, Demaerschalk BM, Caviness JN, Wellik KE, Adler CH, Wingerchuk DM. Sniffing out Parkinson disease: can olfactory testing differentiate parkinsonian disorders? Neurologist 2007;13(6):382–385

39. Liberini P, Parola S, Spano PF, Antonini L. Olfactory dysfunction in dementia associated with Lewy bodies. Parkinsonism Relat Disord 1999;5(Suppl 1):30

40. Williams SS, Williams J, Combrinck M, Christie S, Smith AD, McShane R. Olfactory impairment is more marked in patients with mild dementia with Lewy bodies than those with mild Alzheimer disease. J Neurol Neurosurg Psychiatry 2009;80(6):667–670

41. Katzenschlager R, Lees AJ. Olfaction and Parkinson's syndromes: its role in differential diagnosis. Curr Opin Neurol 2004;17(4):417–423

42. Ferraris A, Ialongo T, Passali GC, et al. Olfactory dysfunction in Parkinsonism caused by PINK1 mutations. Mov Disord 2009;24(16):2350–2357

43. Kertelge L, Brüggemann N, Schmidt A, et al. Impaired sense of smell and color discrimination in monogenic and idiopathic Parkinson's disease. Mov Disord 2010;25(15):2665–2669

44. Silveira-Moriyama L, Guedes LC, Kingsbury A, et al. Hyposmia in G2019S LRRK2-related parkinsonism: clinical and pathologic data. Neurology 2008;71(13):1021–1026

45. Silveira-Moriyama L, Munhoz RP, de J Carvalho M, et al. Olfactory heterogeneity in LRRK2 related Parkinsonism. Mov Disord 2010;25(16):2879–2883

46. Krüger S, Haehner A, Thiem C, Hummel T. Neuroleptic-induced parkinsonism is associated with olfactory dysfunction. J Neurol 2008;255(10): 1574–1579

47. Mueller A, Reuner U, Landis B, Kitzler H, Reichmann H, Hummel T. Extrapyramidal symptoms in Wilson's disease are associated with olfactory dysfunction. Mov Disord 2006;21(9):1311–1316

48. Witt M, Bormann K, Gudziol V, et al. Biopsies of olfactory epithelium in patients with Parkinson's disease. Mov Disord 2009;24(6):906–914

49. Braak H, Braak E. Neuropathological stageing of Alzheimer-related changes. Acta Neuropathol 1991;82(4):239–259

50. Thomann PA, Dos Santos V, Toro P, Schönknecht P, Essig M, Schröder J. Reduced olfactory bulb and tract volume in early Alzheimer's disease—a MRI study. Neurobiol Aging 2009;30(5):838–841

51. Mueller A, Abolmaali ND, Hakimi AR, et al. Olfactory bulb volumes in patients with idiopathic Parkinson's disease—a pilot study. J Neural Transm 2005;112(10):1363–1370

52. Eibenstein A, Fioretti AB, Simaskou MN, et al. Olfactory screening test in mild cognitive impairment. Neurol Sci 2005;26(3):156–160

53. Wilson RS, Arnold SE, Schneider JA, Boyle PA, Buchman AS, Bennett DA. Olfactory impairment in presymptomatic Alzheimer's disease. Ann N Y Acad Sci 2009;1170:730–735

54. Luzzi S, Snowden JS, Neary D, Coccia M, Provinciali L, Lambon Ralph MA. Distinct patterns of olfactory impairment in Alzheimer's disease, semantic dementia, frontotemporal dementia, and corticobasal degeneration. Neuropsychologia 2007; 45(8):1823–1831

55. Moberg PJ, Doty RL. Olfactory function in Huntington's disease patients and at-risk offspring. Int J Neurosci 1997;89(1–2):133–139

56. Larsson M, Lundin A, Robins Wahlin TB. Olfactory functions in asymptomatic carriers of the Huntington disease mutation. J Clin Exp Neuropsychol 2006;28(8):1373–1380

57. Velázquez-Pérez L, Fernandez-Ruiz J, Díaz R, et al. Spinocerebellar ataxia type 2 olfactory impairment shows a pattern similar to other major neurodegenerative diseases. J Neurol 2006;253(9):1165–1169

58. Fernandez-Ruiz J, Díaz R, Hall-Haro C, et al. Olfactory dysfunction in hereditary ataxia and basal ganglia disorders. Neuroreport 2003;14(10):1339–1341

59. Connelly T, Farmer JM, Lynch DR, Doty RL. Olfactory dysfunction in degenerative ataxias. J Neurol Neurosurg Psychiatry 2003;74(10):1435–1437

60. Elian M. Olfactory impairment in motor neuron disease: a pilot study. J Neurol Neurosurg Psychiatry 1991;54(10):927–928

61. Sajjadian A, Doty RL, Gutnick D, Chirurgi RJ, Sivak M, Perl D. Olfactory dysfunction in amyotrophic lateral sclerosis. Neurodegeneration 1994;3:153–157

62. Hummel T, Jahnke U, Sommer U, Reichmann H, Müller A. Olfactory function in patients with idiopathic Parkinson's disease: effects of deep brain stimulation in the subthalamic nucleus. J Neural Transm 2005;112(5):669–676

63. Doty RL, Li C, Mannon LJ, Yousem DM. Olfactory dysfunction in multiple sclerosis. Relation to plaque load in inferior frontal and temporal lobes. Ann N Y Acad Sci 1998;855:781–786

64. Zivadinov R, Zorzon M, Monti Bragadin L, Pagliaro G, Cazzato G. Olfactory loss in multiple sclerosis. J Neurol Sci 1999;168(2):127–130

65. Kohler CG, Moberg PJ, Gur RE, O'Connor MJ, Sperling MR, Doty RL. Olfactory dysfunction in schizophrenia and temporal lobe epilepsy. Neuropsychiatry Neuropsychol Behav Neurol 2001;14(2):83–88

66. Eskenazi B, Cain WS, Novelly RA, Mattson R. Odor perception in temporal lobe epilepsy patients with and without temporal lobectomy. Neuropsychol 1986;24(4):553–562

67. Hummel T, Pauli E, Schüler P, Kettenmann B, Stefan H, Kobal G. Chemosensory event-related potentials in patients with temporal lobe epilepsy. Epilepsia 1995;36(1):79–85

68. Sjöstrand C, Savic I, Laudon-Meyer E, Hillert L, Lodin K, Waldenlind E. Migraine and olfactory stimuli. Curr Pain Headache Rep 2010;14(3):244–251

69. Demarquay G, Royet JP, Giraud P, Chazot G, Valade D, Ryvlin P. Rating of olfactory judgements in migraine patients. Cephalalgia 2006;26(9):1123–1130

70. Welge-Luessen A, Temmel A, Quint C, Moll B, Wolf S, Hummel T. Olfactory function in patients with olfactory groove meningioma. J Neurol Neurosurg Psychiatry 2001;70(2):218–221

71. Green TL, McGregor LD, King KM. Smell and taste dysfunction following minor stroke: a case report. Can J Neurosci Nurs 2008;30(2):10–13

72. Mainland JD, Johnson BN, Khan R, Ivry RB, Sobel N. Olfactory impairments in patients with unilateral cerebellar lesions are selective to inputs from the contralesional nostril. J Neurosci 2005; 25(27):6362–6371

73. Negoias S, Croy I, Gerber J, et al. Reduced olfactory bulb volume and olfactory sensitivity in patients with acute major depression. Neuroscience 2010; 169(1):415–421

74. Moberg PJ, Turetsky BI. Scent of a disorder: olfactory functioning in schizophrenia. Curr Psychiatry Rep 2003;5(4):311–319

12 Clinical Disorders of the Trigeminal System

Johannes Frasnelli, Thomas Hummel, Dennis Shusterman

Introduction

As the respiratory system's sentinel organ, the nose plays a complex role. Similar to the mouth—in which flavor is a blend of taste, olfaction, and piquancy—the nose integrates olfactory and "trigeminal" (irritant) sensations into seamless percepts. Thus it is not unusual to hear a statement such as, "I smelled a pungent odor," even though the observer is combining olfactory (cranial nerve I) and trigeminal (cranial nerve V) sensations in the process (**Fig. 12.1**). Evaluating olfactory and trigeminal function separately in clinical and research settings is challenging. Appreciating the ramifications of trigeminal function—in terms of not only primary sensation, but also mucous membrane and airway reflexes—is equally challenging.

The objective of this chapter is to provide the reader with an appreciation of nasal trigeminal anatomy, physiology, and pathophysiology, including responses to infection, allergy, airborne chemical irritants, and idiopathic inflammation. To this end, the chapter is organized under the following headings: Functional Neuroanatomy; Responsiveness to Physical and Chemical Stimuli; and Clinical Disorders. Where appropriate, clinical vignettes and algorithms have been included to provide a realistic context for the material discussed.

Functional Neuroanatomy of the Trigeminal System

Peripheral and Central Anatomy

> The trigeminal nerve is the sensory nerve that innervates the skin and the mucosa of the face.

The trigeminal nerve (cranial nerve V), with its three major branches: ophthalmic nerve (V1), maxillary nerve (V2), and mandibular nerve (V3), is the largest cranial nerve, and is primarily a sensory nerve (with some motor functions). V1 and V2 together innervate the nasal mucosa; V2 and V3 innervate the oral mucosa. From here, they convey both somatosensory and chemosensory information. The three branches converge on the trigeminal ganglion (Gasserian ganglion), where the cell bodies of the incoming sensory fibers are located. This ganglion is analogous to the dorsal root ganglia of the spinal cord.

From the trigeminal ganglion, neurons project to the trigeminal nucleus (extending from the caudal medulla to the rostral pons) and, after synapsing there, project to lateral (e.g., ventrobasal) and medial (e.g., centromedial and parafascicular) thalamic nuclei. From here, neurons proj-

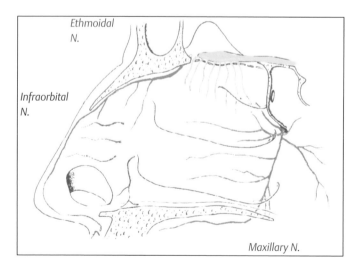

Ethmoidal N.

Infraorbital N.

Maxillary N.

Fig. 12.1 Innervation of the nasal cavity. The olfactory nerve is unique within the central nervous system in that its olfactory receptor neurons, which are in contact with the external environment, undergo continuous regeneration. The ethmoid and infraorbital nerves arise from the ophthalmic (first) division of the trigeminal nerve; the maxillary nerve constitutes the second division. Olfactory nerves and olfactory bulb in yellow (From Hummel T. Olfactory evoked potentials as a tool to measure progression of Parkinson's disease. In: Chase T, Bedard P, eds. Focus on Medicine Vol. 14—New Developments in the Drug Therapy Of Parkinson's Disease. Oxford: Blackwell Science; 1999: 47–53, with permission.)

ect to the somatosensory cortex. In humans, the V1 regions are represented in the inferior portion of the postcentral gyrus, and V3 regions in more superior regions in the central sulcus. In addition to these somatosensory brain regions, chemosensory trigeminal stimuli activate brain regions that are commonly considered olfactory and gustatory regions, such as the insula, the orbitofrontal cortex, and the piriform cortex.[1]

Somatic and Autonomic Functions

> The intranasal trigeminal system acts as a sentinel of the airways by monitoring the nasal mucosal environment, and is involved in detecting and clearing inhaled harmful substances.

The intranasal trigeminal system has several functions, which may be subdivided into four categories.[2] (1) Neurons of the intranasal trigeminal systems release *immediate protective mucosal responses* by axon response mechanisms.[3] (2) The intranasal trigeminal system provides the afferent connections of *brainstem reflex* circuits such as coughing, sneezing, gagging, and vomiting. These reflexes also include parasympathetically mediated secretions, which are locally active, and systemically acting sympathetic vasoconstrictor reflexes.[3] (3) The intranasal trigeminal system modulates *breathing parameters*.[4] (4) The intranasal trigeminal system, together with the olfactory system, *monitors inhaled air* for quality and composition.[5]

Trigeminal Role in Local and Remote Reflexes

> The trigeminal system is involved in local and remote reflexes.

The myelinated (Aδ) and unmyelinated fibers of the mucous membranes are responsive to a variety of physical and chemical stimuli.[6] Stimulation of these nerves (by heat, cold, touch, and chemical irritation) can trigger a variety of local and remote reflexes. Within the nasal mucosa, release of neuropeptides (e.g., substance P) from unmyelinated fibers (the axon reflex) can produce tissue swelling,

produce glandular secretion, and facilitate mast cell degranulation.[7] Central (autonomic) reflexes also participate in the secretory response in the upper airway.[8] Tissue swelling decreases luminal size, thereby increasing nasal airway resistance and the work of nasal breathing. Mucosal swelling also results in decreased patency of upper airway ostia (i.e., the Eustachian tubes and the osteomeatal complex of the paranasal sinuses), and may play a part in the pathogenesis of both otitis media and sinusitis.[9]

In terms of nasal secretory reflexes, so-called gustatory rhinitis—watery rhinorrhea produced by ingestion of hot or spicy foods, which is very common in the population[10]—involves trigeminal nerve afferents and facial nerve (cranial nerve VII) parasympathetic efferents. Depending upon the individual, the strength of the stimulus, and the degree of irritation, this response may also include lacrimation. Gustatory rhinitis can be blocked by local application of anticholinergic agents (e.g., atropine or ipratropium bromide).[11]

Both reflex nasal airflow obstruction and rhinorrhea have been postulated to protect against injurious inhalants. In addition to these purely upper airway reflexes, a variety of nasal reflexes is initiated in the nose but effected at remote sites (**Fig. 12.2**). Coughing and sneezing are the two best-known protective reflexes triggered by airway irritation. Both involve the musculature of the diaphragm and thoracic cage. These reflexes act to expel noxious substances forcefully, thus protecting the airway. Less well-known autonomic reflexes originating in the upper airway can be parasympathetic (cardiac slowing, bronchoconstriction) or sympathetic (epinephrine release from the adrenal medulla, peripheral vasoconstriction).[12]

Despite their protective function, when dysregulated, airway reflexes can become pathological. Chronic cough, for example, can arise from a variety of causes, including pharmacological (e.g., ACE [angiotensin-converting enzyme] inhibitors), inflammatory (e.g., asthma), irritant (postnasal drip; gastroesophageal reflux disease [GERD]; cigarette smoke), infectious, intrinsic lung disease, and behavioral factors.[13] An exaggerated cough reflex—defined functionally as a heightened response to aerosolized capsaicin—has been termed "sensory hyper-reactivity".[14] This diagnosis may characterize a subset of patients who self-identify as "chemically sensitive" and with impaired ability to cope with a variety of environmental exposures.[15]

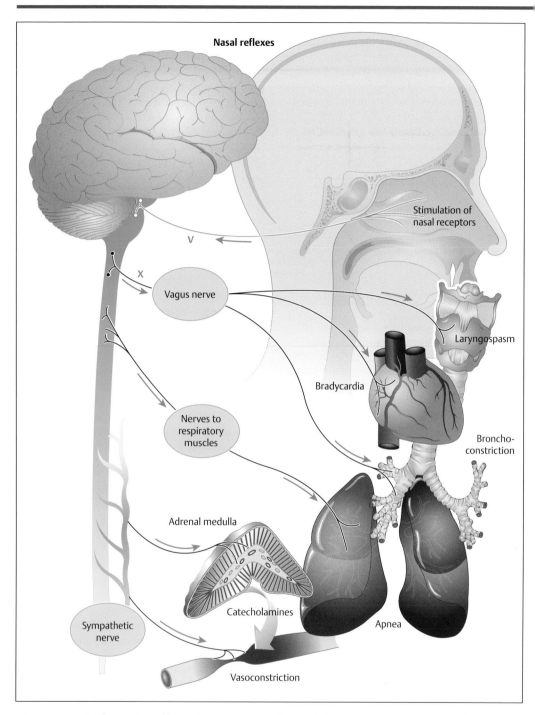

Fig. 12.2 Remote reflexes triggered by nasal trigeminal stimulation. Trigeminovagal reflexes include laryngeal adduction and nasobronchial and reflex bradycardia. (Reproduced with kind permission from Widdicombe JG. Nasal and pharyngeal reflexes: protective and respiratory functions. In: Mathew OP, Sant' Ambrogio G, eds. Respiratory Function of the Upper Airway. New York: Marcel Dekker; 1998:235.)

Responsiveness to Physical and Chemical Stimuli

Receptive Structures

> The trigeminal system is stimulated via the activation of polymodal nociceptors on free nerve endings and solitary chemoreceptor cells.

Polymodal nociceptors respond to thermal and chemical stimuli. Their receptive structures are located on free trigeminal nerve endings throughout the oral and nasal mucosa. Compared with the olfactory nerve, receptor diversity within the trigeminal system is relatively modest, although their activation leads to diverse perceptions such as cooling, burning, stinging, or tingling. With few exceptions (e.g., vanillin and hydrogen sulfide), most volatile substances activate the trigeminal system, especially at higher concentrations.[5] If volatile substances stimulate both the olfactory and the trigeminal system, they are called mixed olfactory–trigeminal stimuli (e.g., benzaldehyde, menthol). At a receptor level, chemical and thermal stimuli activate specific receptors of the trigeminal nerve, most of which are ion channels belonging to the subfamily of transient receptor potential (TRP) receptors. They include TRPV1 (excited by capsaicin,[16] eugenol,[17] acids,[18] and heat[16]), TRPM8 (excited by menthol, eucalyptol, and cool temperatures[19]), and TRPA1 (excited by mustard oil, cold temperatures, and a variety of irritant gases[20]). There is also evidence for non-TRP trigeminal receptors activated by nicotine[21] and acids.[22]

In addition to these receptors on free trigeminal nerve endings, *solitary chemoreceptor cells* have been described in the nasal cavity, although not yet in humans. These cells reach the surface of the nasal epithelium and form synaptic contacts with trigeminal afferent nerve fibers. They are activated by bitter substances via specific receptors. These cells may add to the repertoire of compounds that can activate the intranasal trigeminal system.[23]

The low-threshold *trigeminal mechanoreceptors* responsible for the perception of mechanical stimuli from the nasal mucosa have not yet been identified.[24] Some of the TRP channels mentioned above may serve as mechanoreceptors.

Testing the Intranasal Trigeminal System

The major challenge when testing the intranasal trigeminal system is the intimate connection between olfactory and trigeminal sensory systems. Most trigeminal stimuli also activate the olfactory system,[5] and do so at lower concentrations than those needed for trigeminal activation. Different methods have been developed to overcome this problem, with their own advantages and disadvantages.

Psychophysical Testing Methods

> Psychophysical methods to assess the intranasal trigeminal system include testing of anosmic patients; instructing patients to focus on trigeminal rather than olfactory sensations; or using methods that depend purely or predominantly on trigeminal stimulation.

Anosmic patients can only detect mixed olfactory–trigeminal stimuli by virtue of their trigeminal component. Accordingly, the percentage of patients with anosmia who detect a stimulus correlates to the stimulus' trigeminal impact.[5,25] As patients with anosmia do not perceive olfactory information, the same methods used for measuring an olfactory threshold in subjects with normosmia will result in a trigeminal threshold in subjects with anosmia.[26] However, results from anosmic subjects cannot be generalized to the general population, as anosmia per se leads to reduced trigeminal sensitivity.[27,28] It is important to note that even though trigeminal thresholds are reduced in anosmic subjects, trigeminal compounds can nevertheless be perceived. In fact, the difference in trigeminal sensitivity between anosmic and normosmic subjects is small, and therefore may not be detected when investigating only a small number of subjects. However, it is a clear limiting factor of this approach.

Methods depending on trigeminal stimulation: Some psychophysical tests depend on information from the trigeminal system. The main such method is the lateralization task, in which patients identify the nostril (i.e., right or left) to which a chemical stimulus is applied monorhinally (i.e., to only one nostril). This task is based upon the fact that humans seem unable to localize pure odorants,[29] but can localize mixed olfactory–trigeminal stimuli with high accuracy.[29–32] This method is able to establish the sensitivity of the trigeminal system (e.g., when comparing the sensory acuity of subject groups,[31,33] or when comparing the trigeminal potency of different chemical compounds).[26] In clinical testing, a single concentration of a test compound that is a strong trigeminal stimulus (e.g., menthol) may be used in a semiquantitative screening protocol. The sum of correct identifications is used for further statistical analyses. Alternatively, quantitative thresholds for irritant detection can be generated by employing an ascending concentration series of the test chemical of interest (**Fig. 12.3**).

Some groups take advantage of the fact that the cornea and conjunctiva of the eye are also innervated by the trigeminal nerve and perceive painful sensations, but do not respond to pure olfactory stimuli. As vapor-phase chemical stimuli can evoke sensations of burning or stinging in the cornea, they can be used to assess trigeminal irritation thresholds in the eye if care is taken to avoid costimulation of the nose. Interestingly, for many compounds, irritation thresholds in the eye and nose correlate significantly.[34]

An alternative is to use patients with normosmia who are instructed and trained to *focus on trigeminal sensations* and to disregard simultaneous olfactory sensations. Typically, subjects receive instructions such as, "Have you felt any sensation like burning, stinging, cooling, or tickling?" This method allows for the assessment of trigeminal perception thresholds,[35] but other applications are also possible. The main disadvantage of the method

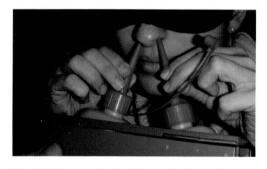

Fig. 12.3 Apparatus for obtaining nasal trigeminal thresholds via the lateralization technique. (Image courtesy of Thomas Hummel, MD.)

is that it can never be completely discounted that patients may be influenced by the olfactory input.

There is also the possibility to use *"pure"* trigeminal stimuli (i.e., stimuli that do not produce an additional chemosensory sensation). However, it is very difficult to exclude a possible concomitant olfactory stimulation. Possible pure trigeminal stimuli include CO_2 and capsaicin. Of note, the CO_2 concentrations necessary to act as an effective trigeminal stimulus are very high (> 100,000 ppm).[36] Thus, CO_2 as a nasal trigeminal stimulus can safely be employed only as a brief (< 3-second) stimulus, or, alternatively, with mouth breathing and velopalatine closure (i.e., isolation of the nasal cavity).

Neurophysiological Methods

Neurophysiological methods to assess the intranasal trigeminal system include the measurement of trigeminal event-related potentials (ERPs) or negative mucosal potentials, or nonspecific imaging techniques such as functional magnetic resonance imaging or positron emission tomography (PET).

Trigeminal ERPs are electroencephalography (EEG)-derived polyphasic signals obtained at the surface of the scalp[37] due to the activation of cortical neurons that generate electromagnetic fields. Trigeminal ERPs are therefore a central nervous representation of the processing of trigeminally mediated sensations. As the EEG is a noisy signal that detects the activity of many cortical neurons as well as non-neuronal activity, ERPs are extracted from the random background activity by averaging responses to single stimuli to improve the signal-to-noise ratio. To avoid effects of habituation, it is necessary to have an interstimulus interval of at least 30 to 40 seconds. Thus, ERP recordings take a long time (in the range of 45 minute to 2 hours), and the patient's concentration has to be maintained by simple tasks, such as a tracking task on a computer screen. ERPs allow the trigeminal system to be investigated with the highest temporal resolution (in the range of milliseconds). However, spatial resolution of ERP is poor. Recording of ERP requires an olfactometer, to ensure the stimulus has a sharp onset, a precisely defined duration, and is free from concomitant mechanical or thermal costimulation, all of which are prerequisites for artifact-free responses.[37] The nomenclature of the trigeminal ERP responses follows that of other sensory domains: a first positive peak (P1) typically occurs at latencies later than 200 milliseconds, followed by a first major negative peak (N1; 400 milliseconds), and the late positive complex (P2/P3; 650 milliseconds).[38] The largest responses are obtained from central and parietal electrodes; measures of interest are usually amplitudes and latencies of the major peaks.

The *negative mucosal potential* (NMP) allows the periphery of the trigeminal system to be assessed.[39] It is the summation of the receptor potentials of chemosensitive nociceptors of the trigeminal nerve,[40] and thus is an electrophysiological correlate of trigeminal activation in the nasal respiratory epithelium,[39] independent of olfactory stimulation. NMPs are recorded by means of an electrode placed on the respiratory mucosa under endoscopic control. Usually, fewer recordings are required for NMP than for ERP. In fact, one single recording may be enough for a meaningful interpretation. Like ERP, NMP recording requires an olfactometer for stimulus presentation. NMPs consist of a slow negative wave with a latency of ~1,000 milliseconds.[41] The largest NMPs, indicating highest sensitivity, are observed at the nasal septum; the lowest, on the nasal floor.[42]

Functional magnetic resonance imaging (fMRI) measures the ratio of oxygenated hemoglobin:deoxygenated hemoglobin, and enables us to observe areas of the brain activated by a task with high spatial resolution (in the millimeter range). fMRI has shown that chemosensory trigeminal stimulation leads to activation patterns that only partly overlap with somatosensory stimuli (e.g., brainstem, thalamus, SI/SII, anterior cingulate[1]). However, chemosensory trigeminal stimuli also activate olfactory regions (e.g., piriform, orbitofrontal, and insular cortex).[1] *PET* assesses the concentration of radioactive markers and allows for distortion-free imaging of the orbitofrontal areas of the brain, but with a weaker spatial and temporal resolution than fMRI. PET-based experiments reported additional activation in the amygdala, claustrum, and lateral hypothalamus after trigeminal chemosensory stimulation.[43] Other imaging methods for the investigation of the intranasal trigeminal system include *magnetoencephalography* and *near-infrared spectroscopy*.

Relationship Between Olfactory and Nasal Trigeminal Stimulation

> The olfactory and the trigeminal systems are intimately connected; interactions between the two sensory systems take place on several levels.

First, many actions—such as food consumption—lead to the *simultaneous stimulation* of different chemosensory systems. When we eat, some substances in the food will activate the olfactory system, others the trigeminal system. Second, the majority of odorants, at least if presented at sufficiently high concentrations, also activate the trigeminal system, and should therefore be considered mixed *olfactory–trigeminal stimuli*, with few exceptions to this rule.[5] Third, it has been shown that the trigeminal and the olfactory system exhibit *central interactions*. If a trigeminal stimulus is presented simultaneously with an olfactory stimulus, its intensity is rated higher than if the trigeminal stimulus is presented on its own. When subjects are, however, focusing on an olfactory stimulus, trigeminal costimulation has the opposite effect. This phenomenon was also evident when stimuli were presented to different nostrils, indicating central nervous interactions.[44] Multisensory integration centers and orbitofrontal areas[45] have been suggested as potential sites for this interaction.

Demographic and Health Conditions Affecting Nasal Trigeminal Function

> Age, olfactory dysfunction, and disease may affect nasal trigeminal function.

Age is the most prominent demographic factor to influence intranasal trigeminal function. Older people exhibit a reduced sensitivity of the intranasal trigeminal system. This can be observed by means of NMP, which indicates that age affects the peripheral responsiveness of the trigeminal system.[46] The presence of nasal allergies, on the other hand, appears to confer heightened sensitivity to at least some trigeminal stimuli.[47] Further, olfactory dysfunction and other diseases also affect trigeminal sensitivity as shown by ERP, NMP, and psychophysical methods.[28]

Nasal Response to Airborne Chemicals

> The intranasal trigeminal system reacts to many different industrial chemicals and naturally occurring substances.

Trigeminally mediated sensory irritation constitutes the most prominent symptom complex in so-called sick building syndrome.[48] Sensory irritation has also been modeled in experimental animals, and provides a critical endpoint for many chemical exposure standards.[49] Both reactive chemicals (e.g., chlorine, formaldehyde) and nonreactive volatile organic compounds are capable of stimulating upper airway nerves. For several chemicals, irritant thresholds in different areas of trigeminal distribution (i.e., nose and eye) have been shown to be closely correlated.[50]

In addition to industrial chemicals, a variety of naturally occurring substances, including capsaicin (chili peppers), eugenol (cloves), menthol (mint), allyl isothiocyanate (mustard oil), and cinnemaldehyde (cinnamon), are intentionally ingested for their trigeminal effects in the oral cavity. These compounds also reach the nose, via either inhalation or the retronasal route. Of note in this context, the sensation of nasal cooling produced by menthol exposure creates an illusion of nasal airflow patency without actually affecting nasal airway resistance.[51] Thus, menthol-containing products are often sold as cold remedies for the subjective relief of nasal blockage, despite their lack of objective physiological effect.

Qualitatively, nasal sensations induced by trigeminal stimulation are diverse, and have been described as stinging, burning, tingling, itching, or cooling. Itching sensations conveyed by the trigeminal nerve are important in the pathophysiology of allergic rhinitis.[52] While a distinction between histamine- and capsaicin-responsive neurons is well appreciated, much of the remaining neurobiology underlying qualitative encoding in the nasal trigeminal system is not yet understood.[53]

Clinical Disorders of the Trigeminal System

Endogenous Disorders

> Endogenous disorders of the trigeminal system include trigeminal neuralgia and migraine.

Trigeminal neuralgia (tic douloureux) is a chronic pain condition affecting the trigeminal nerve. The pain is typically triggered by activation of the trigeminal nerve, which may include smiling, drinking, talking, or shaving, leading to strong behavioral consequences. Usually, trigeminal neuralgia starts with mild symptoms but may become more frequent and more intense over time. Most frequently, trigeminal neuralgia affects women older than 50 years. Possible causes may include contact between the trigeminal nerve and a blood vessel, demyelinating disease, such as multiple sclerosis, or tumors. In patients with trigeminal neuralgia, olfactory and gustatory thresholds have been found to be elevated. However, little change has been noted in sensitivity to thermal, mechanical, and painful stimuli; if changes were found, patients exhibited decreased sensitivity.[54]

Migraine can be a debilitating condition characterized by headaches of varying severity, typically accompanied by nausea and photophobia. While the cause of migraine headache is unknown, the most common theories relate to a disorder of the serotonergic system, or release of calcitonin gene-related peptide from trigeminal nerve fibers in the meninges.[55] Migraine seems to be accompanied by interictal hypersensitivity of the trigeminal system to painful stimulation,[56] which has been interpreted as the result of sensitization in nociceptive pain pathways due to frequent pain experiences[57]; in addition, subclinical pre-attack thermal pain hypersensitivity has been reported.[58] Trigeminal hypersensitivity may also be connected to serotonin depletion.[59] Changes in the olfactory system are less clear. Some studies argue for an increased olfactory sensitivity[60]; others provide evidence for reduced sensitivity in patients with migraine.[56]

Exogenous Disorders

Exogenous disorders of the trigeminal system include herpes zoster ophthalmicus, nasal allergies, the reactive upper airways dysfunction syndrome, vocal cord dysfunction, respiratory or autonomic syndromes triggered by olfactory or trigeminal stimulation, and odor-triggered panic attacks.

Herpes zoster ophthalmicus represents up to 25% of all cases of herpes zoster (caused by human herpesvirus type 3). Most patients present with a periorbital vesicular rash in the affected dermatome. Some patients may also exhibit ocular effects such as conjunctivitis. Poor nutrition and immunocompromised status correlate with outbreaks of herpes zoster; physical or emotional stress and fatigue may also precipitate an episode. To our knowledge, there are no studies on intranasal trigeminal sensitivity in this condition.

Nasal allergies and the trigeminal nerve: The trigeminal nerve is likely to participate in allergies through various mechanisms, including neurogenic inflammation.[3] Research also indicates that the trigeminal system is hyper-reactive in patients with allergies, who are significantly more sensitive than controls to nonallergic triggers,[10] as measured by trigeminal ERP.[61] Further, patients with nasal allergies respond more vigorously in terms of nasal congestion to low concentrations of chlorine gas[62] or acetic acid vapor.[63] In addition to increased nasal sensitivity, the nasal trigeminal system is connected to several other systems and participates in numerous reflexes (e.g., changes in blood pressure or heart rate, mucus secretion in the entire respiratory system, tear secretion, or sneezing).[64] Thus, on multiple levels, the trigeminal system is involved in nasal allergies. It is currently unclear whether trigeminal sensitivity could be used to predict the status of an allergic process or the efficacy of an antiallergic therapy.

Respiratory or autonomic syndromes triggered by olfactory or trigeminal stimulation: Reflex rhinorrhea is quite common after either ingestion of spicy foods or inhalation of cold air. Nasal symptoms triggered by other chemicals (e.g., perfumes and colognes, cleaning products, vehicle exhaust, smoke, and alcohol) or physical factors (e.g., exercise, bright lights) are somewhat less prevalent in the population. Individuals who report multiple nonallergic triggers in the absence of aller-

gic reactivity are considered to have "nonallergic rhinitis." In the absence of another underlying disorder, nonatopic, nasally reactive individuals have been referred to as having "idiopathic rhinitis," "vasomotor rhinitis," "nonallergic, noninfectious perennial rhinitis", or "noninfectious, nonallergic rhinitis". In addition to patients with nonallergic rhinitis, ~40% of individuals with *allergic* rhinitis also report reactivity to nonallergic triggers.[10] Phenotypically, then, so-called nasal hyper-reactivity (defined as nonspecific reactivity to physical and chemical triggers) is a condition that can affect both atopic and nonatopic individuals. Beyond symptom reporting, nasal hyper-reactivity has been defined functionally in a manner analogous to that of bronchial hyper-reactivity (e.g., using challenges with histamine, methacholine, or cold air).[65] Nasal challenge endpoints can include both symptoms (rhinorrhea, nasal blockage) and objective measures (weight of secretions, nasal airway resistance, nasal cross-sectional area). Although challenge testing holds promise, a given individual may exhibit inconsistent reactivity to different test agents, suggesting a complex underlying pathophysiology. Thus, consensus has yet to emerge regarding the clinical utility of these study techniques.[66]

Also analogous to lower airway disease is so-called *reactive upper airways dysfunction syndrome* (RUDS). Similar to irritant-induced asthma, RUDS is a consequence of high-level irritant exposure, with persistent symptoms of airway reactivity (rhinorrhea, nasal obstruction, and nasal hyperesthesia).[67] Although originally defined solely in terms of a one-time, high-level exposure, both irritant-induced asthma and rhinitis have also been reported after repeated exposures to more moderate levels of irritant.[68]

Vocal cord dysfunction (VCD), another upper airway condition of potential reflex origin, is a disorder of laryngeal motility in which the vocal folds inappropriately adduct during inspiration rather than expiration. This results in the sensation of breathlessness, throat pressure, stridor, and hoarseness. A subset of patients with VCD report the onset of symptoms after irritant inhalation, or symptoms triggered by odors and irritants.[69] Pathophysiological mechanisms may include mucosal irritability, motor hyper-reactivity, or cortical factors (e.g., odor processing, conversion reactions). Supporting the possible role of mucosal irritability is the fact that both GERD and postnasal drip from rhinosinusitis are risk factors for developing VCD.[70] Many individuals with VCD are misdiagnosed as having asthma, leading to escalating medication doses with minimal, if any, therapeutic response.

Odor-triggered panic attacks are another nasal irritant–triggered disorder. In this condition, an individual is rendered intolerant to a specific chemical's odor by virtue of a one-time, unexpected, high-level chemical exposure at an irritant concentration (typically far above the odor threshold). Subsequent to such an incident, the chemical's odor is interpreted as a physical threat. Typical panic symptoms include breathlessness, perioral and acrodigital paresthesias, lightheadedness, palpitations, a sense of impending doom (anxiety), and a sense of depersonalization or derealization.[71] If stimulus generalization occurs, the person may report reactivity to a variety of chemical odors. The relationship between asthma and two asthma-like mimics (VCD and panic attacks) is illustrated in **Fig. 12.4**. In all three conditions, symptoms may be triggered by odorant or irritant exposure, and thus are relevant to a discussion of trigeminal function. The three conditions can exist in isolation or in combination in the same patient. Diagnostically, it is important that clinicians consider nonasthma diagnoses when evaluating patients with episodic dyspnea triggered by sensory stimuli, especially with symptoms such as inspiratory dyspnea, upper airway symptoms, or autonomic or central nervous system symptoms. While the diagnostic approach

to asthma is well established, if VCD is suspected, the diagnostic work-up should include flow–volume loops on pulmonary function testing, as well as rhinolaryngoscopy to evaluate for possible paradoxical vocal fold motion.[72] Odor-triggered panic attacks are often treated as a diagnosis of exclusion, after consideration of asthma and VCD. By sharing the differential diagnosis and diagnostic logic with the patient as the work-up begins, the clinician may avoid the defensive response that can often accompany consideration of somatoform diagnoses.

Conclusion

The intranasal trigeminal system constitutes a third chemical sense next to smell and taste, with which it is intimately connected. There are specific methods to assess sensitivity of the trigeminal system. The trigeminal system may be involved in the pathogenesis of several syndromes and diseases.

Acknowledgments

This publication was supported, in part, by a grant to DS from FAMRI (the Flight Attendant Medical Research Foundation); JF is supported by fellowships from FRSQ (Fonds de Recherche en Santé de Québec) and CIHR (Canadian Institutes of Health Research).

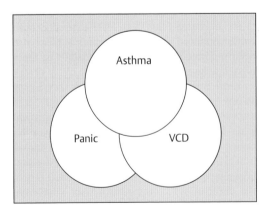

Fig. 12.4 Differential diagnosis of episodic dyspnea triggered by odorants or irritants. VCD, vocal cord dysfunction. (Reproduced with kind permission from Shusterman D. Review of the upper airway, including olfaction, as mediator of symptoms. Environ Health Perspect 2002; 110 (Suppl 4):652, with permission.)

References

1. Albrecht J, Kopietz R, Frasnelli J, Wiesmann M, Hummel T, Lundström JN. The neuronal correlates of intranasal trigeminal function—an ALE meta-analysis of human functional brain imaging data. Brain Res Brain Res Rev 2010;62(2):183–196
2. Ravindran M, Jean Merck S, Baraniuk JN. Functional neuroanatomy of the human upper airway. In: Morris JB, Shusterman DJ, eds. Toxicology of the Nose and Upper Airways. New York: Informa Healthcare; 2010: 65–81
3. Baraniuk JN, Merck SJ. Neuroregulation of human nasal mucosa. Ann N Y Acad Sci 2009;1170: 604–609
4. Walker JC, Kendal-Reed M, Hall SB, Morgan WT, Polyakov VV, Lutz RW. Human responses to propionic acid. II. Quantification of breathing responses and their relationship to perception. Chem Senses 2001;26(4):351–358
5. Doty RL, Brugger WE, Jurs PC, Orndorff MA, Snyder PJ, Lowry LD. Intranasal trigeminal stimulation from odorous volatiles: psychometric responses

from anosmic and normal humans. Physiol Behav 1978;20(2):175–185

6. Silver WL, Finger TE. The anatomical and electrophysiological basis of peripheral nasal trigeminal chemoreception. Ann N Y Acad Sci 2009;1170: 202–205

7. Stjärne P, Lundblad L, Anggård A, Hökfelt T, Lundberg JM. Tachykinins and calcitonin gene-related peptide: co-existence in sensory nerves of the nasal mucosa and effects on blood flow. Cell Tissue Res 1989;256(3):439–446

8. Raphael GD, Baraniuk JN, Kaliner MA. How and why the nose runs. J Allergy Clin Immunol 1991; 87(2):457–467

9. Dubin MG, Pollock HW, Ebert CS, Berg E, Buenting JE, Prazma JP. Eustachian tube dysfunction after tobacco smoke exposure. Otolaryngol Head Neck Surg 2002;126(1):14–19

10. Shusterman D, Murphy MA. Nasal hyperreactivity in allergic and non-allergic rhinitis: a potential risk factor for non-specific building-related illness. Indoor Air 2007;17(4):328–333

11. Jovancevic L, Georgalas C, Savovic S, Janjevic D. Gustatory rhinitis. Rhinology 2010;48(1):7–10

12. Widdicombe JG. Nasal and pharyngeal reflexes: Protective and respiratory functions. In: Mathew OP, Sant' Ambrogio G, eds. Respiratory Function of the Upper Airway. New York: Marcel Dekker; 1988: 233–258

13. Pratter MR. Overview of common causes of chronic cough: ACCP evidence-based clinical practice guidelines. Chest 2006; 129(1, Suppl):59S–62S

14. Millqvist E, Bende M, Löwhagen O. Sensory hyperreactivity—a possible mechanism underlying cough and asthma-like symptoms. Allergy 1998;53(12): 1208–1212

15. Johansson A, Millqvist E, Nordin S, Bende M. Relationship between self-reported odor intolerance and sensitivity to inhaled capsaicin: proposed definition of airway sensory hyperreactivity and estimation of its prevalence. Chest 2006;129(6): 1623–1628

16. Caterina MJ, Schumacher MA, Tominaga M, Rosen TA, Levine JD, Julius D. The capsaicin receptor: a heat-activated ion channel in the pain pathway. Nature 1997;389(6653):816–824

17. Yang BH, Piao ZG, Kim YB, et al. Activation of vanilloid receptor 1 (VR1) by eugenol. J Dent Res 2003; 82(10):781–785

18. Jordt SE, Bautista DM, Chuang HH, et al. Mustard oils and cannabinoids excite sensory nerve fibres through the TRP channel ANKTM1. Nature 2004;427(6971):260–265

19. McKemy DD, Neuhausser WM, Julius D. Identification of a cold receptor reveals a general role for TRP channels in thermosensation. Nature 2002; 416(6876):52–58

20. Bessac BF, Jordt SE. Sensory detection and responses to toxic gases: mechanisms, health effects, and countermeasures. Proc Am Thorac Soc 2010;7(4): 269–277

21. Thuerauf N, Kaegler M, Dietz R, Barocka A, Kobal G. Dose-dependent stereoselective activation of the trigeminal sensory system by nicotine in man. Psychopharmacology (Berl) 1999;142(3):236–243

22. Waldmann R, Champigny G, Bassilana F, Heurteaux C, Lazdunski M. A proton-gated cation channel involved in acid-sensing. Nature 1997;386(6621): 173–177

23. Finger TE, Böttger B, Hansen A, Anderson KT, Alimohammadi H, Silver WL. Solitary chemoreceptor cells in the nasal cavity serve as sentinels of respiration. Proc Natl Acad Sci U S A 2003; 100(15):8981–8986

24. Silver WL, Roe P, Saunders CJ. Functional neuroanatomy of the upper airway in experimental animals. In: Morris JB, Shusterman DJ, eds. Toxicology of the Nose and Upper Airways. New York: Informa Healthcare; 2010: 45–64

25. Frasnelli J, Hummel T, Berg J, Huang G, Doty RL. Intranasal localizability of odorants: influence of stimulus volume. Chem Senses 2011;36(4): 405–410

26. Cometto-Muñiz JE, Cain WS. Trigeminal and olfactory sensitivity: comparison of modalities and methods of measurement. Int Arch Occup Environ Health 1998;71(2):105–110

27. Frasnelli J, Schuster B, Zahnert T, Hummel T. Chemosensory specific reduction of trigeminal sensitivity in subjects with olfactory dysfunction. Neuroscience 2006;142(2):541–546

28. Hummel T, Barz S, Lötsch J, Roscher S, Kettenmann B, Kobal G. Loss of olfactory function leads to a decrease of trigeminal sensitivity. Chem Senses 1996;21(1):75–79

29. Kobal G, Van Toller S, Hummel T. Is there directional smelling? Experientia 1989;45(2):130–132

30. Vonbékésy G. Olfactory analogue to directional hearing. J Appl Physiol 1964;19:369–373

31. Hummel T, Futschik T, Frasnelli J, Hüttenbrink KB. Effects of olfactory function, age, and gender on trigeminally mediated sensations: a study based on the lateralization of chemosensory stimuli. Toxicol Lett 2003;140–141:273–280

32. Wysocki CJ, Cowart BJ, Radil T. Nasal trigeminal chemosensitivity across the adult life span. Percept Psychophys 2003;65(1):115–122

33. Frasnelli J, Hummel T. Interactions between the chemical senses: trigeminal function in patients with olfactory loss. Int J Psychophysiol 2007;65(3):177–181

34. Cometto-Muñiz JE, Cain WS, Hudnell HK. Agonistic sensory effects of airborne chemicals in mixtures: odor, nasal pungency, and eye irritation. Percept Psychophys 1997;59(5):665–674

35. Gudziol H, Schubert M, Hummel T. Decreased trigeminal sensitivity in anosmia. ORL J Otorhinolaryngol Relat Spec 2001;63(2):72–75

36. Shusterman D, Balmes J. Measurement of nasal irritant sensitivity to pulsed carbon dioxide: a pilot study. Arch Environ Health 1997;52(5):334–340

37. Kobal G. Elektrophysiologische untersuchungen des menschlichen geruchssinns. Stuttgart: Thieme Verlag; 1981

38. Hummel T, Kobal G. Chemosensory evoked potentials. In: Doty RL, Müller-Schwarze D, eds. Chemical signals in vertebrates VI. New York: Plenum; 1992:565–569

39. Kobal G. Pain-related electrical potentials of the human nasal mucosa elicited by chemical stimulation. Pain 1985;22(2):151–163
40. Hummel T, Schiessl C, Wendler J, Kobal G. Peripheral electrophysiological responses decrease in response to repetitive painful stimulation of the human nasal mucosa. Neurosci Lett 1996;212(1):37–40
41. Frasnelli J, Schuster B, Hummel T. Interactions between olfaction and the trigeminal system: what can be learned from olfactory loss. Cereb Cortex 2007;17(10):2268–2275
42. Scheibe M, van Thriel C, Hummel T. Responses to trigeminal irritants at different locations of the human nasal mucosa. Laryngoscope 2008;118(1):152–155
43. Savic I, Gulyás B, Berglund H. Odorant differentiated pattern of cerebral activation: comparison of acetone and vanillin. Hum Brain Mapp 2002;17(1):17–27
44. Cain WS, Murphy CL. Interaction between chemoreceptive modalities of odour and irritation. Nature 1980;284(5753):255–257
45. Boyle JA, Frasnelli J, Gerber J, Heinke M, Hummel T. Cross-modal integration of intranasal stimuli: a functional magnetic resonance imaging study. Neuroscience 2007;149(1):223–231
46. Frasnelli J, Hummel T. Age-related decline of intranasal trigeminal sensitivity: is it a peripheral event? Brain Res 2003;987(2):201–206
47. Shusterman D, Murphy MA, Balmes J. Differences in nasal irritant sensitivity by age, gender, and allergic rhinitis status. Int Arch Occup Environ Health 2003;76(8):577–583
48. Cometto-Muñiz JE, Cain WS. Sensory irritation. Relation to indoor air pollution. Ann N Y Acad Sci 1992;641:137–151
49. Kuwabara Y, Alexeeff GV, Broadwin R, Salmon AG. Evaluation and application of the RD50 for determining acceptable exposure levels of airborne sensory irritants for the general public. Environ Health Perspect 2007;115(11):1609–1616
50. Cometto-Muñiz JE, Cain WS. Relative sensitivity of the ocular trigeminal, nasal trigeminal and olfactory systems to airborne chemicals. Chem Senses 1995;20(2):191–198
51. Eccles R. Nasal airway resistance and nasal sensation of airflow. Rhinol Suppl 1992;14:86–90
52. Tai CF, Baraniuk JN. A tale of two neurons in the upper airways: pain versus itch. Curr Allergy Asthma Rep 2003;3(3):215–220
53. Shusterman D. Qualitative effects in nasal trigeminal chemoreception. Ann N Y Acad Sci 2009;1170:196–201
54. Siviero M, Teixeira MJ, de Siqueira JTT, Siqueira SRDT. Somesthetic, gustatory, olfactory function and salivary flow in patients with neuropathic trigeminal pain. Oral Dis 2010;16(5):482–487
55. Villalón CM, Olesen J. The role of CGRP in the pathophysiology of migraine and efficacy of CGRP receptor antagonists as acute antimigraine drugs. Pharmacol Ther 2009;124(3):309–323
56. Grosser K, Oelkers R, Hummel T, et al. Olfactory and trigeminal event-related potentials in migraine. Cephalalgia 2000;20(7):621–631
57. Zohsel K, Hohmeister J, Oelkers-Ax R, Flor H, Hermann C. Quantitative sensory testing in children with migraine: preliminary evidence for enhanced sensitivity to painful stimuli especially in girls. Pain 2006;123(1–2):10–18
58. Sand T, Zhitniy N, Nilsen KB, Helde G, Hagen K, Stovner LJ. Thermal pain thresholds are decreased in the migraine preattack phase. Eur J Neurol 2008;15(11):1199–1205
59. Supornsilpchai W, Sanguanrangsirikul S, Maneesri S, Srikiatkhachorn A. Serotonin depletion, cortical spreading depression, and trigeminal nociception. Headache 2006;46(1):34–39
60. Snyder RD, Drummond PD. Olfaction in migraine. Cephalalgia 1997;17(7):729–732
61. Doerfler H, Hummel T, Klimek L, Kobal G. Intranasal trigeminal sensitivity in subjects with allergic rhinitis. Eur Arch Otorhinolaryngol 2006;263(1):86–90
62. Shusterman D, Murphy MA, Balmes J. Influence of age, gender, and allergy status on nasal reactivity to inhaled chlorine. Inhal Toxicol 2003;15(12):1179–1189
63. Shusterman D, Tarun A, Murphy MA, Morris J. Seasonal allergic rhinitic and normal subjects respond differentially to nasal provocation with acetic acid vapor. Inhal Toxicol 2005;17(3):147–152
64. Baraniuk JN, Kim D. Nasonasal reflexes, the nasal cycle, and sneeze. Curr Allergy Asthma Rep 2007;7(2):105–111
65. Shusterman DJ, Tilles SA. Nasal physiological reactivity of subjects with nonallergic rhinitis to cold air provocation: a pilot comparison of subgroups. Am J Rhinol Allergy 2009;23(5):475–479
66. Gerth van Wijk RG, de Graaf-in 't Veld C, Garrelds IM. Nasal hyperreactivity. Rhinology 1999;37(2):50–55
67. Meggs WJ. RADS and RUDS—the toxic induction of asthma and rhinitis. J Toxicol Clin Toxicol 1994;32(5):487–501
68. Leroyer C, Malo JL, Girard D, Dufour JG, Gautrin D. Chronic rhinitis in workers at risk of reactive airways dysfunction syndrome due to exposure to chlorine. Occup Environ Med 1999;56(5):334–338
69. Perkner JJ, Fennelly KP, Balkissoon R, et al. Irritant-associated vocal cord dysfunction. J Occup Environ Med 1998;40(2):136–143
70. Balkissoon R. Vocal cord dysfunction, gastroesophageal reflux disease, and nonallergic rhinitis. Clin Allergy Immunol 2007;19:411–426
71. Shusterman DJ, Dager SR. Prevention of psychological disability after occupational respiratory exposures. Occup Med 1991;6(1):11–27
72. Tilles SA. Differential diagnosis of adult asthma. Med Clin North Am 2006;90(1):61–76

II Sense of Taste

13   Functional Anatomy of the Gustatory System:
     From the Taste Papilla to the Gustatory Cortex   150

14   Taste Testing   168

15   Taste Disorders   179

16   Burning Mouth Syndrome and Qualitative Taste
     and Smell Disorders   189

17   Structural Imaging in Chemosensory Dysfunction   195

18   Providing Expert Opinion on Olfactory and
     Gustatory Disorders   207

19   Flavor: Interaction Between the Chemical Senses   219

13 Functional Anatomy of the Gustatory System: From the Taste Papilla to the Gustatory Cortex

Tatsu Kobayakawa, Hisashi Ogawa

General Aspects of Taste Sensation

Taste sensation is one of the five sensory modalities, activated by chemical stimuli that react with taste organs on the oral epithelium.

Five basic or fundamental tastes (i.e., taste quality) are described; sweet, salty, sour, bitter, and umami. Sweetness is caused by sucrose or artificial sweeteners such as saccharin; saltiness solely by sodium chloride and lithium chloride; sourness by inorganic and organic acids; bitterness by various substances, such as urea or quinine; and umami by monosodium glutamate and nucleoside monophosphates. Sweet and umami represent energy sources or innate rewards; salty, the balance of minerals; acid, the signal of putridity; and bitter, that of toxins (with some exceptions, such as white lead tasting sweet).

Some specific areas of the tongue or palate have been thought to be most responsive to one particular taste, but this has been proven incorrect and there is large individual variation in the regional specificity of taste responsiveness.[1]

A mixture of two or more tastants sometimes causes increased or decreased taste sensations compared with the sum of taste intensities caused by each of the component tastants alone (mixture facilitation or suppression, respectively).[2] In most cases, this occurs at the peripheral level (e.g., receptor sites). Mixture facilitation is seen in synergistic responses between two different umami substances.[3]

Localization of taste stimuli is poor compared with that of tactile stimulation,[1] and is achieved with the aid of tactile sensation. When chemicals are applied to both sides of the tongue, the intensity of the tastant or the location of the sensation changes,[4] and central mechanisms are probably involved in this.

All aspects of taste sensation are not fully studied in humans. This chapter reviews taste reception in rodents, and neural pathways and coding in monkeys, on which our knowledge of the human gustatory system is largely based. Finally, recent findings from noninvasive studies of human gustatory cortices are reviewed.

Taste Reception

Taste Buds: Taste Receptor Organs

Taste buds (gemmae) are taste receptor organs located on the tongue, palate, and pharynx (**Fig. 13.1**).[5] They are 70 μm in length, and 40 μm in width. Electron microscopy reveals that a taste bud contains 30 to 80 elongated cells together with a few basal cells inside the capsule. Three different types of elongated cells are identified: dark cells or supporting cells (type I; constituting 55 to 75% of taste bud cells), light cells (type II; 15 to 30%), and intermediate cells (type III; 5 to 15%). One or two basal cells (type IV) are also recognized (**Fig. 13.1**).[6] Types I, II and III cells bear microvilli that project from the apical dendrites toward the taste pore (the opening to the oral cavity), and are connected by tight junctions at the apical dendrites so that tastants and salivary fluid cannot access the lateral or basal surface of the cell membrane within the taste bud. The taste pore is filled with mucus, but the tip of the microvilli of some cells projects above this to receive tastants. Type I cells contain secretory granules containing mucous substances. Type III cells possess microfilaments similar to neurons, making synaptic contacts with nerve terminals and various synaptic vesicles at the presynaptic area.[6] Type II cells do not.

Type IV cells, situated at the base of the taste bud, are round with a lobulated nucleus. Some type IV cells express the Sonic hedgehog protein, and may be a transient precursor of types I to III cells and a signal center for the proliferation of progenitor cells in the taste buds.[7] At the basal pore, a few small nerve fibers (intragemminal fibers) enter the taste bud.

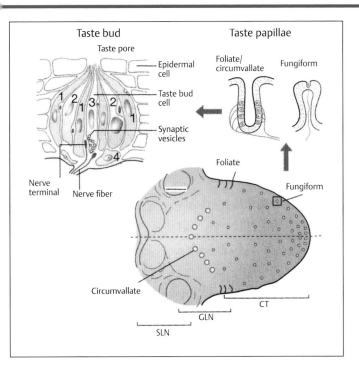

Fig. 13.1 Taste organs. Illustration showing taste buds, the location of taste papillae on the tongue, and their innervation. 1, dark cells; 2, light cells; 3, intermediate cells; 4, basal cells; CT, chorda tympani; GLN, glossopharyngeal nerve; SLN, supralaryngeal nerve. (From Ogawa.[5])

The lifespan of the taste bud cells is very short at around 10.5 days,[8] although a much longer lifespan is noted for some taste receptor cells.[9]

Taste Papillae

There are four kinds of papilla on the tongue. Three of them bear taste buds and are called the taste papillae (**Fig. 13.1**), although taste buds also exist independently in the epidermis of the soft palate or pharynx. Among taste papillae, fungiform papillae (0.7 to 2 mm in diameter) are found on the anterior two-thirds of the tongue and bear an average of 3.5 taste buds on top,[10] although some fungiform papillae (12.8 to 63%) lack taste buds completely.[10] Foliate papillae, consisting of as many as 20 ridges and furrows, are situated on each side of the posterior tongue.[10] Circumvallate papillae, concentrically grooved structures with a diameter of 4 to 8 mm, are located in front of the terminal sulcus. Most people have between 4 and 18 (average of 9.2 ± 1.8) circumvallate papillae.[10] Both foliate and circumvallate papillae bear a large number of taste buds deep in the trench where the taste pores open. Filiform papillae bear no taste buds and are characterized by a cornified layer on the top of the epithelium.

The total number of taste buds on the tongue is up to 4,600 in humans: 24% on fungiform papillae, 28% on foliate papillae, and 48% on circumvallate papillae.[11] More taste buds are located on the posterior tongue than on the anterior tongue.

The density of fungiform papillae on the anterior tongue can be examined. It is high at the tongue tip (24.5 /cm^2; range 2.4 to 80), but low on the median dorsum (8.2 /cm^2; range 0 to 28.3).[11] The number of taste buds varies individually, and, in contrast to previous reports, does not decline with age.[11] Patients who can taste phenylthiocarbamide (PTC) or 6-n-propylthiouracil (PROP) have a larger number of taste buds than those who cannot.[11] The threshold of detection of a certain tastant is lower when a tongue area with a higher density of taste buds is stimulated.[12]

Although it is reported that single fungiform papillae are sensitive to a single basic stimulus,[4] they are often sensitive to a few tastants. About 65% of papillae examined have been found to be sensitive to at least three of four tastants tested, 20% sensitive to a single tastant, and 13% not sensitive at all.[13]

Innervation of Taste Papillae and Taste Buds

Several nerve fibers enter a single fungiform papilla, some of which send collaterals to neighboring papillae. This means that a single taste fiber can innervate several taste papillae.[12] On average, a single fiber innervates one to four papillae.[11]

Fungiform papillae are innervated by the chorda tympani (CTN), a sensory branch of the facial nerve; foliate papillae by both the CTN and a lingual branch of the glossopharyngeal nerve (GLN); and circumvallate papillae by the GLN (**Fig. 13.1**). Taste buds in the soft palate are innervated by the superficial greater petrosal nerve (SGP), another sensory branch of the facial nerve, while those in the pharynx are innervated by the supralaryngeal nerve, a sensory branch of vagal nerve (VN).

Taste Receptors and Taste Transduction

Type II cells in the taste bud express G-protein coupled receptor proteins for sweet, umami, or bitter, while type III cells express ionic taste receptors for salty or sour tastants. Taste signals may be integrated within the taste buds before being transmitted to the taste nerves.

The taste receptors for sweet, bitter, and umami are G protein–coupled receptor proteins (GCRPs). They are seven transmembrane domain receptor proteins with an N-terminal in the extracellular space and a C-terminal associated with G pro-tein in the intracellular space. Taste receptors are believed to be located at the apical microvilli of taste receptor cells (TRCs). They can be classed as type 1 (T1R) or type 2 (T2R). T1Rs are class C GCRPs with a long N-terminal, whereas T2Rs are class A GCRPs with a short N-terminal.[15] T1R1, T1R2, and T1R3 are themselves orphan receptor proteins, but a heterodimer of T1R2 + T1R3 is sweet receptor, and that of T1R1 + T1R3 is umami receptor (**Fig. 13.2**).[15] Twenty-five T2Rs are involved in receiving bitter tastants in humans, and different T2Rs are concerned with different bitter tastants[15] (e.g., T2R4 for denatonium, T2R38 or T2R44 for PTC or PROP, and T2R43 or T2R44 for saccharin). A taste version of metabotropic glutamate receptor type 1 or 4 (taste mGluR1 and mGluR4) is also presumed to be the receptor protein for glutamate, but, unlike T1R1 + T1R3, does not yield synergistic responses to a mixture of glutamate and ribonucleotide.[16] In the mouse, T1Rs and T2Rs are expressed in different TRCs, but almost all T2Rs are expressed in the same TRC.[15]

Salty or sour taste receptors have not been fully elucidated. The degenerin/epithelial sodium channel (EnaC) family has been suggested,[16] with the selective amiloride-sensitive ENaC proposed as a candidate for the salty taste receptor[16] (with no convincing evidence), and a neuronal (degenerin) amiloride-sensitive cation channel, including an acid-sensing ion channel (ASCIC), proposed as a candidate receptor for sour taste.[17,18] A heterodimer of polycystic kidney disease protein 1L3 and 2L1 (PKD2L1) has also been proposed as the sour receptor,[15,16] and its involvement in human sour taste has been reported.[14,15]

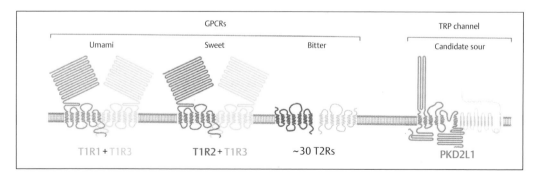

Fig. 13.2 Taste receptor proteins. GPCR, G protein–coupled receptor protein; T1R, taste receptor type 1; T2R, taste receptor type 2; TRP channel, transient receptor potential channel; PKD2L1, polycystic kidney disease protein 2L1. (From Chandrashekar et al.[15])

GCRPs are expressed in type II cells, whereas ionic channel receptors for acid or salt are located in type III cells.[14,15] Therefore, type II cells are now called receptor cells and type III cells are presynaptic cells.

Taste Transduction

Sodium or lithium ions enter ENaCs to depolarize taste cells, an action that is partly inhibited by amiloride. Protons (H⁺) activate ASCIC or PKD2L1 to open an ionic channel and depolarize cells.

Sweet, bitter, or umami substances react with GCRPs, leading to activation of a G protein (gustducin in T2Rs[15]), which triggers an intracellular cascade common to TRCs expressing either T1R or T2R: activation of phospholipase Cβ2; production of inositol-1,4,5-triphosphate; calcium ion release from intracellular calcium stores; and finally stimulation of transient receptor potential (TRP) protein TRPM5 to depolarize cells (**Fig. 13.3**).[15,16] Transduction of sweet tastant is blocked by gymnemic acids.

Type II cells release adenosine triphosphate from pannexin 1 hemichannels, into the intracellular space, which activates type III cells with purinergic receptors and probably taste nerve fibers by paracrine secretion (**Fig. 13.3**).[17] Type III cells activate taste fiber terminals via synapses. Thus, type III cells as well as taste fibers are able to respond to organic tastants.[17] Chemicals such as serotonin or glutamate have been suggested as synaptic transmitters between type III cells and nerve terminals.[18,19]

Temperature dependence of taste transduction has been noted in taste psychophysics[20] and the physiology of taste fibers.[21] Most taste responses have an optimal temperature of 30°C, except sodium chloride, which has an optimal temperature of 10°C or lower, suggesting the presence of an energy barrier for chemical reactions between tastants and receptors. However, it is partially ascribed to the temperature dependence of TRPM5.[22]

Responsiveness of Taste Receptor Cells

Electrophysiology has shown that TRCs generate depolarizing receptor potentials in response

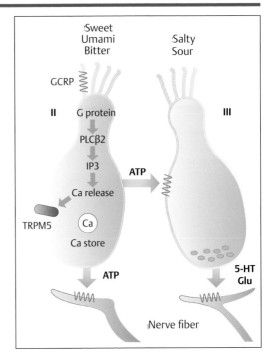

Fig. 13.3 Intracellular and intercellular signaling in taste bud cells. II, type II cell; III, type III cell; 5-HT, serotonin; ATP, adenosine triphosphate; GCRP, G protein–coupled receptor protein; Glu, glutamate; IP3, inositol-3 phosphate; PLCβ2, phospholipase C β2; TRPM5, transient receptor potential protein M5; Ca, calcium ions.

to tastants,[23] but can also produce sodium spikes because of the presence of sodium channels.[24] In mice, type II cells differentially respond to umami, sweet, or bitter, while type III cells respond to salt or sour tastants.[16]

Peripheral Taste Nerves

Course of Taste Nerves

The CTN and SGP take a peripheral course toward the taste buds, together with the lingual branch (LN) or palatal branch of the trigeminal nerve. They take a complex central course to the medulla to terminate in the solitary tract nucleus (NTS) (**Fig. 13.4**).

The CTN travels to the tympanic cavity, where it runs near the auditory ossicles. It then enters the facial canal to form the geniculate ganglion, and to fuse with the SGP to form the intermediate nerve of Wrisberg (IMN), which joins the facial nerve.

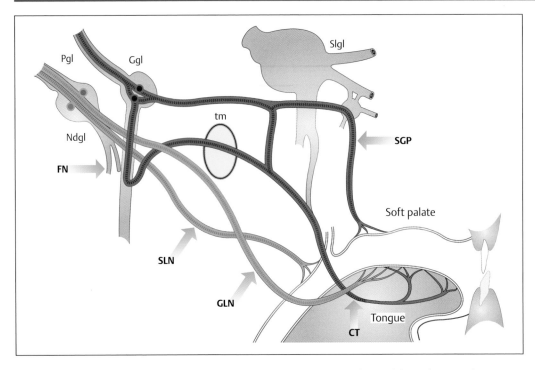

Fig. 13.4 Course of peripheral taste nerves. FN, facial nerve; Ggl, geniculate ganglion; Ndgl, nodosal ganglion; Pgl, petrosal ganglion; SGP, superficial greater petrosal nerve; tm, tympanic membrane; Slgl, semilunar ganglion; SLN, superior laryngeal nerve; GLN, glossopharyngeal nerve; CT, chorda tympani.

After leaving the soft palate, the SGP traverses the sphenopalatine ganglion to the tympanic cavity, with its cell body in the geniculate ganglion. The IMN enters the cranium, diverges from the facial nerve, and enters the solitary tract in the medulla. A somatosensory branch innervating the pinna joins the facial nerve in the canal. The GLN runs just underneath the pharyngeal epithelium to innervate foliate or circumvallate papillae. The GLN forms the petrosal ganglion, and the VN forms the nodosal ganglion. The latter two enter the cranium to the solitary tract. In humans, all three taste nerves enter the solitary tract before terminating in the NTS, while in monkeys the IMN and GLN do not.[25]

The IMN, GLN, and supralaryngeal nerves contain large and small somatosensory fibers. The IMN and GLN also contain autonomic nerve fibers innervating salivary glands. The conduction velocity of taste fibers is similar to that of myelinated or unmyelinated fibers.[26]

Response Profile of Taste Nerve Fibers: Neural Taste Information

Single taste fibers are responsive to a single or a few basic tastants depending on the species of animal. In monkeys and mice, single taste fibers generally respond to a single basic taste, but in rats and cats they respond to multiple basic tastes. The responsiveness of taste fibers to various tastants is often expressed in terms of the tastant that produces the largest response of the four or five basic tastes (best-stimulus category).[27] When tastants are arranged in the order of sweet, salt, sour, and bitter along the abscissa, and response magnitudes are plotted on the ordinate, the response profile of single taste fibers has a single peak in each best-stimulus category in the CTN and GLN.[27]

In monkeys, single CTN fibers are most responsive to sweet, salty, or sour substances, but rarely to bitter or umami substances, whereas single GLN fibers best respond to sweet, bitter, and umami substances (**Fig. 13.5**).[28–30] In rats, umami mixtures

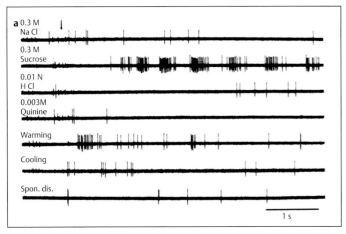

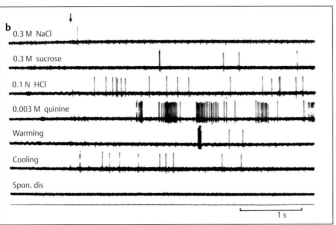

Fig. 13.5a–d Responses of single chorda tympani fibers. NaCl, sodium chloride; HCl, hydrochloric acid. (Reproduced with kind permission from Sato et al[28] for **a**, **b** and **d**; and Sato et al[29] for **c**.)

a Sucrose-best fiber.

b Quinine-best fiber.

Fig. 13.5 c–d ▷

evoke synergistic effects in the CTN (the sweet-responsive fibers in particular[31]) but not in the GLN. In rodents, the whole SGP bundle is more responsive to sweet substances than the CTN.[32] However, single-fiber analysis does not confirm this finding. Most single fibers in the supralaryngeal nerve are responsive to water in rabbits or rats, and this response is inhibited by addition of ions.[33] The CTN of primates also yields responses to water.[34]

> Each of the taste nerves innervates different regions of the oral cavity, conveying various characteristics of taste signals. They take their own courses to the central nervous system where they may be damaged during surgical procedures, e.g., surgery of the middle ear.

Central Pathways: Taste Relay Nucleus and Related Structures

Nucleus of the Solitary Tract

Anatomy

The NTS is located at the dorsal medulla. The anterior portion lies ventral to the dorsal vestibular nucleus and the posterior portion fuses with the contralateral counterpart to make the nucleus communicans near the obex, the posterior end of the rhomboid fossa. In monkeys, the NTS is histologically subdivided into the lateral and medial subnucleus.[25] The anterior portion, made of the lateral subnucleus, is the first relay of the central

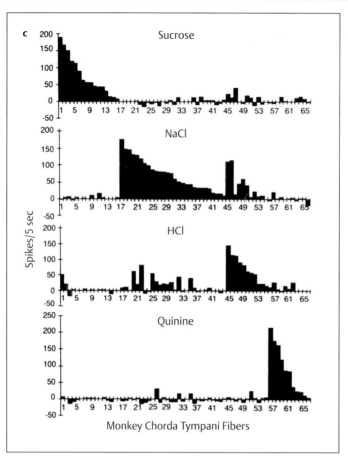

◁ continued

c Response profile of total 50 fibers.

Fig. 13.5 d ▷

gustatory pathway. The IMN enters the NTS posterior to the entry of the facial nerve, followed by the GLN, and the VN most posteriorly.[25] The IMN and GLN terminate at the lateral subnucleus, while the VN terminates at both subnuclei.[25] The lateral subnucleus probably contains taste neurons. The human NTS is subdivided into ten subnuclei, among which the interstitial subnucleus corresponds to the lateral subnucleus in monkey.[25] Somatosensory components of taste nerves, including the facial nerve innervating the pinna, terminate at the nucleus of the spinal tract of the trigeminus.

Efferent Connections

In monkeys, neurons in the anterior NTS send axons ipsilaterally through the central tegmental tract to terminate directly in the thalamic taste relay, a parvicellular part of the ventromedial posterior nucleus (VPMpc) (**Fig. 13.6**).[25]

No projection is seen to the parabrachial nucleus from the lateral subnucleus, but from the medial subnucleus receiving visceral afferents.[25] Thus, in subhuman primates, the parabrachial nucleus is probably not involved in taste sensation. In rats, the rostral portion of the NTS projects to the reticular formation in the medulla, which is involved in the ingestion reflex and mastication.[35] No report has been published on pathways to the thalamus through the reticular formation.

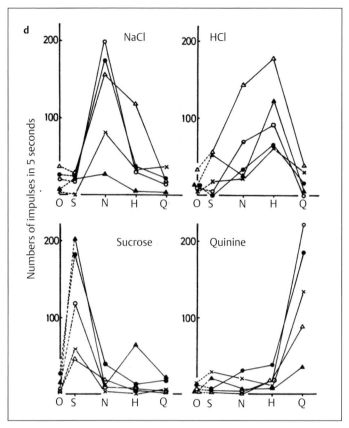

◁ continued

d Response profiles of a few single fibers in each best-stimulus category.

Physiological Features

Taste neurons have been recorded from the NTS in macaque monkeys.[36] However, detailed study has been limited to rats, in which taste neurons are found among neurons responding to tactile or high-threshold mechanical stimulation. Taste neurons respond best to sweet, salty, or sour tastants, as in the CTN, but rarely to bitter tastants, with some responsive to mechanical stimulation.[37] Taste neurons from the anterior tongue respond best to salt, but those from both the tongue and the nasoincisor duct in the palate respond best to sweet tastants.[25,38] Taste neurons with a receptive field (RF) at the rostral part of the oral cavity tend to be located in the more rostral portion of the nucleus. Taste neurons responding to salty or sour tastants often have RFs in the anterior tongue, and those to sweet tastants have RFs in both the anterior tongue and the nasoincisor duct, in which many taste buds are found in rodents.[38] Some taste neurons have RFs in the posterior tongue or soft palate.[38]

Some taste neurons respond to several olfactory stimuli[39] in rats, probably by way of trigeminal nerve innervation of the nasal cavity.

The Ventral Posteromedial Nucleus of the Thalamus, a Parvicellular Part

Anatomy

The VPMpc lies between the VPM proper and the medial lemniscus at the ventral posterior part of the thalamus, and is packed with small-sized cells. The gustatory part is the medial half,[25] comprising the second relay of the gustatory pathway in primates.

Afferent Connections

In monkeys, the VPMpc receives afferents ipsilaterally from the lateral subnucleus of the NTS, and also ipsilaterally from the parabrachial nucleus.[25]

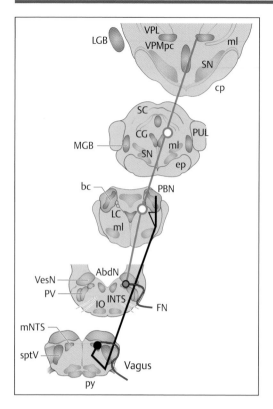

Fig. 13.6 Gustatory pathway from the solitary tract nucleus (NTS) to a parvocellular part of the ventromedial posterior nucleus (VPMpc). The central gustatory pathway starts from the lateral subnucleus of the NTS and goes up through the central tegmental path to the VPMpc, which is contrast to the visceral pathway that goes up from the medial subnucleus of the NTS to the parabrachial nucleus (PBN). AbdN, abducence nucleus; bc, brachium conjunctivum; CG, central gray; cp, cerebral peduncle; FN, facial nerve; IO, inferior olive; LC, locus coeruleus; LGB, lateral geniculate body; lNTS, lateral subnucleus of the NTS; MGB, medial geniculate body; ml, medial lemniscus; mNTS, medial subnucleus of the NTS; PUL, pulvinar nucleus; PV, principal nucleus of the trigeminus; py, pyramidal tract; SC, superior colliculus; SN, substantia nigra; sptV, spinal tract of the trigeminus; VPL, ventral posterolateral thalamic nucleus; VPMpc, parvocellular part of the ventral posteromedial thalamic nucleus; VesN, vestibular nucleus.

The VPMpc is reciprocally connected with the reticular formation of thalamus in rats,[40] and is found in specific nuclei in the thalamus in other animals. The gustatory part of the thalamic reticular formation is ventral to the caudal end of the somatosensory part, rostral to both the visual and auditory parts.[40]

In rats, the gustatory cortex and VPMpc are thought to form the thalamocortical reverberating circuits involving the reticular formation and containing inhibitory neurons.[41]

Efferent Connections

Neurons in the gustatory part of the VPMpc project to two gustatory cortices, at the exposed part of the frontal operculum and at the rostral end of the Sylvian sulcus in monkeys.[25]

Physiological Features

In humans and monkeys, taste responses are recorded from the VPMpc.[25] Detailed studies have been carried out in rats.[25,36,42] Thalamic neurons are

spontaneously active, but yield a small response to tastants. Their RFs are larger than those of NTS neurons, covering the whole tongue or anterior tongue.[42]

> The central taste pathway from the NTS, the first relay, to the VPMpc runs directly and ipsilaterally through the central tegmental path. Then the VPMpc sends axons to the two primary gustatory cortices: the frontal extent of Area 3, and Area G within the Sylvian sulcus.

Gustatory Cortices in Subhuman Primates

Primary Cortex

Anatomy and Afferent Connections

The primary gustatory cortices in monkeys have been identified by the evoked potential method[43,44] and by tracer methods.[25,44]

Two primary gustatory cortices are recognized: (1) The precentral extension of Area 3 (precentral Area 3) to which the CTN, LN, and GLN project bilaterally with ipsilateral predominance;[43,44] and (2) Area G[45] at the rostral end in the inside of the Sylvian sulcus to which the CTN and GLN, but not the LN, project ipsilaterally.

Area G lies at the transition between Areas 1 and 2 at the frontal operculum and granular insula (**Fig. 13.7**),[44,45] and is the granular area, characterized with well-developed outer and inner granular layers (layers II and IV) and with Gennari stria at layer IV.[44,45] Cytochrome oxidase activity distinguishes Area G from the surrounding areas.[44] Studies using tracer show the projections of the VPMpc to both Area G and precentral Area 3.[25] The axons of VPMpc neurons may be bifurcated to project to both areas.[43] Areas 1 and 2 may also be included in the primary gustatory areas, as the deposition of a large concentration of tracers in the VPMpc has identified terminals in Areas 1 and 2 (Pritchard, personal communication, September 1994).

Efferent Connections

The precentral Area 3 projects to the precentral operculum (PrCO) and Area 12, the lateral part of the orbitofrontal cortex,[46,48] whereas Area G projects to Area 12 and the orbitofrontal operculum (OFO) (**Fig. 13.7**).[47,48] In rats, the gustatory cortex is connected to the contralateral counterpart through the corpus callosum.[49]

Physiological Features

Areas G and 3 contain many mechanoreceptive neurons, such as chewing movement–related neurons or tactile neurons with RFs in the mouth.[50] Among these mechanoreceptive neurons, taste neurons are found.[36,44,50] Areas G and 3 contain neurons with different taste response characteristics[51]: neurons in Area G tend to respond differentially to hedonically positive (sweet or salty) or negative (sour or bitter) tastants, but those in Area 3 do not. In each best category, some taste neurons display response profiles with two modes at the best stimulus and another one, by producing the largest responses to the two tastants and a difference in response between the two (**Fig. 13.8**). For example, some sucrose-best neurons show larger responses to quinine but smaller ones to NaCl or HCl. These findings suggest that the primary cortex is concerned with taste contrast, as in rats.[52] Neurons most responsive to monosodium glutamate are also found in Areas 3 and G (**Fig. 13.8**),[36] probably representing umami.

Studying the gustatory cortices in behaving monkeys revealed that almost all of the neurons in both Area 3 and Area G respond to the same chemical cues with consistent response patterns irrespective of changes in behavioral responses, such as lever pressing to gain a reward[53]; this indicates that the neurons in the primary cortices are real taste neurons.

Higher Order Cortex and Other Areas

Anatomy

The PrCO, Area 12, and probably the OFO, receiving afferents from the primary areas,[46,47] are higher order gustatory areas. They are dysgranular neocortex. Taste neurons are also found in Area 13

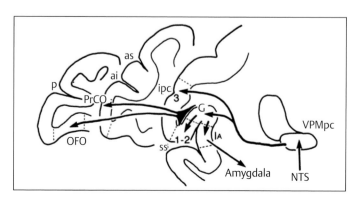

Fig. 13.7 Gustatory pathway from VPMpc to the primary gustatory cortex and to higher order gustatory cortex. G, area G; IA, agranular part of the insula; OFO, orbitofrontal operculum; PrCO, precentral operculum; ai, arcuate sulcus, inferior branch; as, arcuate sulcus, superior branch; ipc, inferior precentral sulcus; p, principal sulcus; ss, Sylvian sulcus; 1–2, area 1–2; 3, area 3. Other abbreviations, see the legend for Fig. 13.6. (From Ogawa et al.[48])

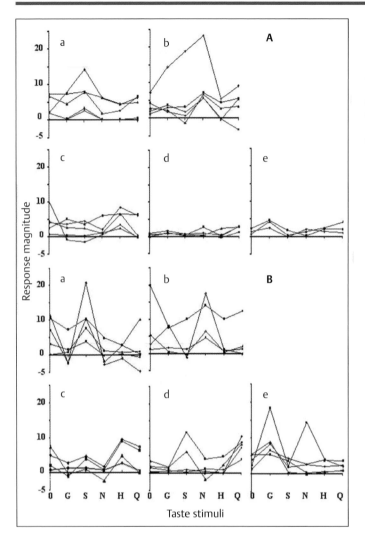

Fig. 13.8 Response profiles of taste neurons in Areas 3 and G. Responses (number of impulses per second) are plotted against taste stimuli. **A** Area 3; **B** Area G; **a** sucrose best; **b** NaCl best; **c** HCl best; **d** quinine best; **e** glutamate best; 0, spontaneous discharge rate; G, glutamate; H, hydrochloric acid; N, sodium chloride; Q, quinine; S, sucrose.

in the medial part of the orbitofrontal cortex, the limbic cortex.[25] Area 12 and dysgranular insula project to the amygdala.[36,44,54]

Response Features

Neurons in Area 12 respond to taste stimuli and other modalities such as somatosensory, visual, and olfactory stimuli.[36,44] Pleasant stimuli are effective. Neurons in Area 12 show sensory-specific satiety, with taste responses facilitated by hunger to a certain stimulus but suppressed by satiety to it. Hypothalamic signals may gate taste inputs to Area 12.[36]

In behaving monkeys, almost all of the neurons in Area 12 and half the neurons in the PrCO respond to the same chemical cues, with the response pattern reversed after changes in behavioral response (**Fig. 13.9**). These areas do not represent taste, but rather behavioral context, or what the monkey wants to do in response to cues.[53]

Neurons in the amygdala tend to respond to aversive stimuli. Neurons in the amygdala or temporal pole differentially respond to food or nonfood.[55] The amygdala is also involved in learned taste aversion in rats.[56] Ablation of the lower part of the parietal cortex and the temporal pole in monkeys yields hyperorality, or Kluever–Bucy syndrome.[54]

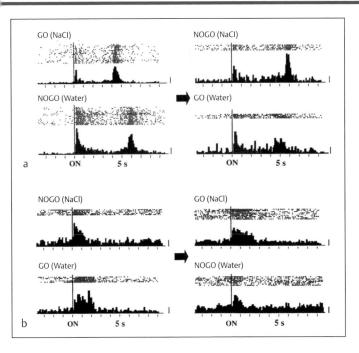

Fig. 13.9a, b Responses of cortical neurons to cues in monkey engaged in a delayed version of the NaCl–water discrimination GO/NOGO task. The task was reversed before and after the arrow. (From Ifuku et al.[53])

a Neuron consistently responding to NaCl or water irrespective of task reversal, representing chemical nature of cues (Area G).

b Neuron changing response to cues according to the task, representing the behavioral context (Area 12).

> Taste neurons in the two primary areas show invariant taste responsiveness irrespective of behavioral context, while those in higher-order Area 12, show changes in responsiveness depending on behavioral context. The latter also shows sensory-specific satiety.

Gustatory Cortices in Humans

Primary Cortex

The location of the primary gustatory cortex (PGA) in the human cerebral cortex has been argued for many decades. Börnstein studied patients with ageusia after bullet wounds involving the parietal lobe, and located a gustatory cortical area in Area 43 or the Roland operculum.[57] Penfield and Jasper,[58] on the other hand, suggested taste representation in the circuminsular cortex superior to the circular sulcus near the foot of the central sulcus and extending to the insular cortex, even though the relation to secondary sensory areas is not certain. Both reports suggest that the gustatory cortex lies at the foot of the central sulcus, but differ as to whether it is at the lateral surface or buried in the cerebral cortex. As described on p. 158, two primary gustatory cortices are recognized in squirrel and macaque monkeys.

Recent developments in imaging techniques have yielded various noninvasive methods (e.g., functional magnetic resonance imaging [fMRI], positron emission tomography [PET], and magnetoencephalography [MEG]) that allow us to measure the brain activity in healthy living human subjects. fMRI measures changes in blood flow by detecting the contrast in magnetic susceptibility between oxyhemoglobin and deoxyhemoglobin. PET measures the density of oxygen-15-water ($H_2^{15}O$) in blood, by detection of gamma rays caused by electron–positron annihilation. Both methods mainly measure changes in metabolism associated with neural activity, which provides better spatial resolution than detecting activated regions. MEG or electroencephalography (EEG), however, measure changes in magnetic fields or electric potential, respectively, on the surface of the skull, caused by electrical activation in clusters of neurons. MEG and EEG, therefore, provide better temporal resolution of cortical activation. Additionally, MEG is superior to EEG for localizing cortical activity because of the uniformity of magnetic permeability in a skull, compared with the large distortion of electric signals for EEG.

As the PGA is the first cortical area receiving projections from the thalamus, MEG is the most suitable method of identifying the PGA. MEG

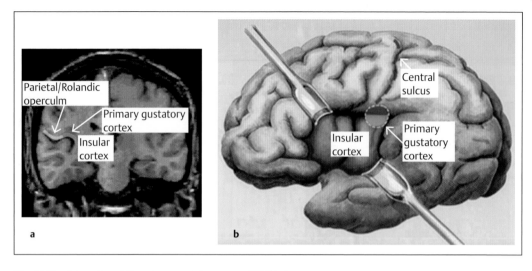

Fig. 13.10a, b Location of the primary gustatory cortex (PGA) in humans.

a Coronal section shows that one of the PGAs (human Area G) locates at a transition area between the insular cortex and parietal or Rolandic operculum.

b Illustrates the PGA when the insular cortex is exposed by clamps.

experiments revealed that taste stimuli evoked the first cortical activation at two regions: First, the lower end of the central sulcus, probably corresponding to the frontal extension of Area 3 in primates; and, second, the transition area between the parietal or Rolandic operculum and the posterior part of the insula, probably corresponding to Area G near the anterior end of the lateral sulcus in primates (human Area G), as shown in **Fig. 13.10**. Activation of the former was found to continue to Area 43 in an fMRI study. The former, including Area 43 and the foot of the central sulcus, probably corresponds to Börnstein's gustatory area, and the human Area G (inside the lateral sulcus) to that of Penfield and Jasper. The onset latency was ~150 milliseconds for sodium chloride and 250 milliseconds for saccharin (artificial sweet substance) in the latter area; these latencies in the former area are much shorter (90 milliseconds for sodium chloride).[59] Compared with the location of the PGA in primates,[43,44] that of human beings moves posteriorly, traversing the central sulcus to the parietal cortex. Such movement of sensory areas on the cerebral cortex with phylogenetic evolution is also known in other areas, such as the visual cortex. Factor analysis of correspondences suggested that gustatory stimuli activated the insular region, and somatogustatory stimuli activated the Rolandic opercula, including a part of the sensory homun-

culus dedicated to the tactile representation of oral structures.[60]

Some reports[61,62] insist that the frontal operculum and anterior insula are PGA in humans on the grounds that the PGA of primates is located in these cortical areas. As fMRI or PET measure metabolic changes in the brain and have poor temporal resolution, it is difficult to establish whether the PGA is located in parietal areas with fMRI or PET study alone. MEG study[59] revealed that the frontal operculum and anterior insula were activated after Area G with longer latency (286 milliseconds). It is reasonable, therefore, to assume that these frontal areas are higher areas related to taste perception rather than PGA.

The PGA is involved in taste concentration coding. The amplitude of activity in the PGA had good linearity according to the logarithm of four sodium chloride concentrations, as shown in **Fig. 13.11a**.[63] The latency, however, did not change with changes in concentrations. **Fig. 13.11b** shows, however, that psychological perceived intensity has a partial discrepancy from cortical activation in PGA at high concentration. The interpretation for this phenomenon will be described in the next section.

In addition, the PGA is characterized by sensitivity to the repetition of taste stimulation, as found in other primary sensory cortices, such as the primary visual cortex in which changes in

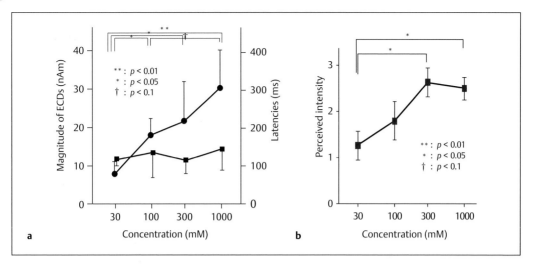

Fig. 13.11a, b Relation of magnetoencephalography activity in the primary gustatory cortex and perceived intensity to various concentrations of taste stimulation.

a The amplitude (circle) of equivalent current dipole (ECD) increases with increase in sodium chloride concentration from 30 mM to 1M, but the onset latency (square) does not. Taste stimulus was presented to the tip of the tongue.

b Psychological perceived intensity evaluated in the same experiment also increases with increases in tastant concentration. Psychological perceived intensity was measured using visual analog scale from 0 to 5.

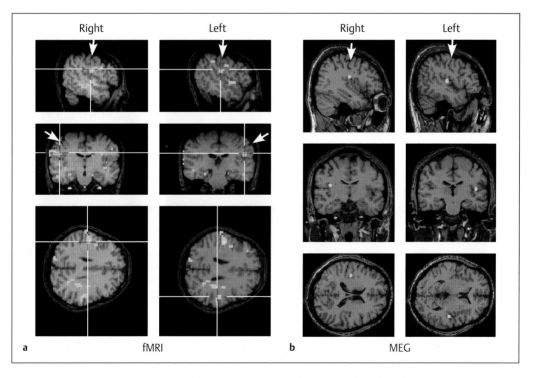

Fig. 13.12a, b Location of the primary gustatory cortex (PGA) revealed by functional magnetic resonance imaging (fMRI) (a) and magnetoencephalography (MEG) (b). Yellow regions indicate taste-activated areas. In the fMRI study, a short pulse of sodium chloride solution was repetitively applied to the tongue tip of participants during the stimulation period. Arrows indicate the central sulcus.

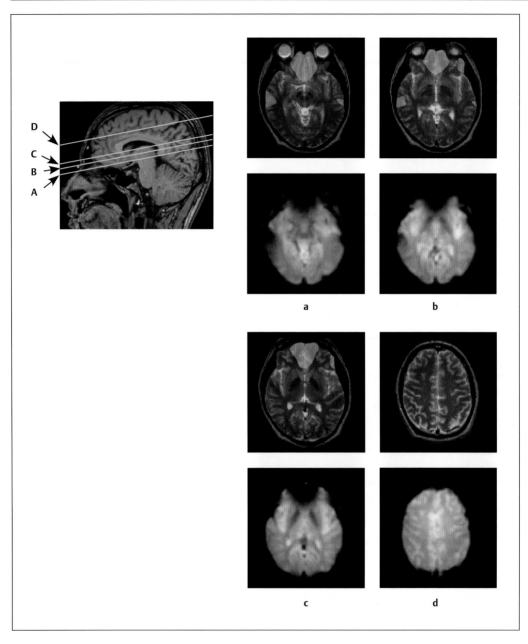

Fig. 13.13a–d Attenuation of 3-T magnetic resonance signals in the orbitofrontal cortex. Upper and lower lines of images indicate anatomical (T2-weighted images) and functional images (echo planar images) obtained from the horizontal plane through the lines (**a–d**) shown at the left sagittal section. Lines (**A–C**) run through the orbitofrontal cortex (OFC), but (**D**) does not. Yellow masked areas in anatomical images demonstrate the areas in which no or feeble magnetic resonance signal was detected in echo planar images. Thus, the rostromedial part of the OFC is "signal black out" because of the heterogeneity of magnetic susceptibility caused by the paranasal cavity.

regional cerebral blood flow (rCBF) are observed by repetitive stimuli or checker-board reversal.[64] Although many studies have reported weak or rare activation of the PGA by long-lasting taste stimuli, significant changes of rCBF at the PGA were also observed by frequent taste stimuli,[65] as shown in **Fig. 13.12a**, and the location revealed by fMRI is consistent with MEG results (**Fig. 13.12b**).

Laterality of the gustatory pathway from the tongue to the PGA in humans has been debated for a long time. It is still a matter of ongoing controversy, having been reported as being ipsilateral,[66] contralateral,[67] and bilateral.[68] Experiments using patients with unilaterally transected chorda tympani during middle ear cholesteatoma operations have revealed that unilateral (right-sided) stimulation evoked bilateral cortical activation in the PGA with a short latency difference between the two hemispheres,[69] suggesting bilateral neural projection in humans.

Higher Order Cortex

Many fMRI and PET studies reported gustatory activation in cortices in peri-insular regions, frontal operculum, orbitofrontal cortex, the amygdala, and cingulate gyrus. In particular, the orbitofrontal cortex is related to higher order taste functions such as food reward,[70,71] palatability,[72] sensory-specific satiety,[73] and integration with olfaction.[74,75] In fMRI measurement using echo planar methods, however, the heterogeneity of magnetic susceptibility caused by the paranasal cavity strongly attenuates the magnetic resonance signal[76] from the rostral and medial part of orbitofrontal cortex, as shown in **Fig. 13.13**. The amygdala has been referred to as the region related to hunger or satiety,[77] food reward, or valence (palatability).[78]

The neural mechanism for taste intensity evaluation is unknown, even though this is a fundamental function of food evaluation. As described above, psychological perceived intensity had a partial discrepancy with cortical activation in PGA when the tastant was presented to the tip of participant's tongue. Correlation analysis of psychological intensity and the whole amplitude of magnetic field revealed that three latency periods from stimulus onset are significant in the process of intensity evaluation. Dipole analysis revealed that the PGA was observed in the first activation (shortest latency ~150 milliseconds), the hippocampus and cingulate gyrus in the second latency

(~400 milliseconds) simultaneously, and, again, the PGA and midfrontal gyrus for the last latency (~800 milliseconds).[79] These results show that lots of cortical areas are dynamically related to the simple intensity evaluation of taste.

Other higher taste functions, such as reward, palatability, memory, and integration, are also supposed to be developed by such dynamic cortical networks. The role of cortical networks in such function remains to be studied.

> Location of the primary gustatory cortex was suggested to be the transition area between the parietal operculum and posterior part of the insula. The frontal operculum, orbitofrontal cortex, amygdala, and cingulate gyrus would be related to higher functions such as food reward, palatability, sensory-specific satiety, or integration with olfaction.

References

1. Snyder DJ, Prescott J, Bartoshuk LM. Modern psychophysics and the assessment of human oral sensation. Adv Otorhinolaryngol 2006;63:221–241
2. Kroeze JHA. Is taste mixture suppression a peripheral or central event? In: Laing DG, Cain WS, McBride RL, Ache BW, eds. Reception of Complex Smells and Tastes. Sydney: Academic; 1989: 225–243
3. Yamaguchi S. The synergistic taste effect of monosodium glutamate and disodium 5′inosinate. J Food Sci 1967;32:473–478
4. Von Bekesy G. Sensory Inhibition. Princeton: Princeton University Press; 1967
5. Ogawa H. Taste and smell. In: Ozawa S, Fukuda K, eds. Standard Textbook of Physiology. 7th ed. Tokyo: Igakushoin; 2009: 294–302 [in Japanese]
6. Murray RC. The ultrastructure of taste buds. In: Friedmann I, ed. The Ultrastructure of Sensory Organs. Amsterdam: North Holland Publishing Company; 1973: 1–81
7. Miura H, Kusakabe Y, Harada S. Cell lineage and differentiation in taste buds. Arch Histol Cytol 2006;69(4):209–225
8. Beidler LM, Smallman RL. Renewal of cells within taste buds. J Cell Biol 1965;27(2):263–272
9. Hamamichi R, Asano-Miyoshi M, Emori Y. Taste bud contains both short-lived and long-lived cell populations. Neuroscience 2006;141(4):2129–2138
10. Witt M, Reutter K, Miller IJ Jr. Morphology of the peripheral taste system. In Doty RL, ed. Handbook of Olfaction and Gustation. 2nd ed. New York: Marcel Dekker, Inc; 2003:651–677
11. Miller IJJr, Bartoshuk LM. Taste perception, taste bud distribution, and spatial relationships. In: Getchell TV, Bartoshuk LM, Doty RL, Snow JBJ Jr,

eds. Smell and Taste in Health and Disease. New York: Raven Press; 1991:205–233

12. Doty RL, Bagla R, Morgenson M, Mirza N. NaCl thresholds: relationship to anterior tongue locus, area of stimulation, and number of fungiform papillae. Physiol Behav 2001;72(3):373–378

13. Bealer SL, Smith DV. Multiple sensitivity to chemical stimuli in single human taste papillae. Physiol Behav 1975;14(6):795–799

14. Bachmanov AA, Beauchamp GK. Taste receptor genes. Annu Rev Nutr 2007;27:389–414

15. Chandrashekar J, Hoon MA, Ryba NJP, Zuker CS. The receptors and cells for mammalian taste. Nature 2006;444(7117):288–294

16. Niki M, Yoshida R, Takai S, Ninomiya Y. Gustatory signaling in the periphery: detection, transmission, and modulation of taste information. Biol Pharm Bull 2010;33(11):1772–1777

17. Huang YA, Dando R, Roper SD. Autocrine and paracrine roles for ATP and serotonin in mouse taste buds. J Neurosci 2009;29(44):13909–13918

18. Tomchik SM, Berg S, Kim JW, Chaudhari N, Roper SD. Breadth of tuning and taste coding in mammalian taste buds. J Neurosci 2007;27(40):10840–10848

19. Vandenbeuch A, Tizzano M, Anderson CB, Stone LM, Goldberg D, Kinnamon SC. Evidence for a role of glutamate as an efferent transmitter in taste buds. BMC Neurosci 2010;11(77):77

20. Bartoshuk LM, Rennert K, Rodin J, Stevens JC. Effects of temperature on the perceived sweetness of sucrose. Physiol Behav 1982;28(5):905–910

21. Yamashita S, Sato M. The effects of temperature on gustatory response of rats. J Cell Physiol 1965; 66(1):1–17

22. Damann N, Voets T, Nilius B. TRPs in our senses. Curr Biol 2008;18(18):R880–R889

23. Ozeki M. Conductance change associated with receptor potentials of gustatory cells in rat. J Gen Physiol 1971;58(6):688–699

24. Kinnamon SC, Roper SD. Passive and active membrane properties of mudpuppy taste receptor cells. J Physiol 1987;383:601–614

25. Pritchard TC, Norgren R. Gustatory system. In: Paxinos G, Mai JK, eds. The Human Nervous System. 2nd ed. Amsterdam: Elsevier; 2004:1171–1196

26. Iggo A, Leek BF. The afferent innervation of the tongue of the sheep. In: Hayashi T, ed. Olfaction and Taste II. Oxford: Pergamon Press; 1967: 493–507

27. Frank ME. An analysis of hamster afferent taste nerve response functions. J Gen Physiol 1973; 61(5):588–618

28. Sato M, Ogawa H, Yamashita S. Response properties of macaque monkey chorda tympani fibers. J Gen Physiol 1975;66(6):781–810

29. Sato M, Ogawa H, Yamashita S. Gustatory responsiveness of chorda tympani fibers in the cynomolgus monkey. Chem Senses 1994;19(5):381–400

30. Hellekant G, Danilova V, Ninomiya Y. Primate sense of taste: behavioral and single chorda tympani and glossopharyngeal nerve fiber recordings in the rhesus monkey, Macaca mulatta. J Neurophysiol 1997;77(2):978–993

31. Sato M, Yamashita S, Ogawa H. Potentiation of gustatory response to monosodium glutamate in rat chorda tympani fibers by addition of 5'-ribonucleotides. Jpn J Physiol 1970;20(4): 444–464

32. Harada S, Yamamoto T, Yamaguchi K, Kasahara Y. Different characteristics of gustatory responses between the greater superficial petrosal and chorda tympani nerves in the rat. Chem Senses 1997; 22(2):133–140

33. Shingai T. Water fibers in the superior laryngeal nerve of the rat. Jpn J Physiol 1980;30(2):305–307

34. Ogawa H, Yamashita S, Noma A, Sato M. Taste responses in the macaque monkey chorda tympani. Physiol Behav 1972;9(3):325–331

35. Nasse J, Terman D, Venugopal S, Hermann G, Rogers R, Travers JB. Local circuit input to the medullary reticular formation from the rostral nucleus of the solitary tract. Am J Physiol Regul Integr Comp Physiol 2008;295(5):R1391–R1408

36. Rolls TE, Scott TR. Central taste anatomy and neurophysiology. In: Doty RL, ed. Handbook of Olfaction and Gustation. 2nd ed. New York, Basel: Marcel Dekker, Inc; 2003:679–704

37. Ogawa H, Imoto T, Hayama T. Responsiveness of solitario-parabrachial relay neurons to taste and mechanical stimulation applied to the oral cavity in rats. Exp Brain Res 1984;54(2):349–358

38. Hayama T, Ito S, Ogawa H. Responses of solitary tract nucleus neurons to taste and mechanical stimulations of the oral cavity in decerebrate rats. Exp Brain Res 1985;60(2):235–242

39. Van Buskirk RL, Erickson RP. Odorant responses in taste neurons of the rat NTS. Brain Res 1977; 135(2):287–303

40. Hayama T, Hashimoto K, Ogawa H. Anatomical location of a taste-related region in the thalamic reticular nucleus in rats. Neurosci Res 1994; 18(4):291–299

41. Ogawa H, Nomura T. Response properties of thalamocortical relay neurons responsive to natural stimulation of the oral cavity in rats. Ann N Y Acad Sci 1987;510:532–534

42. Nomura T, Ogawa H. The taste and mechanical response properties of neurons in the parvicellular part of the thalamic posteromedial ventral nucleus of the rat. Neurosci Res 1985;3(2):91–105

43. Burton H, Benjamin RM. Central projections of the gustatory system. In: Beidler LM, ed. Handbook of Sensory Physiology Vol. IV Chemical Senses 2, Taste. Berlin: Springer-Verlag; 1971:148–164

44. Ogawa H. Gustatory cortex of primates: anatomy and physiology. Neurosci Res 1994;20(1):1–13

45. Sanides F. The architecture of the cortical taste nerve areas in squirrel monkey (Saimiri sciureus) and their relationships to insular, sensorimotor and prefrontal regions. Brain Res 1968;8(1):97–124

46. Cipolloni PB, Pandya DN. Cortical connections of the frontoparietal opercular areas in the rhesus monkey. J Comp Neurol 1999;403(4):431–458

47. Baylis LL, Rolls ET, Baylis GC. Afferent connections of caudolateral orbitofrontal cortex taste area of the primate. Neuroscience 1995;64(3):801–812

48. Ogawa H, Ifuku H, Ohgushi M, Nakamura T, Hirata S. Gustatory discrimination behavior and neuronal activity in the gustatory cortex of primates. FFI [In Japanese with English summary] Journal 2007;212:762–774

49. Hayama T, Ogawa H. Callosal connections of the cortical taste area in rats. Brain Res 2001; 918(1–2):171–175

50. Ito S, Ogawa H. Neural activities in the fronto-opercular cortex of macaque monkeys during tasting and mastication. Jpn J Physiol 1994;44(2):141–156

51. Hirata S, Nakamura T, Ifuku H, Ogawa H. Gustatory coding in the precentral extension of area 3 in Japanese macaque monkeys; comparison with area G. Exp Brain Res 2005;165(4):435–446

52. Ogawa H, Hasegawa K, Otawa S, Ikeda I. GABAergic inhibition and modifications of taste responses in the cortical taste area in rats. Neurosci Res 1998; 32(1):85–95

53. Ifuku H, Hirata S, Nakamura T, Ogawa H. Neuronal activities in the monkey primary and higher-order gustatory cortices during a taste discrimination delayed GO/NOGO task and after reversal. Neurosci Res 2003;47(2):161–175

54. Small DM. Central gustatory processing in humans. Adv Otorhinolaryngol 2006;63:191–220

55. Ono T, Tamura R, Nishino H, Nakamura K. Neural mechanisms of recognition and memory in the limbic system. In: Ono R, Squire LR, Raiche ME, et al, eds. Brain Mechanisms of Perception and Memory. New York, Oxford: Oxford University Press; 1993: 330–369

56. Bermudez-Rattoni F, Yamamoto T. Neuroanatomy of CTA: lesions studies. In: Bures J, Bermucez-Rattoni F, Yamamoto T, eds. Conditioned Taste Aversion. Memory of a Special Kind. Oxford: Oxford University Press; 1997: 28–45

57. Börnstein WS. Cortical representation of taste in man and monkey: II. The localization of the cortical taste area in man and a method of measuring impairment of taste in man. Yale J Biol Med 1940; 13(1):133–156

58. Penfield W, Jasper H. III–VIII Gustatory sensation. In: Penfield W, Jasper H, eds. Epilepsy and the Functional Anatomy of the Human Brain. Boston: Little, Brown and Company; 1954:147–149

59. Kobayakawa T, Ogawa H, Kaneda H, Ayabe-Kanamura S, Endo H, Saito S. Spatio-temporal analysis of cortical activity evoked by gustatory stimulation in humans. Chem Senses 1999;24(2): 201–209

60. Cerf-Ducastel B, Van de Moortele PF, MacLeod P, Le Bihan D, Faurion A. Interaction of gustatory and lingual somatosensory perceptions at the cortical level in the human: a functional magnetic resonance imaging study. Chem Senses 2001; 26(4):371–383

61. O'Doherty J, Rolls ET, Francis S, Bowtell R, McGlone F. Representation of pleasant and aversive taste in the human brain. J Neurophysiol 2001;85(3):1315–1321

62. Small DM, Zald DH, Jones-Gotman M, et al. Human cortical gustatory areas: a review of functional neuroimaging data. Neuroreport 1999;10(1):7–14

63. Kobayakawa T, Saito S, Gotow N, Ogawa H. Representation of salty taste stimulus concentrations in the primary gustatory area in humans. Chemosens Percept 2008;1:227–234

64. Barnikol UB, Amunts K, Dammers J, et al. Pattern reversal visual evoked responses of V1/V2 and V5/MT as revealed by MEG combined with probabilistic cytoarchitectonic maps. Neuroimage 2006;31(1):86–108

65. Ogawa H, Wakita M, Hasegawa K, et al. Functional MRI detection of activation in the primary gustatory cortices in humans. Chem Senses 2005; 30(7):583–592

66. Shikama Y, Kato T, Nagaoka U, et al. Localization of the gustatory pathway in the human midbrain. Neurosci Lett 1996;218(3):198–200

67. Lee BC, Hwang SH, Rison R, Chang GY. Central pathway of taste: clinical and MRI study. Eur Neurol 1998;39(4):200–203

68. Onoda K, Ikeda M. Elucidation of taste disorders caused by central lesions. JMAJ 2003;46:296–301

69. Onoda K, Kobayakawa T, Ikeda M, Saito S, Kida A. Laterality of human primary gustatory cortex studied by MEG. Chem Senses 2005;30(8):657–666

70. O'Doherty JP, Deichmann R, Critchley HD, Dolan RJ. Neural responses during anticipation of a primary taste reward. Neuron 2002;33(5):815–826

71. Felsted JA, Ren X, Chouinard-Decorte F, Small DM. Genetically determined differences in brain response to a primary food reward. J Neurosci 2010;30(7):2428–2432

72. Kringelbach ML, O'Doherty J, Rolls ET, Andrews C. Activation of the human orbitofrontal cortex to a liquid food stimulus is correlated with its subjective pleasantness. Cereb Cortex 2003;13(10): 1064–1071

73. O'Doherty J, Rolls ET, Francis S, et al. Sensory-specific satiety-related olfactory activation of the human orbitofrontal cortex. Neuroreport 2000; 11(4):893–897

74. Small DM, Prescott J. Odor/taste integration and the perception of flavor. Exp Brain Res 2005;166(3–4):345–357

75. de Araujo IE, Rolls ET, Kringelbach ML, McGlone F, Phillips N. Taste-olfactory convergence, and the representation of the pleasantness of flavour, in the human brain. Eur J Neurosci 2003;18(7): 2059–2068

76. Wilson JL, Jenkinson M, de Araujo I, Kringelbach ML, Rolls ET, Jezzard P. Fast, fully automated global and local magnetic field optimization for fMRI of the human brain. Neuroimage 2002;17(2):967–976

77. Haase L, Cerf-Ducastel B, Murphy C. Cortical activation in response to pure taste stimuli during the physiological states of hunger and satiety. Neuroimage 2009;44(3):1008–1021

78. O'Doherty J, Rolls ET, Francis S, Bowtell R, McGlone F. Representation of pleasant and aversive taste in the human brain. J Neurophysiol 2001;85(3):1315–1321

79. Kobayakawa T, Saito S, Gotow N. Temporal characteristics of neural activity associated with perception of gustatory stimulus intensity in humans. Chemosens Percept 2012;5(1):80–86

14 Taste Testing

Tino Just, Masafumi Sakagami

General Remarks on Gustatory Testing

In the general population, isolated taste disturbances are rare. Using two different psychophysical taste tests, hypogeusia was found in ~5% of a group of 761 healthy subjects.[1] Complete ageusia is very rare. Taste testing in clinical practice is mainly restricted to departments of otorhinolaryngology and neurology, or to taste and smell centers involved in the treatment of diseases that may cause taste disorders. Ear, nose, and throat (ENT)-related causes of taste disturbance include middle ear surgery, tonsillectomy, oropharyngeal surgery (including oncological treatment), and procedures associated with lingual compression.[2]

Taste in humans begins on the tongue, where taste cells of different gustatory papillae (fungiform, foliate, and circumvallate papillae with taste buds) detect contact-chemical cues. The three different morphological types of taste-detecting papillae are topographically arranged on the tongue. Fungiform papillae are located on the anterior two-thirds of the tongue, while foliate papillae and circumvallate papillae are found on the lateral edges and on the posterior third of the tongue, respectively. Sensitivity to all tastes (sweet, sour, salty, bitter, and umami) is found in all areas of the human tongue,[3] and there is no evidence that there is a tongue map.[4] However, some studies have revealed that some tongue regions are more sensitive to natural stimuli than others.[5,6] Similar findings were reported in electrogustometric studies.[7,8] In electrogustometry (electric stimulation of small regions of the tongue) in healthy humans, electric thresholds are higher on the tongue edge than on the tongue tip.[8] This should be kept in mind when comparing gustatory results in healthy humans with those in patients with taste disorders.

This chapter describes common clinical taste tests, including questionnaires mainly in Europe and Japan.

> Isolated taste disturbances are rare.

Patient History

In more than two-thirds of patients, a detailed patient history provides diagnostic evidence of disturbances of the olfactory and gustatory system.[9] In most cases, patients suffering from smell and taste loss have isolated smell disorders or a combined olfactory and gustatory impairment rather than an isolated taste disturbance.[10] Loss of smell presenting as taste loss, with normal findings on gustatory testing, is described as a "flavor disturbance."[10] Taste and flavor are generally used as synonyms. Retronasal olfaction has a strong influence on flavor perception and supports the need for a standardized psychophysical taste and smell test, rather than relying on the patients' symptoms alone. Additionally, patients with anosmia have poorer sensitivity to all taste qualities than normosmics.[11]

Another aspect that is important to consider is innervation of the gustatory system. On both sides, different nerves (the chorda tympani for the anterior two-thirds of the tongue and the glossopharyngeal nerve for the posterior part of the tongue) provide a gustatory supply for the tongue; the petrosal nerve supplies the soft palate.[12] Somatosensory supply is provided by the trigeminal nerve. Patients reporting numbness or tactile dysgeusia[13] of the tongue are often unaware whether the trigeminal or the gustatory system is affected.

The following aspects need to be clarified in the patient history:

- Surgery in the head and neck region[14]: middle ear,[15,16] including stapes, surgery[17]; dental procedures; tonsillectomy[18]; oropharyngeal surgery; oncological therapy; procedures with lingual compression, such as surgery in general anesthesia; microlaryngoscopy[18]; tracheal intubation; and surgery of the nasal septum or paranasal cavities
- Trauma
- Medication: numerous drugs[19] and toxic agents[20] are known to cause taste disturbances
- Infections: influenza-like infections of the upper respiratory airways may cause loss of smell and tend to lead to taste disturbances, but may also cause flavor disturbances; infections

within the oral cavity, and also of the middle ear, may damage the gustatory system[21]
- Burning mouth syndrome (primary and secondary): oral symptoms such as burning, tingling, pain, and dryness may affect the gustatory and trigeminal system of the oral cavity[22]
- Systemic diseases: renal insufficiency, diabetes, diseases of the lower digestive tract, metabolic disorders, Sjögren syndrome[23]
- Neurological or psychiatric diseases

Questionnaire

Taste disorders are less common than olfactory impairments and most actually reflect olfactory disorders. Taste disorders are classified as qualitative or quantitative.[24] The latter includes ageusia (inability to taste) and hypogeusia (decreased ability to taste). Quantitative taste disorders are less frequent than qualitative taste disorders and can be total (all tastes involved), partial (affecting several tastes), or specific (only one or a select few tastes). Qualitative disorders, or dysgeusia, describe a distorted ability to taste, and include parageusia (unpleasant taste sensation, usually metallic, on taste stimulation) and phantogeusia (often permanent taste in the mouth, e.g., metallic or salty, for which no external stimulus can be found).

The accuracy of self-reporting in detecting taste disorders is poor.[25] The relatively low prevalence of taste disorders in the general population, and the tendency to confuse olfactory loss with taste impairment, contributes to this low accuracy.[25] However, questionnaires have been shown to be accurate in detecting patients with *no* taste disorders: patients who reported no problems with the ability to taste sweet, sour, bitter, and salty demonstrated normal taste sensitivity.

In contrast to qualitative taste disorders, quantitative taste disorders can be measured by psychophysical taste tests.

Psychophysical Taste Testing

Many psychophysical taste tests have been introduced to assess peripheral gustatory sensitivity. In general, two test tools can be distinguished. The first tool uses natural stimuli to measure the ability to taste sweet, sour, salty, bitter, and umami.

This tool may be used as a whole-mouth method or as regional taste test to detect side differences.

The second tool uses electric currents applied to the tongue surface to elicit taste perceptions, and is named electrogustometry (EGM). EGM is an excellent method for measuring side differences in patients with taste disorders, provided that electric thresholds can be measured. It is assumed that electrogustometry also costimulates the trigeminal system. Recent studies revealed that gustatory and trigeminal fibers act together peripherally.[26,27] In clinical practice, particularly in patients with symptoms such as numbness and burning of the tongue, it can be helpful to assess both the gustatory and the trigeminal system. Therefore, a somatosensory test will also be presented.

In this section, we describe widely accepted taste tests and categorize them as tests using natural chemicals (sweet, sour, salty, bitter, and umami), or those using non-natural stimuli (electric current). Chemical taste tests are further divided into whole-mouth tests or regional tests.

Taste Tests with Natural Chemicals

Whole-mouth Test

Three-drop Method

This taste test using liquid taste solutions was first introduced by Henkin et al[28] A modified test procedure and normative data from the clinical taste test were presented in 2007 by Gudziol and Hummel.[29] With a 10-μL pipette, a series of three drops of a liquid solution (one drop of tastant and two drops of solvent) is placed in a pseudorandomized order on the midline of the patient's extended tongue. After swishing the drop in the closed mouth, the subject is asked to identify its taste quality. Four verbal gustatory descriptors are presented (sweet, sour, salty, and bitter). A multiple forced-choice procedure is used. Eight triplets are presented to the patient in ascending order, starting with the lowest concentration. Between each triplet presentation, rinsing the mouth with tap water is allowed. Steps of increased concentration are presented until the subject recognizes the taste solution correctly in two consecutive trials. Thus, scores for each taste quality range between 1 and 9. To obtain the overall gustatory test result, the scores of all taste qualities are added to provide a total score. Age- and gender-related normative data are available for each taste quality and for the total score (whole mouth).[29]

Tasting Tablets and Wafers

An alternative procedure is to use tablets of four tastants[30] (sweet, sour, salty, and bitter) instead of liquid solutions. Four tasteless tablets and tablets with six concentrations of four tastants (sucrose, citric acid, sodium chloride, and caffeine) are presented. They are administered in ascending and pseudorandomized order, starting with the lowest concentration. The taste test provides a good test–retest reliability ($r = 0.69$, $p < 0.001$). Similar results were achieved with wafers.[31] The flavored wafers can be used for a regional or whole-mouth taste test.[31] The main advantage of taste tests with tablets or wafers over liquid solutions is the long shelf-life of the test kits. The main disadvantage is the lack of age- and gender-related normative data.

Regional Tests

Taste Strips

The taste strip test is a well-established quantitative test using impregnated taste strips. This test was first introduced in 2003.[32] Filter paper strips (taste strips) with four concentrations of four tastants (sucrose, citric acid, sodium chloride, and quinine hydrochloride) are used (**Table 14.1**). The strips are placed on the left or right side of the anterior third of the extended tongue. Before taste testing and between each applica-

tion, the mouth is rinsed with water. Taste strips are presented in a randomized and ascending order, starting with the lowest concentration of each tastant and alternating the side of presentation. This procedure results in 32 trials (16 trials of each tongue side). Leaving the tongue extended, the patient has to identify the taste quality using gustatory descriptors (sweet, sour, salty, bitter) in a multiple forced-choice procedure. Besides side-related scores, overall gustatory sensitivity is calculated by adding up the scores of both sides to create a total score. With the taste strip method, a test–retest reliability of $r = 0.68$ was achieved (three-drop method $r = 0.69$).[32] Age- and gender-related normative data for the taste strip test were presented in 2009.[33] This test is useful in routine clinical practice. The aim of further studies is to add monosodium glutamate (umami taste) and to extend the validated test.

Filter Paper Disc Method

The filter paper disc (FPD) test (**Fig. 14.1**) is a qualitative clinical tasting test developed by Tomita et al[34] It measures four (sweet, sour, salty, and bitter) taste qualities at five different concentrations (**Table 14.1**). The FPD test uses a round filter paper disc, 5 mm in diameter, impregnated with a drop of tastant solution. Sucrose is used for the sweet taste, sodium chloride for the salty taste, tartaric acid for the sour taste, and quinine hydrochloride for the bitter taste. The impregnated filter paper discs are placed at the same points on the tongue as for EGM. The taste solutions are presented in ascending order from the lowest concentration. The taste qualities and area, however, are presented

Table 14.1 Taste solutions and concentrations of the various taste tests

	Sweet	Sour	Salty	Bitter
Taste strips[32]	Sucrose (0.05, 0.1, 0.2, 0.4 g/mL)	Citric acid (0.05, 0.09, 0.165, 0.3 g/mL)	Sodium chloride (0.016, 0.04, 0.1, 0.25 g/mL)	Quinine hydrochloride (0.0004, 0.0009, 0.0024, 0.006 g/mL)
Filter paper disc[34]	Sucrose (0.3, 2.5, 10, 20, 80%)	Tartaric acid (0.02, 0.2, 2, 4, 8%)	Sodium chloride (0.3, 1.25, 5, 10, 20%)	Quinine hydrochloride (0.001, 0.02, 0.1, 4%)
Liquid solutions[36]	Sucrose (0.03, 0.1, 0.4, 2 g/mL)	Citric acid (0.01, 0.05, 0.1, 0.15 g/mL)	Sodium chloride (0.025, 0.075, 0.15, 0.36 g/mL)	Quinine hydrochloride (0.0002, 0.0005, 0.001, 0.01 g/mL)

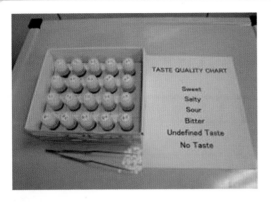

Fig. 14.1 Filter paper disc test.

in a randomized order. The bitter taste should be presented last. When different taste solutions are presented, the mouth needs to be rinsed with water. Patients have to identify the taste from a list of four descriptors (sweet, salty, sour, and bitter) while their tongue is extended. When patients cannot identify the taste clearly, they can choose "Undefined taste" or "No taste," unlike in the taste strip or three-drop methods. The scores of the FPD test range from 1 to 5 for each taste quality, and the regions are lateralized. When the taste can be perceived in the third concentration, taste function is assessed as "within normal limits." When the taste is not identified in the fifth concentration, the score is calculated as "6." The average score for people over 60 years old is ~1 point higher than that for young people. The FPD score for the area innervated by the greater petrosal nerve is particularly influenced by age. When high scores are observed in this area, this finding might be of little significance. The age-related changes start at the age of 30 years.

Tomita et al[34] demonstrated a significant correlation between EGM and FPD tests in an area innervated by the chorda tympani nerve in patients with facial palsy. Ellegård et al[35] reported that there was a significant correlation between EGM threshold and the whole-mouth perception of all tastes, and it was no stronger for sour taste perception than for other taste qualities.

Liquid Solutions

Regional taste tests are also available with liquid tastants.[36] For lateralized assessment of gustatory sensitivity, ~20 µL of liquid tastants (sucrose, citric acid, sodium chloride, and quinine hydrochloride) are administered using a glass probe on both sides of the anterior third of the extended tongue (**Table 14.1**). The administration of the test is similar to taste strips, apart from the descriptors available for answering ("no taste" was added) and the concentrations of the gustatory stimuli. The test–retest reliability of this test is $r = 0.77$. Age- and gender-related normative data are available.

Electrogustometry

The first electrogustometer for clinical use, together with preliminary results from 140 patients, was reported in 1959.[37–39] Krarup replaced the taste solution for taste testing with an inadequate taste stimulus, an electric current.

The existence of electrical taste is common knowledge. When a stimulus produced from a direct-current stainless steel node is applied to the tongue, a taste sensation similar to that of licking metal (metallic taste) is perceived. The electrogustometer (RION TR-06 model, Rion Co., Ltd, Tokyo, Japan) (**Fig. 14.2**) is widely used for the quantitative assessment of lateralized gustatory function in Japan. It has also been used for a variety of clinical purposes, including evaluation of peripheral nervous function in patients with facial palsy, peripheral nervous damage in diabetes, damage to the chorda tympani after middle ear surgery, and other conditions. The electrogustometer comprises an anode, a cathode, and a switch to initiate the stimulation. The neutral electrode must be applied to the neck of the patients to avoid passing an electric current through their heart. Patients with a pacemaker or a cochlear implant should not, in theory, be examined using this method.

The magnitude of the electric stimulation can be varied continuously on a logarithmic scale employing the method of Tomita et al.[34] According to the scale, 8 µA, which is the arithmetic mean value for normal subjects, is defined as 0 dB. The lowest current level is 4 µA (–6 dB) and the highest is 400 µA (34 dB). The score scale-out is defined as 36 dB. Before the assessment, patients are told that electric taste is not a tactile sensation but a metallic taste, and are presented with a 10 to 20 dB current, which can be perceived easily. Direct-current anodic stimulation, ascending in 2-dB steps, is then applied to regions innervated by three gustatory nerves (greater petrosal, glossopharyngeal, and chorda tympani nerves, lateralized) using 5-mm-diameter stainless steel electrodes.

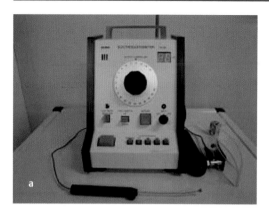
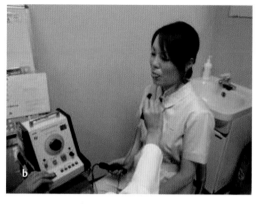

Fig. 14.2a, b Electrogustometer RION TR-06 model used for research and diagnosis in Japan.

a Electrogustometer.

b Electrogustometer in use.

To assess the chorda tympani nerve, the measured point is at the edge of the tongue, ~2 cm away from the center of the tongue tip. In the area innervated by the glossopharyngeal nerve, stimuli are presented on the circumvallate papillae. If patients show a strong gag reflex, it is possible to switch to the foliate papillae near the palatine arch. For the area innervated by the greater petrosal nerve on the palate, we measure at a point 1 cm above the arch of the palate and 1 cm lateral to the center (**Fig. 14.3**).

The TR-06 electrogustometer allows the presentation of low-current stimuli of different durations (0.5, 1.0, and 1.5 seconds). The duration is set at 0.5 seconds in our clinic. It was reported by Loucks and Doty[40] that the duration of the stimulus influences gustatory thresholds. However, because of habituation or adaptation to the stimulus, a longer duration did not necessarily lead to greater sensitivity. In addition, taste sensation adapts to repeated stimulation, so 1.5-second intervals are needed. The normal values of electric taste are 0 ± 8, 4 ± 14, and 10 ± 22 dB, in regions of the chorda tympani nerve, glossopharyngeal nerve, and greater petrosal nerve, respectively. It is normal for the difference between left and right sides to be under 6 dB for each area. When the electrical stimulus is over 20 dB at the anterior tongue, patients can perceive algesthesia on the tongue surface or diffused into the neck. As mentioned above, EGM also stimulates the trigeminal system. However, the taste threshold is different from the trigeminal threshold. We need to confirm which patients can perceive degustation or algesthesia. The threshold of electrical taste increases with

age. Nakazato et al[41] reported that the thresholds of regions innervated by the chorda tympani and glossopharyngeal nerves in people were higher in those over 60 years old, and people in their 70s or older demonstrated a significantly higher electrical taste threshold in regions innervated by the greater petrosal nerve. The authors reported that the thresholds of electrical taste were unaffected

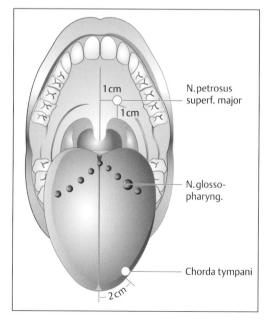

Fig. 14.3 The location for the assessment of each taste nerve (quoted from ref. 34). N. petrosus superf. major, greater superficial petrosal nerve; N. glossopharyng., glossopharyngeal nerve.

by smoking or dentures. In addition, thresholds in women are lower than those in men.

Somatosensory Test

Taste and intraoral somatosensation are closely related. Taste receptors of the tongue papillae are close to mechanoreceptors, nociceptors, and thermoreceptors. Some taste stimuli may also induce tactile, thermal sensations, such as tingling and burning.[42] Some tastants, such as salts and acids, may activate somatosensory receptors, and can produce burning and tingling.[43]

The capsaicin threshold test has been established to measure somatosensory perception in humans.[8] This test uses capsaicin-impregnated filter paper strips similar to taste strips.[32] The filter paper strips are impregnated with five concentrations of capsaicin (0.0001 to 1%). The strips are placed midline on the tongue tip for whole-mouth testing, for which the mouth is closed, or on the tongue edge of both sides for lateralized testing, for which the tongue is extended. Thresholds related to sensory perception and intensity are measured. The test appears applicable to basic research,[22,27] but so far not for clinical use. There are no age- or gender-related normative data for the test. Thresholds depend mainly on food habits, in particular ingestion of spicy or hot food.

> Diagnosis of taste disturbance includes questionnaire administration and psychophysical taste testing (whole-mouth taste test and regional taste and somatosensory tests).

Objective Measurements

Gustatory Event-related Potentials

Gustatory-evoked potentials elicited by gaseous stimuli (acetic acid for sour; chloroform for sweet; thujone for bitter; ammonium chloride for salty) were first reported in 1985.[44] Now, commercial devices are available that allow objective assessment of taste-eliciting gustatory event-related potentials in humans. The custom-made gustometer (gustometer 002, Burghart Messtech-

nik, Wedel, Germany) (**Fig. 14.4**) enables the presentation of up to five different tastants (highly concentrated solutions of salt, citric acid, sugar, quinine, or glutamate). A continuous water flow avoids thermal or mechanical stimulation. An initial study has demonstrated the usefulness of this method in clinical practice, but as yet only the taste quality sour (citric acid) has been used.[45] Further research is needed to establish all taste qualities.

Magnetic Resonance Imaging

The neural processes of taste perception and taste intensity may be visualized with functional magnetic resonance imaging (fMRI). So far, two studies have been published that investigated neural representation of taste intensity after sweet and bitter stimulation[46] and after sweet and salty stimulation.[47] Several brain regions are involved in the differentiation of sweet and bitter taste intensities: the cerebellum, putamen, pons, amygdala, and middle insula.[46] Similar results were reported by Spetter et al[47] They found that taste intensity is represented in the middle insula, but amygdala activation was only found by stimulation with saltiness. Sweet taste intensity was not represented in the amygdala. So far, fMRI has been used to explore scientific questions. In the future, fMRI may become a potential tool for objective taste testing in clinical practice.

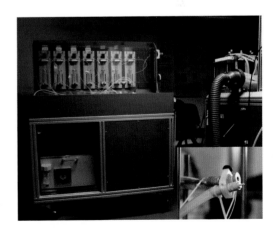

Fig. 14.4 Gustometer for clinical assessment of gustatory function using event-related potentials (gustometer 002, Burghart Messtechnik, Wedel, Germany); inset shows the nozzle element for stimulus presentation.

In Vivo Imaging of the Taste Buds

Attempts to visualize the peripheral gustatory organ in vivo were first published in 2004.[48] The authors used a confocal laser scanning microscope (**Fig. 14.5**) to identify a single fungiform papilla on the human tongue[49] and to measure the volume of the taste buds over time.[50]

To facilitate serial investigations of the same papilla, reference papillae are defined. These are fungiform papillae with a characteristic shape or arrangement of surface taste pores (**Fig. 14.6**).

Preliminary studies demonstrated differences in taste bud volume over time in healthy humans.[49,50] Volumetric data of taste buds from a patient with hypogeusia and with side-differing measurements in gustatory testing seem to differ from those in healthy subjects.[51] Further studies are needed to establish the potential of this novel in vivo method for diagnosis of taste disturbances.

In the future, objective methods may become a potential tool to assess taste processing objectively and to visualize peripheral taste organs and neural processes of taste perception.

Case Reports

Case 1

A 40-year-old woman underwent tympanoplasty for cholesteatoma on the right side. Her chorda tympani nerve (CTN) was transected during the surgery. This nerve confers general sensations on the tongue surface.[26,27] After surgery, the patient complained of taste disorder and tongue numbness in the region of right CTN innervation. Her taste functions before and after surgery are shown in **Table 14.2**. Although the symptoms began to disappear 2 weeks after surgery, the elevated EGM threshold continued for more than 2 years.

Saito et al[52] reported that an elevated EGM threshold in patients with CTN injury is not necessarily related to their symptoms. They also reported that CTN regeneration was observed in 42.3% of patients with a transected CTN. In another study, the symptoms disappeared more than 2 years after surgery in 88.9% of the patients with a transected CTN, regardless of the absence of EGM threshold recovery in 54.5%.[16] Subjective taste is expressed as a whole-mouth taste sensation. Inhibition of glossopharyngeal nerve function is released, which compensates for CTN damage. Therefore, a discrepancy in recovery between the symptoms and EGM threshold is often observed. EGM is available for localizing the site of anatomical deficit following damage to the CTN.

Case 2

A 55-year-old woman had a severe motor vehicle accident. Head magnetic resonance imaging and computed tomography (CT) showed bilateral frontal brain and cerebellum injury and occipital fracture (**Fig. 14.7**). Although there was no temporal bone fracture on head CT, she had facial palsy on the right side. Owing to the aggravation of cerebral hematoma and edema, she underwent craniotomy

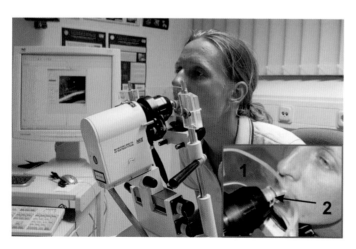

Fig. 14.5 Clinical setting for in vivo examination of the gustatory organs: parabolic Plexiglas disc. Inset: contact element of the water immersion objective lens: 1, parabolic Plexiglas disc; 2, contact element of the water immersion objective lens. (From Just et al.[54])

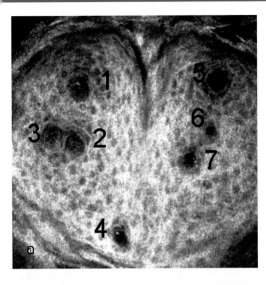

Fig. 14.6a, b Laser scanning photomicrographs of fungiform papillae.

a En-face confocal laser scanning photomicrograph of a single butterfly-shaped fungiform papilla with six taste pores (labeled 1–7) visible on the surface (400 × 400 μm).

b Cross section of confocal laser scanning photomicrograph of a fungiform papilla. The height of the taste bud is ~40 μm.

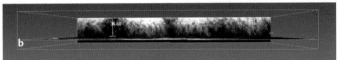

Table 14.2 Pre- and postoperative results of electrogustometry and filter paper disc testing in Case 1

	Preoperative		Postoperative				
			2 weeks after surgery		2 years after surgery		
	Operated side	Contralateral side	Operated side	Contralateral side	Operated side	Contralateral side	
EGM (dB)	-6	-2	34	-2	28	-2	
FPD score (average)	1.5	2	6	2.5	5.5	2.75	

EGM, electrogustometry; FPD, filter paper disc.

to remove the hematoma 2 hours after the accident. She presented with ageusia and anosmia 4 months after the accident. Although the impaired detection threshold was mild, identification threshold impairment was severe on olfactory function testing. Her taste testing results at the first examination and 2 years later are shown in **Table 14.3**. At the first examination, her EGM threshold was approximately within normal limits to mild impairment, except on the right anterior side, which was innervated by the damaged facial nerve at that time. However, a severely impaired perception of taste was observed on FPD testing. There were discrepancies between detection and iden-

tification thresholds in both smell and taste testing. Reiter et al[53] reported that detection threshold levels were useful in evaluating the receptor cell function, whereas identification scores might be more specific for brain injury. They also reported that spontaneous recovery from post-traumatic ageusia occurred more frequently than that from post-traumatic anosmia.

The patient's ageusia and anosmia were treated with nasal steroid drops and oral zinc sulfate, respectively. Although anosmia did not recover at all, ageusia was mostly improved in this case. The patient's facial palsy also recovered completely.

A marked difference between the two kinds of taste test is observed in patients with several encephalopathies, for example, stroke, cerebral tumor, head trauma, and other cerebral conditions. These conditions may affect cognitive gustatory functions, but detection function is often preserved. This finding of dissociation can also indicate early damage to the turnover of taste receptors. Electrical taste can sometimes be perceived even when FPD test results are inconclusive. Theoretically, an electric current is a stronger stimulus than chemical tastant. As in this case, taste function tends to recover. Therefore, both qualitative and quantitative taste testing methods, such as EGM and FPD tests, are needed to confirm the diagnosis.

References

1. Welge-Lüssen A, Dörig P, Wolfensberger M, Krone F, Hummel T. A study about the frequency of taste disorders. J Neurol J Neurol 2011;258(3):386–392
2. Landis BN, Lacroix JS. Postoperative/posttraumatic gustatory dysfunction. Adv Otorhinolaryngol 2006; 63:242–254
3. Smith DV, Margolskee RF. Making sense of taste. Sci Am 2001;284(3):32–39

Table 14.3 Pre- and post-therapy results of electrogustometry and filter paper disc testing in Case 2

| | | EGM (dB) | | FPD score | | | | | | | |
| | | | | Sweet | | Salty | | Sour | | Bitter | |
		R	L	R	L	R	L	R	L	R	L
	Chorda tympani nerve	36	0	6	6	6	6	6	6	6	6
Pre-therapy	Glossopharyng. nerve	20	18	6	6	6	6	5	5	5	5
	Greater petrosal nerve	26	24	6	6	6	6	6	6	6	6
	Chorda tympani nerve	6	-4	4	2	5	2	6	2	3	3
Post-therapy	Glossopharyng. nerve	20	14	4	4	5	4	5	5	4	4
	Greater petrosal nerve	18	22	4	4	4	4	4	4	5	4

EGM, electrogustometry; FPD, filter paper disc.

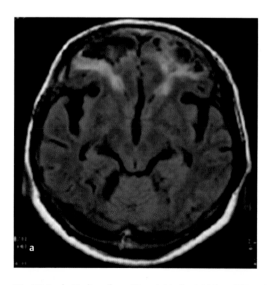
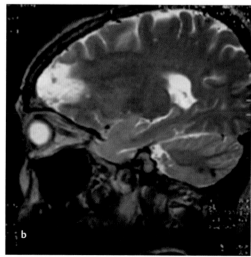

Fig. 14.7a, b Findings from T1-weighted axial (a) and T2-weighted sagittal (b) MRI immediately after the incident in Case 2. Cerebral edema and contusions are seen in the frontal lobe.

4. Chandrashekar J, Hoon MA, Ryba NJP, Zuker CS. The receptors and cells for mammalian taste. Nature 2006;444(7117):288–294

5. Doty RL, Bagla R, Morgenson M, Mirza N. NaCl thresholds: relationship to anterior tongue locus, area of stimulation, and number of fungiform papillae. Physiol Behav 2001;72(3):373–378

6. Kiesow F. Beitrag zur physiologischen Psychologie des Geschmackssinnes (1894): Kessinger Publishing; 2009

7. Miller SL, Mirza N, Doty RL. Electrogustometric thresholds: relationship to anterior tongue locus, area of stimulation, and number of fungiform papillae. Physiol Behav 2002;75(5):753–757

8. Just T, Pau HW, Steiner S, Hummel T. Assessment of oral trigeminal sensitivity in humans. Eur Arch Otorhinolaryngol 2007;264(5):545–551

9. Temmel AF, Quint C, Schickinger-Fischer B, Klimek L, Stoller E, Hummel T. Characteristics of olfactory disorders in relation to major causes of olfactory loss. Arch Otolaryngol Head Neck Surg 2002;128(6):635–641

10. Fujii M, Fukazawa K, Hashimoto Y, et al. Clinical study of flavor disturbance. Acta Otolaryngol Suppl 2004;(553):109–112

11. Gudziol H, Rahneberg K, Burkert S. Anosmics are more poorly able to taste than normal persons. [Article in German] Laryngorhinootologie 2007; 86(9):640–643

12. Ikeda M, Ikui A, Tomita H. Gustatory function of the soft palate. Acta Otolaryngol Suppl 2002; (546):69–73

13. Chen JM, Bodmer D, Khetani JD, Lin VV. Tactile dysgeusia: a new clinical observation of middle ear and skull base surgery. Laryngoscope 2008; 118(1):99–103

14. Landis BN, Lacroix JS. Taste disorders. B-ENT 2009;5(Suppl 13):123–128

15. Sakagami M, Sone M, Tsuji K, Fukazawa K, Mishiro Y. Rate of recovery of taste function after preservation of chorda tympani nerve in middle ear surgery with special reference to type of disease. Ann Otol Rhinol Laryngol 2003;112(1):52–56

16. Nin T, Sakagami M, Sone-Okunaka M, Muto T, Mishiro Y, Fukazawa K. Taste function after section of chorda tympani nerve in middle ear surgery. Auris Nasus Larynx 2006;33(1):13–17

17. Miuchi S, Sakagami M, Tsuzuki K, Noguchi K, Mishiro Y, Katsura H. Taste disturbance after stapes surgery—clinical and experimental study. Acta Otolaryngol Suppl 2009;(562):71–78

18. Tomofuji S, Sakagami M, Kushida K, Terada T, Mori H, Kakibuchi M. Taste disturbance after tonsillectomy and laryngomicrosurgery. Auris Nasus Larynx 2005;32(4):381–386

19. Griffin JP. Drug-induced disorders of taste. Adverse Drug React Toxicol Rev 1992;11(4):229–239

20. Reiter ER, DiNardo LJ, Costanzo RM. Toxic effects on gustatory function. Adv Otorhinolaryngol 2006; 63:265–277

21. Terada T, Sone M, Tsuji K, Mishiro Y, Sakagami M. Taste function in elderly patients with unilateral middle ear disease. Acta Otolaryngol Suppl 2004;(553):113–116

22. Just T, Steiner S, Pau HW. Oral pain perception and taste in burning mouth syndrome. J Oral Pathol Med 2010;39(1):22–27

23. Negoro A, Umemoto M, Fujii M, et al. Taste function in Sjögren's syndrome patients with special reference to clinical tests. Auris Nasus Larynx 2004;31(2):141–147

24. Landis BN, Just T. Taste disorders. An update. [Article in German] HNO 2010;58(7):650–655

25. Soter A, Kim J, Jackman A, Tourbier I, Kaul A, Doty RL. Accuracy of self-report in detecting taste dysfunction. Laryngoscope 2008;118(4):611–617

26. Perez R, Fuoco G, Dorion JM, Ho PH, Chen JM. Does the chorda tympani nerve confer general sensation from the tongue? Otolaryngol Head Neck Surg 2006;135(3):368–373

27. Just T, Steiner S, Strenger T, Pau HW. Changes of oral trigeminal sensitivity in patients after middle ear surgery. Laryngoscope 2007;117(9):1636–1640

28. Henkin RI, Gill JR, Bartter FC. Studies on taste thresholds in normal man and in patients with adrenal cortical insufficiency: The role of adrenal cortical steroids and of serum sodium concentration. J Clin Invest 1963;42(5):727–735

29. Gudziol H, Hummel T. Normative values for the assessment of gustatory function using liquid tastants. Acta Otolaryngol 2007;127(6):658–661

30. Ahne G, Erras A, Hummel T, Kobal G. Assessment of gustatory function by means of tasting tablets. Laryngoscope 2000;110(8):1396–1401

31. Hummel T, Erras A, Kobal G. A test for the screening of taste function. Rhinology 1997;35(4):146–148

32. Mueller C, Kallert S, Renner B, et al. Quantitative assessment of gustatory function in a clinical context using impregnated "taste strips." Rhinology 2003;41(1):2–6

33. Landis BN, Welge-Luessen A, Brämerson A, et al. "Taste Strips"—a rapid, lateralized, gustatory bedside identification test based on impregnated filter papers. J Neurol 2009;256(2):242–248

34. Tomita H, Ikeda M, Okuda Y. Basis and practice of clinical taste examinations. Auris Nasus Larynx 1986;13(Suppl 1):S1–S15

35. Ellegård EK, Goldsmith D, Hay KD, Stillman JA, Morton RP. Studies on the relationship between electrogustometry and sour taste perception. Auris vNasus Larynx 2007;34(4):477–480

36. Pingel J, Ostwald J, Pau HW, Hummel T, Just T. Normative data for a solution-based taste test. Eur Arch Otorhinolaryngol 2010;267(12):1911–1917

37. Krarup B. Electrogustometry: A new method for clinical taste examination. Acta Otolaryngol 1958;49:294–395

38. Krarup B. On the technique of gustatory examinations. Acta Otolaryngol Suppl 1958;140:195–200

39. Krarup B. Electrogustometric examinations in cerebellopontine tumors and on taste pathways. Neurology 1959;9(1):53–61

40. Loucks CA, Doty RL. Effects of stimulation duration on electrogustometric thresholds. Physiol Behav 2004;81(1):1–4

41. Nakazato M, Endo S, Yoshimura I, Tomita H. Influence of aging on electrogustometry thresholds. Acta Otolaryngol Suppl 2002;(546):16–26

42. Green BG, Hayes JE. Capsaicin as a probe of the relationship between bitter taste and chemesthesis. Physiol Behav 2003;79(4–5):811–821

43. Green BG, Gelhard B. Salt as an oral irritant. Chem Senses 1989;14:259–271

44. Kobal G. Gustatory evoked potentials in man. Electroencephalogr Clin Neurophysiol 1985;62(6):449–454

45. Hummel T, Genow A, Landis BN. Clinical assessment of human gustatory function using event related potentials. J Neurol Neurosurg Psychiatry 2010;81(4):459–464

46. Small DM, Gregory MD, Mak YE, Gitelman D, Mesulam MM, Parrish T. Dissociation of neural representation of intensity and affective valuation in human gustation. Neuron 2003;39(4):701–711

47. Spetter MS, Smeets PA, de Graaf C, Viergever MA. Representation of sweet and salty taste intensity in the brain. Chem Senses 2010;35(9):831–840

48. Just T, Zeisner C, Stave J, Pau HW. Confocal laser-scanning microscopy to analyse the epithelium of the tongue. [Article in German] Laryngorhinootologie 2004;83(2):108–112

49. Just T, Srur E, Stachs O, Pau HW. Volumetry of human taste buds using laser scanning microscopy. J Laryngol Otol 2009;123(10):1125–1130

50. Srur E, Stachs O, Guthoff R, Witt M, Pau HW, Just T. Change of the human taste bud volume over time. Auris Nasus Larynx 2010;37(4):449–455

51. Srur E, Pau HW, Just T. Changes in taste bud volume during taste disturbance. Auris Nasus Larynx 2011;38(4):512–515

52. Saito T, Manabe Y, Shibamori Y, et al. Long-term follow-up results of electrogustometry and subjective taste disorder after middle ear surgery. Laryngoscope 2001;111(11 Pt 1):2064–2070

53. Reiter ER, DiNardo LJ, Costanzo RM. Effects of head injury on olfaction and taste. Otolaryngol Clin North Am 2004;37(6):1167–1184

54. Just T, Pau HW, Bombor I, Guthoff RF, Fietkau R, Hummel T. Confocal microscopy of the peripheral gustatory system: comparison between healthy subjects and patients suffering from taste disorders during radiochemotherapy. Laryngoscope 2005;115(12):2178–2182

15 Taste Disorders

Basile N. Landis, Josef G. Heckmann

Summary

Taste disorders are frequently encountered in specialized outpatient clinics. However, they occur less often than olfactory disorders. Most patients with taste disorders suffer considerably, which can present as gustatory loss, or decreased or changed gustatory perception. Within this chapter, we present the different causes, diagnostic procedures, and possible therapies for taste disorders.

Introduction

Talking about taste always requires clarification between the medical term taste and "taste" as it is used in daily language. Taste used in everyday language means the sensations one experiences during eating or drinking. This is composed of texture, retronasal smell, and "pure" taste inputs. The physiological definition of taste is restricted to the five qualities sweet, sour, salty, bitter, and umami (the taste of glutamate). As a consequence, most people confuse olfaction and gustation. For example, most patients with olfactory dysfunction complain of smell and taste alteration, while testing reveals that olfaction but not the five basic tastes are affected.[1]

In clinical practice, patients rarely present with taste disorders restricted to the five basic tastes. The reason for this low incidence is not clear. One explanation could be that many taste disorders are transient, and patients only seek medical advice for long-lasting or permanent taste disorders. Another explanation could be that many patients with taste disorders have concomitant, more troublesome health problems (e.g., facial paresis, stroke) and forget to mention the taste disorder. Taste assessment is far from a routine procedure, and the low incidence of taste deficits may simply reflect the fact that this sense is rarely tested. Finally, taste is represented by three cranial nerves per side, making taste innervation redundant. This could lead to a higher resistance of taste to trauma and injury, thus explaining the few taste disorders observed in clinical practice. An intact sense of taste is significant in the regulation of nourishment, the recognition of poisonous and rotten food, and even for the experience of the hedonic aspects of a common meal.

Recent routine taste testing in a large sample of the general population showed that measurable taste impairment is more frequent than previously thought. In a cohort of 761 healthy individuals aged 5 to 89 years, reduced taste function was measured in 5%, despite the fact that these individuals considered their taste capacity to be normal. Most of these cases were hypogeusia; ageusia was observed rarely.[2] While taking the patient's history, it is therefore important to ask specific questions such as, "Do you have problems tasting sweet, sour, salty, or bitter flavors?" The isolated question, "Do you have taste problems?" is too vague and will be answered too often with no, even when taste problems exist.[3]

Taste problems can be an important sign or symptom in daily clinical practice, as several case vignettes report. Severe taste disorders can occur after laryngoscopy,[4] stroke,[5] temporal bone fracture,[6] dissection of the brain-supplying arteries,[7] in celiac disease,[8] or even as a paraneoplastic symptom.[9] Such severe taste disorders can lead to anorexia, weight loss, and impairment of well-being. An isolated impairment of gustatory sensitivity to salt was recently identified as a risk factor for arterial hypertension.[10]

> There is confusion between smell and taste symptoms. Taste disorders can be the first symptom of underlying pathologies.

Typical Clinical Findings

Taste disorders do not have a distinct pathognomonic clinical finding that can be identified easily. The clinical presentations are rather heterogeneous, and here we try to describe the different types of gustatory disorders that can be present and how they can be diagnosed.

179

Patient History

The patient's history, as in many medical problems, is key to understanding the disorder. When it comes to taste disorders, it must be remembered that patients do not always rate their gustatory function correctly.[11] Sometimes patients do not even notice taste deficiency.[12] Thus, asking about taste function is mandatory but unreliable, and becomes meaningful only with concurrent testing. When taking a history, emphasis should be put on specific questions about tasting the different qualities, production of saliva, swallowing and chewing capacity, orofacial pain, former infections or surgery in the head and neck region (especially the middle ear), diseases of the salivary glands, hearing or vestibular impairment, and oral hygiene. In addition, drug intake (and when this intake began), comorbidities (e.g., diabetes, thyroid dysfunction, Sicca syndrome [Sjögren disease], cancer), and former radiochemotherapy should be ascertained.[13]

Classification of Taste Disorders

Taste disorders can be clinically classified as quantitative or qualitative disorders. The most important quantitative taste disorders are ageusia, a complete loss of taste, and hypogeusia, a diminished taste. The most important qualitative taste disorders are dysgeusia and parageusia, characterized by a distorted sense of taste or an ongoing bad taste even in the absence of a taste stimulant. The dysgeusia taste is often described as bitter, sour, or metallic. Phantogeusia is a gustatory hallucination and is encountered in patients with epilepsy or psychotic disorders. Difficulty identifying a tastant that has been properly perceived is termed taste agnosia. It is assumed that the anteromedial temporal lobe has an important role in recognizing taste quality.[14] Despite the dichotomous classification in clinical practice, quantitative and qualitative taste disorders often coexist. The main difference between qualitative and quantitative taste disorders is that the latter can be tested objectively and assessed psychophysically, whereas qualitative disorders cannot yet be assessed by any available technique. Qualitative taste disorders are comparable to tinnitus in hearing: a frequent, bothersome complaint that may occur with or without hypoacousis and cannot be measured. Qualitative taste disorders (dysgeusia, phantogeusia, parageusia) are much more frequently encountered in a clinical setting than quantitative taste disorders (**Table 15.1**). An alternative way to classify taste disorders is to distinguish between central or peripheral taste disorders (**Fig. 15.1**) according to the site of the lesion. Finally, taste disorders can be classified according to their cause (**Table 15.2**). Congenital ageusia has never been reported to the best of our knowledge (unlike congenital anosmia, which is frequent[15]). Selective taste deficiencies such as ageusia for a single taste quality seem to be rare (except for bitter). Only a few reports of these exist, and it is not clear if this is a result of under-reporting or the particular biological importance of an intact taste function preventing such isolated and congenital ageusia.[16,17]

Table 15.1 Clinical classification of taste disorders (dysgeusia)

Disorder	Description
Quantitative taste disorders—measurable, rare, not always noticed by the patient	
Ageusia	Complete loss of taste
Hypogeusia	Diminished taste capacity
Hypergeusia	Increased taste sensitivity
Qualitative taste disorders—not measurable, frequent, noticed by the patient	
Parageusia	Triggered taste distortion (e.g., metallic taste when eating)
Phantogeusia	Permanent taste distortion, gustatory hallucination
Dysgeusia	Taste disorder, often used for qualitative taste disorders
Complex taste disorders	
Taste agnosia	Difficulty classifying or naming a taste although it is properly perceived

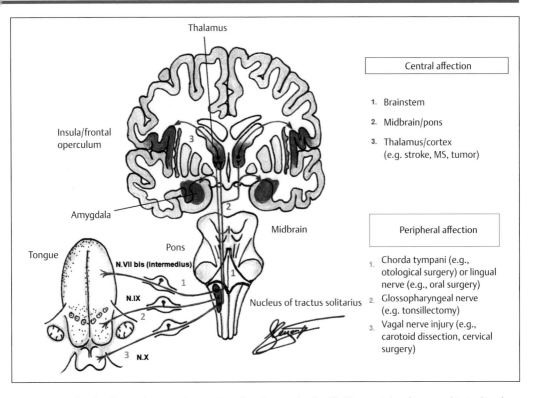

Fig. 15.1 Peripheral and central taste pathways. Taste disorders can be classified into peripheral or central taste disorders. MS, multiple sclerosis.

Table 15.2 Taste disorders classified according to their presumed etiology

Vascular etiology	Ischemic and hemorrhagic stroke
Traumatic	Contusion, skull-base fractures, cranial nerve damage
Toxicity: chemical	Toxins, drugs
Metabolic	Diabetes mellitus
Toxicity: physical	Heat, coldness, radiation, altitude sickness
Neoplastic	Space-occupying lesions
Inflammatory: infectious	Borreliosis, HIV, hepatitis C, rabies
Inflammatory: autoimmune	Multiple sclerosis, Guillain–Barré syndrome
Systemic autoimmune disorders	Sjögren syndrome, Wegener granulomatosis
Paraneoplastic disorders	Autoimmune mechanisms (molecular mimicry)
Neurodegenerative disorders	Alzheimer disease, Parkinson disease, and related disorders, Creutzfeldt–Jakob disease
Genetic disorders	Machado–Joseph disease, familial dysautonomia

HIV, human immunodeficiency virus.

A careful patient history, testing of each modality, and clinical work-up is important for patients with taste disorders.

Pathophysiology

Often, we do not know the exact pathological mechanism underlying taste disorders, which is reflected by the classification systems. Two of the three classification systems presented here are clinical and observational classifications without any explanation about the underlying mechanism. We observe patients with medication side effects, but barely know any molecular details about the disorders. In contrast, the pathological mechanism seems clear in situations where a lesion is visible or documented (as seen in **Fig. 15.1**). In these cases, the taste pathway is directly injured.

Etiology of Taste Disorders

To determine etiology of taste disorders the following differential diagnostic approach has been shown to be useful:

- Is the taste disorder caused by drugs or toxins?
- Is the taste disorder caused by local factors in the oral cavity, for instance atrophy of the mucosa, physical or chemical injuries, alteration of the composition of saliva, or otorhinolaryngological or dental diseases (e.g., *Candida albicans*)?
- Is the taste disorder caused by a disease of the peripheral nervous system?
- Is the taste disorder caused by a disease of the central nervous system?
- Is the taste disorder caused by a systemic disease?
- Did the taste disorder occur after any distinct event (e.g., infection, surgery, etc.)?

Taste Disorder Caused by Lesions of the Peripheral Nervous System

Taste disorders caused by peripheral nervous system disease can occur because of an isolated or combined lesion of one of the cranial nerves VII, IX, or X, such as occur in polyneuritis cranialis or Guillain–Barré syndrome.[18] Taste disorders can also occur in polyneuropathy.

Taste disorders affect 31 to 46% of patients with acute facial palsy, with no difference in incidence between the idiopathic form (Bell palsy) and borrelia-caused palsy. Compared with clinical signs and symptoms, and especially analysis of cerebrospinal fluid, taste results were of poor clinical value in differentiating among the causes of facial palsy.[19] Isolated peripheral cranial nerve lesions with resulting taste disorder have a wide differential diagnosis, including dissection of the brain-supplying arteries and local or systemic diseases affecting peripheral nerves. Further, lesions of the skull base or cerebellopontine angle, as well as traumatic skull fractures, might lead to taste disorders.[20] However, the most frequent cause of isolated peripheral taste disorder is surgical (iatrogenic) damage to one of the taste nerves (**Fig. 15.1**). The procedures most frequently associated with taste disorders are otological surgery with damage to the chorda tympani,[21] tonsillectomy and microlaryngoscopy[22] with damage to the lingual branch of the glossopharyngeal nerve, and oral or dental surgery with damage to the lingual nerve.[23] Unless the nerve is accidentally severed, most cases of surgically induced taste disorders are transient because peripheral nerves regenerate. This process takes a long time and patients often suffer from dysgeusia for many months or years.

In polyneuropathy, prominent taste disorders can occur and have been reported in cases of diphtheria, porphyries, systemic lupus erythematosus, or amyloidosis.[13] In a recent observational study of 53 patients with polyneuropathy, 43% demonstrated significant taste disorder on taste strip testing. The disorder was more severe in patients with diabetic polyneuropathy.[24] There are also reports of some degree of taste disorder in patients with trigeminal neuropathy, based on the fact that gustatory nerve fibers run via the trigeminal nerve.[25] This raises an interesting issue about interaction between the chemical senses. As mentioned, trigeminal lesions seem to influence taste function subclinically. The converse also seems to be true, with taste loss affecting lingual trigeminal function.[26] Likewise, olfactory impairment influences taste function subclinically.[27] Taken together, these observations make interpretation of selective chemosensory disorders difficult.

Generally, taste disorders due to peripheral nerve disease are accompanied by additional signs and symptoms such as pain, altered oral perceptions, and foreign body feelings in the pharynx or oral cavity; swallowing disorders; palpable masses; or palatal or facial palsy. Taste disorders can occur after dental procedures,[28] after surgical treatment of vestibular Schwannoma,[29] or following manipulation of the lingual nerve. In the case of carotid gustatory syndrome, a transient metallic taste perception emerges after compression of the carotid artery, probably due to a misconnection within the glossopharyngeal nerve between afferent impulses from carotid baroreceptors and sensory impulses from taste fibers.[30]

Taste Disorders Caused by Lesions of the Central Nervous System

Central taste disorders are caused by lesions along the taste pathway, which starts at the solitary tract nucleus (NTS) and ends at the cortical taste-representing zones (**Fig. 15.1**). An isolated occurrence of a gustatory symptom alone, however, is rare, and additional clinical signs are usually present and dominant in the acute phase of disease. For this reason, taste disorders are not often reported by patients with central lesions, and are only detected if clinicians seek them specifically.[31]

Different approaches can be taken to centrally caused taste disorders. From a topographical point of view, taste disorders can be attributed to lesions of the brainstem, the thalamus, or cortical areas. In brainstem lesions, the taste disorder is mainly ipsilateral (hemihypogeusia or hemiageusia) and is due to a lesion of the NTS or pons.[32] Taste disorders caused by thalamic lesions manifest contralaterally, ipsilaterally, or even bilaterally.[31,33] This phenomenon indicates that there are ascending crossing and noncrossing fibers from the brainstem to the thalamus. In bilateral thalamic lesions, anhedonic aspects can be prominent, leading to gustatory indifference and changes in eating behavior.[20]

Taste disorders due to cortical lesions are difficult to identify from the history or clinical neurological examination. Recent studies have shown that gustatory function is represented in the parietal, insular, anteromedial temporal, and orbitofrontal cortex.[34] Lesions in these regions can lead to epileptic gustatory sensations (phantogeusia,

gustatory aura) or to general taste disorders with impairment of the total taste perception.

In terms of etiology, taste disorders due to cerebrovascular and neurodegenerative diseases are most frequent. In an observational study in cooperative stroke patients, 30% revealed significant taste impairment and 6% had a lateralized taste disorder. Predictors for such impairment are male gender, high National Institutes of Health Stroke Scale score, coexistent swallowing disorder, and a partial anterior circulation infarct.[31] Similar results were obtained in a study of 120 consecutive postmenopausal women with acute stroke, 21 to 40% of whom demonstrated impairment of gustatory capacity without signs of lateralization.[35] In both studies, a substantial remission was observed. Even in cases of minor stroke, taste disorders can occur and lead to a change in food intake behavior.[36]

In neurodegenerative diseases, taste disorders are more frequent and severe. Taste testing should be performed on patients with Parkinson disease, in particular, because taste, like olfaction, might be diminished.[37-39] A taste disorder was recently reported even in patients with mild cognitive impairment and graded as severe as that in Alzheimer patients.[40]

Taste disorders in patients with multiple sclerosis have been reported,[41,42] and circumscribed taste abnormalities can be seen in patients with brainstem plaques.[43,44] Recently, it was emphasized that inflammation and demyelination along the gustatory pathway can cause significant taste disorders, which fortunately remit completely following steroid therapy.[45]

Anecdotal evidence also suggests that amyotrophic lateral sclerosis,[46] myasthenia gravis,[47] or central nervous dermoid cysts may be preceded by dysgeusia.[48] In some cases, dysgeusia as a paraneoplastic symptom has been reported as the first sign of lung cancer.[49] Other prominent taste disorders have been reported in single cases of altitude disease, familial dysautonomia, Machado–Joseph disease, new variant Creutzfeldt–Jakob disease, and even rabies.[13]

Taste Disorders in Neurological Diseases with no Distinct Localization

Taste disorders can occur in neurological conditions that cannot be precisely classified as central or peripheral, as in most cases of systemic or metabolic diseases or deficiency syndromes. Thus, in diabetes—a systemic disease with several neurological complications—a general reduction in taste capacity has been reported.[50,51] Cancer patients often reveal severe taste disorders with a strong negative impact on quality of life. Etiologically, cytotoxic therapy is the most common cause.[52] In immunological connective tissue diseases (e.g., Morbus Wegener or Sicca syndrome), chemosensory disturbances are often encountered.[53,54] Phantogeusia is predominantly seen in patients with psychotic disorders, whereas anorexia patients show a general taste impairment that is associated with food unpleasantness.[55] Taste disorders after allogeneic stem cell transplantation are associated with the cytotoxic drugs that are necessary in this complex treatment regimen, whereas chronic graft-versus-host disease or hyposalivation are of less importance.[56] Further, any kind of metabolic disorder (e.g., kidney or liver insufficiency) may initially present as taste disorder.[57]

Taste disorders have been detected in sewage and toxic waste workers, probably due to toxic agents in their working environment.[58] It is known that ammonia, isodecane, hairdressing chemicals, and gasoline can lead to toxically mediated taste disturbances.[59] Smoking significantly increases the risk of olfactory dysfunction but does not affect the risk of taste disorder.[60]

Overall, it should be remembered that taste disorders are more frequent in these generalized diseases, even if there is no known underlying mechanism. These systemic diseases—as well as age per se—increase susceptibility to taste disorders.[61] Interestingly, there are recent reports on taste phenomena in patients with synesthesia. Some individuals with synesthesia perceive specific taste impressions while listening to certain pieces of music.[62,63]

> The taste fibers from three cranial nerves converge from the periphery to a single nucleus in the brainstem. Large parts of the taste pathway are ipsilateral, but there is partial crossing and bilateral projection at the level of the thalamus and insula. Taste disorders can be classified into those with peripheral causes or those with central nervous system causes.

Drug-induced Taste Disorders

One major cause of taste disorders is medication side effects. Patients often perceive a relationship between a new taste disorder and the intake of a drug. In the Drug Interactions and Side Effects Index, more than 200 drugs are listed as capable of causing chemosensory taste disturbances. A recent review of drug-induced taste disorders, based on data from the Physician's Desk Reference, summarizes 22 drug classes that cause altered taste or smell perceptions.[64] **Table 15.3** lists drug classes and typical agents capable of causing taste disorders.

The mechanisms that contribute to taste disorders are not well understood. One theory is that drugs affect the physiological process of tasting by altering receptor affinity or signal transduction. Furthermore, a change in saliva flow rate may play a role. Also, the excretion of the drug or its metabolites into the saliva may cause an unpleasant or distorted taste. Other proposed mechanisms of drug-induced taste disorders include the following: the accumulation of silver in nerve fibers; a change in the influx of calcium and other ions; ion chelation and the loss of tissue-bound zinc; altered bradykinin metabolism; disturbed second-messenger synthesis; general catabolism; and altered metabolism of prostaglandins.[65] Most of these hypotheses remain speculation, supported by little biochemical or physiological evidence. Finally, it is important to note that drug-induced taste disorders are not limited to medication. Some fruits have the capacity to induce a transient taste distortion,[66] and, very recently, pine nuts have been claimed to induce dysgeusia lasting for several weeks.[67]

> Any kind of drug—and also some foods—can cause dysgeusia. The onset and disappearance of symptoms may be considerably delayed in relation to drug/food intake and discontinuation.

Postviral and Idiopathic Taste Disorders

Most taste disorders seen in specialized centers either follow an upper respiratory tract infection or are of unknown etiology. These are generally described as idiopathic taste disorders and prob-

Table 15.3 Drug-induced taste disorders (modified according Doty et al[64])

Drug group	Class or agent
Antihypertensives and cardiac medications	Amiodarone, propafenone, ACE inhibitors, diuretics, losartan, spironolactone, β-blockers, calcium antagonists, lipid-lowering agents (atorvastatin, fluvastatin, lovastatin, pravastatin)
Psychiatric medications	Benzodiazepines, tricyclic antidepressants, lithium, antipsychotics (clozapine, trifluoperazine), hypnotics (zolpidem, eszopiclone), CNS stimulants (amphetamine, dexamphetamine, methylphenidate)
Neurological medications	Antiepileptic drugs (carbamazepine, phenytoin, lamotrigine, topiramate), antimigraine drugs (sumatriptan, naratriptan, rizatriptan), antiparkinsonian agents (levodopa), anticholinergics, acetazolamide, baclofen, dantrolene
Anti-infectious agents	Antibacterials (ampicillin, ciprofloxacin, azithromycin, metronidazole, tetracycline), antifungals (griseofulvin, terbinafine), antivirals (aciclovir, ganciclovir, pirodavir, oseltamivir)
Antineoplastics	Platin derivatives, alkylating drugs, vincristine, methotrexate
Anti-inflammatory agents	Dexa- and beclometasone, budesonide, gold, penicillamine
Thyroid drugs	Carbimazole, levothyroxine, thiamazole, propylthiouracil

CNS, central nervous system; ACE, angiotensin-converting enzyme.

ably constitute a highly heterogeneous group. Idiopathic taste disorders are usually qualitative but can also present with quantitative complaints. Fortunately, most idiopathic taste disorders—and especially qualitative disorders—seem to improve over the years. Mood state seems to be related to resolution rates,[68] which suggests that some of these idiopathic dysgeusia cases may be induced by depressive states.

> Idiopathic taste disorders are the most commonly diagnosed causes of dysgeusia. This probably reflects the poor clinical knowledge we currently have of taste disorders.

Diagnosis

As for all medical disciplines, the first step toward therapy is the diagnosis. As discussed, a detailed history, extensive testing (see Chapter 14), and thorough neurological, dental, and otolaryngological examination is required.

After these steps, most diagnoses are clear. However, how do we proceed with the remaining patients, in whom no suspected cause can be isolated? There is currently no evidence-based scheme for how these patients should be managed. We do not claim our proposed approach to further

diagnostic procedures to be the only valid one, but we hope to give some useful clinical recommendations. First, imaging, ideally head and brain magnetic resonance imaging, should at least rule out the possibility of any neoplasia. Blood screening for liver, renal, and thyroid function, immune and inflammatory markers, hematological parameters, and glucose metabolism may suggest if further investigation of any systemic disorders is required. The necessity for vitamin and metal analysis is debatable in a population highly unlikely to suffer from malnourishment. Drug discontinuation and oral swabs for *Candida* screening might be helpful, although there is no published evidence to support this. Follow-up sometimes reveals new factors that help identify the underlying cause.

> It is important to seek a diagnosis. After a history and appropriate testing, blood tests to screen for deficiencies, and imaging of the brain/cranial nerves, may be helpful.

Therapy of Taste Disorders

A specific therapy for taste disorder is not available. In some small randomized studies, zinc has shown significant benefit in patients with idiopathic taste disorders. Patients treated with zinc demonstrated a significant improvement in taste capacity accompanied by a significant improvement in general well-being and a decrease in depression.[69] In another study, the intake of zinc led to an improvement in tasting in both patients with zinc deficiency and patients with normal zinc levels.[70] The ratio of apo:holo-activities of angiotensin-converting enzyme may be a predictor of improvement in these cases. In a further study, a zinc-containing drug (polaprezinc), administered at 68 mg daily for 12 weeks, led to an improvement in tasting compared with placebo. The noted side effects were mild.[71]

There are therapeutic recommendations for steroids and vitamin A, although their efficacy is not proven.[13] In a small cohort, branched-chain amino acid supplementation improved taste capacity in patients with hepatitis C, accompanied by an increase of the level of zinc.[72]

In cases of burning-mouth syndrome and dysgeusia, supportive measures, such as stimulation with an ice cube and medication for the treatment of neuropathic pain (e.g., antidepressants, gabapentin, pregabalin), can be tried.[13,73–76] In patients with taste disorders after chemotherapy or radiotherapy, a self-care program can be of value, for example omitting strongly smelling or tasting meals, drinking more water, optimizing oral hygiene, and eating small meals more frequently.[77]

> Therapy for taste disorders depends on the diagnosed cause of the dysgeusia. Most cases improve spontaneously.

Acknowledgments

We thank Dr. Hergen Friedrich for the drawing of **Fig. 15.1**.

References

1. Deems DA, Doty RL, Settle RG, et al. Smell and taste disorders, a study of 750 patients from the University of Pennsylvania Smell and Taste Center. Arch Otolaryngol Head Neck Surg 1991;117(5):519–528
2. Welge-Lüssen A, Dörig P, Wolfensberger M, Krone F, Hummel T. A study about the frequency of taste disorders. J Neurol 2011;258(3):386–392
3. Gent JF, Goodspeed RB, Zagraniski RT, Catalanotto FA. Taste and smell problems: validation of questions for the clinical history. Yale J Biol Med 1987;60(1):27–35
4. Woschnagg H, Stöllberger C, Finsterer J. Loss of taste is loss of weight. Lancet 2002;359(9309):891
5. Nakajima M, Ohtsuki T, Minematsu K. Bilateral hypogeusia in a patient with a unilateral paramedian thalamic infarction. J Neurol Neurosurg Psychiatry 2010;81(6):700–701
6. Landis BN, Guinand NO. Selective taste disorder after temporal bone fracture. J Clin Neurosci 2009;16(4):605
7. Theys T, Kho KH, Siemons W, Thijs V. Neurological picture. A matter of taste. J Neurol Neurosurg Psychiatry 2009;80(2):139–140
8. Schattner A. A 70-year-old man with isolated weight loss and a pellagra-like syndrome due to celiac disease. Yale J Biol Med 1999;72(1):15–18
9. Marinella MA. Paraneoplastic salt dysgeusia. South Med J 2008;101(12):1275–1276
10. Volkov VS, Poseliugina OB, Nilova SA, Vinogradova TS, Rokkina SA, Svistunov OP. Impaired gustatory sensitivity of the tongue to table salt as a risk factor of arterial hypertension. [Article in Russian] Klin Med (Mosk) 2010;88(1):15–18
11. Soter A, Kim J, Jackman A, Tourbier I, Kaul A, Doty RL. Accuracy of self-report in detecting taste dysfunction. Laryngoscope 2008;118(4):611–617
12. Landis BN, Beutner D, Frasnelli J, Hüttenbrink KB, Hummel T. Gustatory function in chronic inflammatory middle ear diseases. Laryngoscope 2005; 115(6):1124–1127
13. Heckmann JG, Lang JC, Hüttenbrink KB, Hummel T. Facialis (vii)—Schmeckstörungen. In: Hopf HC, Kömpf D, eds. Erkrankungen der hirnnerven. Stuttgart: Thieme Verlag; 2006:149–158
14. Small DM, Bernasconi N, Bernasconi A, Sziklas V, Jones-Gotman M. Gustatory agnosia. Neurology 2005;64(2):311–317
15. Abolmaali ND, Hietschold V, Vogl TJ, Hüttenbrink KB, Hummel T. MR evaluation in patients with isolated anosmia since birth or early childhood. AJNR Am J Neuroradiol 2002;23(1):157–164
16. Henkin RI, Shallenberger RS. Aglycogeusia: the inability to recognize sweetness and its possible molecular basis. Nature 1970;227(5261):965–966
17. Lugaz O, Pillias AM, Faurion A. A new specific ageusia: some humans cannot taste L-glutamate. Chem Senses 2002;27(2):105–115
18. Odaka M, Yuki N, Nishimoto Y, Hirata K. Guillain–Barré syndrome presenting with loss of taste. Neurology 2002;58(9):1437–1438
19. Hufschmidt A, Shabarin V, Yakovlev-Leyendecker O, Deppe O, Rauer S. Prevalence of taste disorders in idiopathic and *B. burgdorferi*-associated facial palsy. J Neurol 2009;256(10):1750–1752
20. Heckmann JG, Heckmann SM, Lang CJ, Hummel T. Neurological aspects of taste disorders. Arch Neurol 2003;60(5):667–671
21. Saito T, Manabe Y, Shibamori Y, et al. Long-term follow-up results of electrogustometry and subjective taste disorder after middle ear surgery. Laryngoscope 2001;111(11 Pt 1):2064–2070
22. Heiser C, Landis BN, Giger R, et al. Taste disturbance following tonsillectomy—a prospective study. Laryngoscope 2010;120(10):2119–2124

23. Hotta M, Endo S, Tomita H. Taste disturbance in two patients after dental anesthesia by inferior alveolar nerve block. Acta Otolaryngol Suppl 2002; 122(546):94–98

24. Heckmann JG, Höcherl C, Dütsch M, Lang C, Schwab S, Hummel T. Smell and taste disorders in polyneuropathy: a prospective study of chemosensory disorders. Acta Neurol Scand 2009;120(4):258–263

25. Grisold W, Nussgruber V. Comments on neurological aspects of taste disorders. Arch Neurol 2004;61(2):297–298, author reply 298

26. Perez R, Fuoco G, Dorion JM, Ho PH, Chen JM. Does the chorda tympani nerve confer general sensation from the tongue? Otolaryngol Head Neck Surg 2006;135(3):368–373

27. Landis BN, Scheibe M, Weber C, et al. Chemosensory interaction: acquired olfactory impairment is associated with decreased taste function. J Neurol 2010;257(8):1303–1308

28. Klasser GD, Utsman R, Epstein JB. Taste change associated with a dental procedure: case report and review of the literature. Tex Dent J 2008;125(8):678–687

29. Sahu RN, Behari S, Agarwal VK, Giri PJ, Jain VK. Taste dysfunction in vestibular schwannomas. Neurol India 2008;56(1):42–46

30. Shibasaki H, Tomi H. Carotid gustatory syndrome in a patient with Holmes–Adie syndrome. J Neurol Neurosurg Psychiatry 1990;53(4):359

31. Heckmann JG, Stössel C, Lang CJ, Neundörfer B, Tomandl B, Hummel T. Taste disorders in acute stroke: a prospective observational study on taste disorders in 102 stroke patients. Stroke 2005; 36(8):1690–1694

32. Landis BN, Leuchter I, San Millán Ruíz D, Lacroix JS, Landis T. Transient hemiageusia in cerebrovascular lateral pontine lesions. J Neurol Neurosurg Psychiatry 2006;77(5):680–683

33. Onoda K, Ikeda M. Gustatory disturbance due to cerebrovascular disorder. Laryngoscope 1999;109(1): 123–128

34. Rolls ET. Taste, olfactory, and food texture processing in the brain, and the control of food intake. Physiol Behav 2005;85(1):45–56

35. Kim JS, Choi-Kwon S, Kwon SU, Kwon JH. Taste perception abnormalities after acute stroke in postmenopausal women. J Clin Neurosci 2009;16(6): 797–801

36. Green TL, McGregor LD, King KM. Smell and taste dysfunction following minor stroke: a case report. Can J Neurosci Nurs 2008;30(2):10–13

37. Lang CJ, Leuschner T, Ulrich K, Stössel C, Heckmann JG, Hummel T. Taste in dementing diseases and parkinsonism. J Neurol Sci 2006;248(1–2):177–184

38. Shah M, Deeb J, Fernando M, et al. Abnormality of taste and smell in Parkinson's disease. Parkinsonism Relat Disord 2009;15(3):232–237

39. Sienkiewicz-Jarosz H, Scinska A, Kuran W, et al. Taste responses in patients with Parkinson's disease. J Neurol Neurosurg Psychiatry 2005;76(1):40–46

40. Steinbach S, Hundt W, Vaitl A, et al. Taste in mild cognitive impairment and Alzheimer's disease. J Neurol 2010;257(2):238–246

41. Rollin H. Gustatory disturbances in multiple sclerosis. [Article in German] Laryngol Rhinol Otol (Stuttg.) 1976;55(8):678–681

42. Cohen L. Disturbance of taste as a symptom of multiple sclerosis. Br J Oral Surg 1965;3:184–185

43. Combarros O, Sánchez-Juan P, Berciano J, De Pablos C. Hemiageusia from an ipsilateral multiple sclerosis plaque at the midpontine tegmentum. J Neurol Neurosurg Psychiatry 2000;68(6):796

44. Uesaka Y, Nose H, Ida M, Takagi A. The pathway of gustatory fibers of the human ascends ipsilaterally in the pons. Neurology 1998;50(3):827–828

45. Benatru I, Terraux P, Cherasse A, Couvreur G, Giroud M, Moreau T. Gustatory disorders during multiple sclerosis relapse. [Article in French] Rev Neurol (Paris) 2003;159(3):287–292

46. Petzold GC, Einhäupl KM, Valdueza JM. Persistent bitter taste as an initial symptom of amyotrophic lateral sclerosis. J Neurol Neurosurg Psychiatry 2003;74(5):687–688

47. Nakazato Y, Ito Y, Naito S, Tamura N, Shimazu K. Dysgeusia limited to sweet taste in myasthenia gravis. Intern Med 2008;47(9):877–878

48. Kocaeli H, Korfali E, Doğan S, Savran M. Sylvian cistern dermoid cyst presenting with dysgeusia. Acta Neurochir (Wien) 2009;151(5):561–563

49. Panayiotou H, Small SC, Hunter JH, Culpepper RM. Sweet taste (dysgeusia). The first symptom of hyponatremia in small cell carcinoma of the lung. Arch Intern Med 1995;155(12):1325–1328

50. Naka A, Riedl M, Luger A, Hummel T, Mueller CA. Clinical significance of smell and taste disorders in patients with diabetes mellitus. Eur Arch Otorhinolaryngol 2010;267(4):547–550

51. Gondivkar SM, Indurkar A, Degwekar S, Bhowate R. Evaluation of gustatory function in patients with diabetes mellitus type 2. Oral Surg Oral Med Oral Pathol Oral Radiol Endod 2009;108(6):876–880

52. Epstein JB, Barasch A. Taste disorders in cancer patients: pathogenesis, and approach to assessment and management. Oral Oncol 2010;46(2):77–81

53. Kamel UF, Maddison P, Whitaker R. Impact of primary Sjogren's syndrome on smell and taste: effect on quality of life. Rheumatology (Oxford) 2009;48(12):1512–1514

54. Göktas O, Cao Van H, Fleiner F, Lacroix JS, Landis BN. Chemosensory function in Wegener's granulomatosis: a preliminary report. Eur Arch Otorhinolaryngol 2010;267(7):1089–1093

55. Szalay C, Abrahám I, Papp S, et al. Taste reactivity deficit in anorexia nervosa. Psychiatry Clin Neurosci 2010;64(4):403–407

56. Boer CC, Correa ME, Miranda EC, de Souza CA. Taste disorders and oral evaluation in patients undergoing allogeneic hematopoietic SCT. Bone Marrow Transplant 2010;45(4):705–711

57. Vreman HJ, Venter C, Leegwater J, Oliver C, Weiner MW. Taste, smell and zinc metabolism in patients with chronic renal failure. Nephron 1980;26(4):163–170

58. Dzaman K, Wojdas A, Rapiejko P, Jurkiewicz D. Taste and smell perception among sewage treatment and landfill workers. Int J Occup Med Environ Health 2009;22(3):227–234

59. Smith WM, Davidson TM, Murphy C. Toxin-induced chemosensory dysfunction: a case series and review. Am J Rhinol Allergy 2009;23(6):578–581

60. Vennemann MM, Hummel T, Berger K. The association between smoking and smell and taste impairment in the general population. J Neurol 2008;255(8):1121–1126

61. Schiffman SS. Effects of aging on the human taste system. Ann N Y Acad Sci 2009;1170:725–729

62. Carmichael G. Hearing taste and colouring text. Lancet Neurol 2005;4(5):274

63. Beeli G, Esslen M, Jäncke L. Synaesthesia: when coloured sounds taste sweet. Nature 2005; 434(7029):38

64. Doty RL, Shah M, Bromley SM. Drug-induced taste disorders. Drug Saf 2008;31(3):199–215

65. Ackerman BH, Kasbekar N. Disturbances of taste and smell induced by drugs. Pharmacotherapy 1997;17(3):482–496

66. Kurihara K, Beidler LM. Taste-modifying protein from miracle fruit. Science 1968; 161(3847):1241–1243

67. Picard F, Landis BN. Pine nut-induced dysgeusia: an emerging problem! Am J Med 2010;123(11):e3

68. Deems DA, Yen DM, Kreshak A, Doty RL. Spontaneous resolution of dysgeusia. Arch Otolaryngol Head Neck Surg 1996;122(9):961–963

69. Heckmann SM, Hujoel P, Habiger S, et al. Zinc gluconate in the treatment of dysgeusia—a randomized clinical trial. J Dent Res 2005;84(1):35–38

70. Takaoka T, Sarukura N, Ueda C, et al. Effects of zinc supplementation on serum zinc concentration and ratio of apo/holo-activities of angiotensin converting enzyme in patients with taste impairment. Auris Nasus Larynx 2010;37(2):190–194

71. Sakagami M, Ikeda M, Tomita H, et al. A zinc-containing compound, Polaprezinc, is effective for patients with taste disorders: randomized, double-blind, placebo-controlled, multi-center study. Acta Otolaryngol 2009;129(10):1115–1120

72. Nagao Y, Matsuoka H, Kawaguchi T, Sata M. Aminofeel improves the sensitivity to taste in patients with HCV-infected liver disease. Med Sci Monit 2010;16(4):PI7–PI12

73. Fujiyama R, Ishitobi S, Honda K, Okada Y, Oi K, Toda K. Ice cube stimulation helps to improve dysgeusia. Odontology 2010;98(1):82–84

74. Heckmann SM, Kirchner E, Grushka M, Wichmann MG, Hummel T. A double-blind study on clonazepam in patients with burning mouth syndrome. Laryngoscope 2012;122(4):813–816

75. Cho GS, Han MW, Lee B, et al. Zinc deficiency may be a cause of burning mouth syndrome as zinc replacement therapy has therapeutic effects. J Oral Pathol Med 2010;39(9):722–727

76. Scardina GA, Ruggieri A, Provenzano F, Messina P. Burning mouth syndrome: is acupuncture a therapeutic possibility? Br Dent J 2010;209(1):E2

77. Rehwaldt M, Wickham R, Purl S, et al. Self-care strategies to cope with taste changes after chemotherapy. Oncol Nurs Forum 2009;36(2):E47–E56

16 Burning Mouth Syndrome and Qualitative Taste and Smell Disorders

Miriam Grushka, Victor Ching, Joel Epstein, Antje Welge-Luessen, Thomas Hummel

Burning Mouth Syndrome

> Burning mouth syndrome can be extremely disturbing. Causes are multiple. Treatment is not established. It is often associated with taste loss.

Introduction

Burning mouth syndrome (BMS) is characterized by a burning sensation in the intraoral mucosal membranes and perioral areas in the absence of clinical and laboratory findings to account for the pain.[1–3] Diagnosis is often made on a clinical basis. Sensations associated with BMS have been variously described as "burning," "annoying," "granular or sandy," or "dryness and swelling."[2] Frequently, patients do not report pain when eating, sleeping, or on waking, but the sensation gradually increases throughout the day to peak in late afternoon and early evening.[1,2] Up to two-thirds of patients with BMS also complain of dysgeusia,[4,5] described as the presence of a constant "foul," bitter, or metallic taste sensation, which may be at least as disturbing as the burning pain itself.[1]

Prevalence

The prevalence of BMS has been reported to be between 0.7 and 5% in the general population (including Canadian studies[1,6]), with the variation probably due to study methodology (survey or clinical assessment) and location.[1,6–8] BMS is most commonly reported by female patients in the fifth to seventh decade of life,[4,9,10] and investigations have often focused on menopausal and postmenopausal populations.[11–14] The high proportion of postmenopausal patients with BMS has led to interest in the role of estrogen in chronic orofacial pain,[15] and whether changes in estrogen levels can precipitate BMS.

Etiology

There is an increasing consensus that BMS is an idiopathic neuropathic pain condition.[9,16] However, there is no consensus on the etiology or whether developing BMS can be attributed to a single precipitating event.[4,12] Recent evidence has suggested that both central[17–20] and peripheral neuropathic changes[10,21–23] are present in patients with BMS. A recent study by Lauria et al[10] assessed superficial nerve changes on biopsy of the anterior two-thirds of the tongue in 12 patients diagnosed with BMS. Compared with control subjects, patients with BMS demonstrated a significantly lower density of unmyelinated epithelial nerve fibers and subpapillary nerve fibers, with evidence of diffuse axonal derangement in the patients with BMS.[10] The changes were caused by a primary axonopathy rather than a neuronopathy. Like other small-fiber neuropathies, the severity of the symptoms did not correlate with the density of epithelial nerve fibers.[10] Previous studies have shown that these epithelial nerve fibers synapse with the taste buds in the fungiform papillae, and such changes may be the basis for both the dysgeusia and the pain experienced by some patients with BMS.[22,24,25]

Most clinicians recognize the existence of secondary BMS—pain related to an organic cause such as a systemic disease—and primary BMS, which is the neuropathic phenomenon.[26] An interesting question is whether there is overlap between the two: is the development of neuropathic changes associated with primary BMS related to a local or systemic disease? Suarez and Clark[26] report that BMS is more frequent in women with systemic diseases. Recent literature on Sjögren syndrome, a common autoimmune disease affecting more women than men, indicates that peripheral neuropathies are among the most common non-gland manifestations.[27] The prevalence of peripheral neuropathy is unknown, but has been estimated at 5 to 20%.[27] Although the general prevalence of small-fiber neuropathy, such as that described by Lauria,[10] is unknown, one study assessing skin

189

biopsies found that mean intraepidermal nerve fiber innervation was considerably lower in patients with Sjögren syndrome than in age- and sex-matched controls.[28] This is similar to the findings of reduced epithelial nerve density reported by Lauria et al[10] Like treatment of BMS, treatment of neuropathy associated with Sjögren syndrome can include antiepileptic drugs (AED) and antidepressants used as adjuvant analgesics.[27]

Recent literature has also suggested that BMS may be caused by mast-cell activation disorder.[29] However, it is likely that the study, based on three cases, describes secondary BMS rather than primary BMS, given that these cases did not respond to AED and antidepressant medication but responded dramatically to nonsteroidal anti-inflammatory drugs and histamine-acting medications.[29] Therefore, it is more likely that mast-cell disorders are part of the differential diagnosis for BMS rather than a cause for primary BMS.[29]

Another suggestion has been an association between zinc deficiency and the pathogenesis of BMS.[30] Cho et al reported that zinc deficiency was present in ~27% of patients with BMS, and that pain scores in such patients who were treated with zinc replacement improved significantly compared with those of a control group.[30] An animal model has suggested that zinc deficiency causes histological changes in the tongue, but it is uncertain how this is associated with neuropathy.[30]

It has been suggested that neuropathic pain begins peripherally and progresses to central sensitization. Jääskeläinen, who has done much of the quantitative sensory testing work in BMS, suggests that BMS encompasses changes in both the peripheral trigeminal nerve and in central pathways.[18] While conventional imaging such as magnetic resonance imaging may fail to detect trigeminal pathology, it may be evident on sensory testing.[18] On testing heat sensation thresholds and pain in BMS, changes were found in the mouth as well as distal locations, suggesting that BMS may be associated with disseminated small-fiber nerve changes.[18] Centrally, blink-reflex testing suggests a role for the striatal dopaminergic system in BMS pain.[18] Overall, sensory data suggest that both peripheral and central nervous system (CNS) changes are present, but do not pinpoint the location of specific changes in the somatosensory system.[18,26]

Taste Changes

Bartoshuk's group have demonstrated the convergence of taste sensation and pain both clinically and experimentally.[30,31] The chorda tympani nerve (cranial nerve VII) leaves the tongue with the lingual nerve (cranial nerve V) and travels through the pterygomandibular space. The inferior alveolar nerve (cranial nerve V), which conveys sensation from the lower teeth, also passes through this same space. Often, anesthesia of the inferior alveolar and lingual nerves required for dental procedures abolishes touch, pain, and also taste sensations on the injected side. The chorda tympani and lingual nerves separate and the chorda tympani passes through the middle ear. Researchers[30,32–34] have demonstrated that anesthesia of the chorda tympani behind the tympanic membrane intensifies tastes from the area innervated by the glossopharyngeal nerve (cranial nerve IX)—the posterior aspect of the tongue on the opposite side—supporting a model of central inhibition between the chorda tympani and glossopharyngeal nerves. According to Bartoshuk's group, reduced input into the CNS from one taste nerve releases inhibition of other tastes, resulting in these tastes being intensified.[30]

Tie et al[35] found that anesthesia of the chorda tympani can intensify capsaicin-induced pain on the contralateral anterior tongue, suggesting the presence of central inhibitory interactions between taste and oral pain. Furthermore, the intensification of pain was found to be related to an individual's genetic ability to taste 6-n-propylthiouracil (PROP), an extremely bitter compound, with the greatest intensification found in "supertasters" (mainly females) who report the most bitter sensation from PROP testing.[36]

Based on these taste–pain interactions, it is believed that some cases of BMS could be the result of taste damage, to either the chorda tympani, with release of inhibition in the glossopharyngeal nerve (taste alterations, alterations in touch and pain), or the trigeminal nerve (changes in touch and pain). Consistent with this model, taste damage has been found in many patients with BMS. Notably, the intensity of peak oral pain was found to correlate with the density of fungiform papillae, with the greatest density being found in patients with BMS who were primarily supertasters.[31,37]

According to Bartoshuk's group,[30] if taste damage produces a sufficient loss of the inhibition normally exerted on central structures mediating oral pain, then centrally acting medications that are known to impact on pain, such as pregabalin, may ameliorate the loss of inhibition and relieve the pain of BMS.

Spatial Taste Testing

Taste on the tongue is innervated by the branches of the facial nerve (cranial nerve VII) and the glossopharyngeal nerve (cranial nerve IX), which serve different regions of the tongue. Often, changes to taste in patients with BMS may occur in one area but not another.[7] As a result, taste damage presents as a regional phenomenon and rarely as a whole-mouth phenomenon.[38]

Therefore, spatial taste testing is performed to assess perceived taste intensity for sweet, sour, salty, and bitter solutions applied with cottons swabs, filter paper, or drops at the anterior tongue tip and the circumvallate papillae, on both left and right sides. Patients rate the quality and intensity of the stimuli using a validated psychometric scale, the general labeled magnitude scale—a modified numeric scale.[39]

Treatment

Therapy for BMS involves the use of centrally acting medications for neuropathic pain, such as tricyclic antidepressants, benzodiazepines, or gabapentinoids,[40] and recently paroxetine.[41] To our knowledge, pregabalin has yet to be studied in BMS, but, in view of its success in the treatment of neuropathic conditions, this medication might provide an additional approach to the treatment of both pain and taste disturbances associated with BMS. Limited trials to date support the use of low-dose clonazepam (0.25 to 0.75 mg) or tricyclic antidepressants (10 to 40 mg), including amitriptyline, desipramine, nortriptyline, imipramine clomipramine, or the selective serotonin reuptake inhibitor paroxetine. Clonazepam is a benzodiazepine used either topically or systemically,[2,42,43] which appears to have excellent efficacy in the relief of BMS symptoms. In view of only partial or lack of response in some patients with BMS, gabapentin has been used in combination with clonazepam with apparent anecdotal success.[1] Topical medications, including clonidine and capsaicin, may be considered for application to local sites. Systemic use of capsaicin has also been suggested,[44] as has α-lipoic acid with or without psychotherapy.[45] Zinc supplementation for patients with diagnosed zinc deficiency has also been proposed, with significant relief reported.[30]

Qualitative Taste Disorder: Dysgeusia

> Qualitative taste disorders result from similar causes to quantitative taste disorders. The major difference is that dysgeusias are difficult to measure, although they may produce severe discomfort in daily life. Treatment is problematic.

The term dysgeusia is used to describe certain distortions in taste: either that patients perceive any taste as bitter, salty, sour, metallic, or astringent; or that patients suffer from a more-or-less continuous taste sensation, such as the continuous presence of bitter taste. These taste distortions are also termed qualitative taste disorders. Accordingly, these "colorful" cases may include patients with normal gustatory function from a quantitative point of view, but they can be extremely distressing for patients, resulting in weight loss and symptoms of depression.[46] Sweet dysgeusia deserves special mention because it has often been reported to occur with neoplasms in the thorax and also with myasthenia gravis (e.g., refs. 47, 48). Other than that, causes of qualitative taste disorders are similar to those of quantitative taste loss. Many drugs that can potentially cause taste problems have been identified.[49,50] Among many others, AEDs[51] and antihypertensives[52] should be considered as potential causes of gustatory dysfunction. Lesions of the peripheral nervous system may also be responsible, for example after dental surgery or tonsillectomy; dysgeusia can also occur as part of syndromes affecting the facial (most frequent), glossopharyngeal, or vagal nerves, e.g., idiopathic cranial nerve VII palsy (Bell palsy).[53] Other causes of cranial nerve lesions have to be considered (e.g., neuroborreliosis or zoster, processes in the cerebellopontine angle,[49,53] or dissection of cervical arteries).[54] Central causes of dysgeusia include lesions along the taste pathway from the brainstem to its cortical representation. Brainstem taste disorders (ipsilateral disturbance) may be due to demyelinating processes, ischemia or hemorrhage, or vascular lesions.[55] Thalamic lesions are also known to result in taste disorders,[56] and cortical taste disorders have been described in epilepsy.[57] Therapeutic approaches are similar to those for quantitative taste loss (see p. 185). Studies of zinc in patients with idiopathic dysgeusia reported significant improvement[58,59]; however, such improvement was not seen in cancer patients with dysgeusia related to radiotherapy of the oropharynx.[60]

Qualitative Smell Disorder: Parosmia and Phantosmia

> Parosmia and phantosmia are almost always accompanied by smell loss. As with dysgeusia, they cannot be quantified, which emphasizes the significance of the medical history. A simple assessment relates to the frequency and intensity of the symptoms and their consequences for daily life.

Some patients not only suffer from quantitative olfactory disorders, but also experience qualitative olfactory dysfunction. These odor distortions can be roughly divided into parosmias (also called "troposmia") and phantosmias.[61] When patients report parosmia, they perceive inhaled odorants to have a different smell from how they remember it. Phantosmia, on the other hand, indicates the perception of an odor when no odorous source is present. Both parosmic and phantosmic sensations are typically described as unpleasant, e.g., "burned," "foul," "rotten," "fecal," or "chemical" smells.[61–63] While phantosmia appears to be a relatively rare symptom, parosmia is a frequent finding in patients with olfactory systems in a state of regeneration or degeneration.[64] Its frequency has been estimated to range from 10 to 60% among patients with olfactory dysfunction.[62,64,65]

The pathogenesis of parosmia and phantosmia is unclear. Both peripheral and central causes have been discussed[61,66] that may be considered to lead to olfactory distortions.[63] Psychiatric causes need to be excluded (e.g., olfactory reference syndrome).[67] One of the most attractive explanations

of parosmia relates to the loss of olfactory receptor neurons (ORNs), for example, after trauma or upper respiratory tract infection (URTI). If not all ORNs were lost, patients would still be able to perceive an odor, but because of the lack of certain neurons, they would be unable to encode a specific odor quality. Thus, they would be unable to form a complete "picture" of the odorant.[61] Consequently, patients would misinterpret the sensory input in the form of parosmias. On the other hand, parosmia could also be a central nervous problem. Specifically, because of unknown pathologies, the integrative or interpretative centers in the brain could form a distorted picture.[61,68] Consistent with this is the fact that in patients with parosmia, gray matter volume loss has been demonstrated in the left anterior insula and in other areas involved in olfactory processing, such as the right anterior insula, the anterior cingulate cortex, the hippocampus (bilaterally), and the left medial orbitofrontal cortex.[69]

With regard to phantosmia,[61] it has been hypothesized that abnormally active ORNs or a loss of inhibitory neurons could lead to distorted sensations.[70] A central cause is also hypothesized for phantosmia, where hyperactive brain cells might create the impression of an odorous sensation. Some patients with qualitative olfactory disorders do not report a history of URTI or head trauma, but indicate spontaneous onset of the symptoms.[61] Qualitative olfactory dysfunction is typically, but not always, associated with quantitative olfactory loss. While the debate is far from over, parosmia may be seen as an indicator of a changing olfactory system. Phantosmia may be a sign of deafferentation.

It is known that most qualitative olfactory impairments gradually improve.[61,64] Patients therefore appreciate knowing that there is a high chance that the condition will improve or disappear with time. Appropriate counseling and watchful waiting is therefore recommended. In extremely severe cases, endoscopic surgical excision of olfactory epithelium has been suggested as a possible therapeutic approach.[61,71] Although other treatments have been reported, none has yet been established in routine clinical practice. For example, excellent results have been reported by Zilstorff using local cocaine treatment.[63] Other treatment approaches are similar to those described for quantitative olfactory loss.

References

1. Grushka M, Epstein JB, Gorsky M. Burning mouth syndrome. Am Fam Physician 2002;65(4):615–620
2. Woda A, Navez ML, Picard P, Gremeau C, Pichard-Leandri E. A possible therapeutic solution for stomatodynia (burning mouth syndrome). J Orofac Pain 1998;12(4):272–278
3. Danhauer SC, Miller CS, Rhodus NL, Carlson CR. Impact of criteria-based diagnosis of burning mouth syndrome on treatment outcome. J Orofac Pain 2002;16(4):305–311
4. Grushka M. Clinical features of burning mouth syndrome. Oral Surg Oral Med Oral Pathol 1987; 63(1):30–36
5. Eguia Del Valle A, Aguirre-Urizar JM, Martinez-Conde R, Echebarria-Goikouria MA, Sagasta-Pujana O. Burning mouth syndrome in the Basque Country: a preliminary study of 30 cases. Med Oral 2003; 8(2):84–90
6. Klausner JJ. Epidemiology of chronic facial pain: diagnostic usefulness in patient care. J Am Dent Assoc 1994;125(12):1604–1611
7. Grushka M, Sessle BJ. Burning mouth syndrome. Dent Clin North Am 1991;35(1):171–184
8. Basker RM, Sturdee DW, Davenport JC. Patients with burning mouths. A clinical investigation of causative factors, including the climacteric and diabetes. Br Dent J 1978;145(1):9–16
9. Zakrzewska JM. The burning mouth syndrome remains an enigma. Pain 1995;62(3):253–257
10. Lauria G, Majorana A, Borgna M, et al. Trigeminal small-fiber sensory neuropathy causes burning mouth syndrome. Pain 2005;115(3):332–337
11. Bergdahl M, Bergdahl J. Burning mouth syndrome: prevalence and associated factors. J Oral Pathol Med 1999;28(8):350–354
12. Tammiala-Salonen T, Hiidenkari T, Parvinen T. Burning mouth in a Finnish adult population. Community Dent Oral Epidemiol 1993;21(2):67–71
13. Wardrop RW, Hailes J, Burger H, Reade PC. Oral discomfort at menopause. Oral Surg Oral Med Oral Pathol 1989;67(5):535–540
14. Ben Aryeh H, Gottlieb I, Ish-Shalom S, David A, Szargel H, Laufer D. Oral complaints related to menopause. Maturitas 1996;24(3):185–189
15. Cairns BE. The influence of gender and sex steroids on craniofacial nociception. Headache 2007;47(2):319–324
16. Patton LL, Siegel MA, Benoliel R, De Laat A. Management of burning mouth syndrome: systematic review and management recommendations. Oral Surg Oral Med Oral Pathol Oral Radiol Endod 2007;103 Suppl:S39.e1–13
17. Jääskeläinen SK, Rinne JO, Forssell H, et al. Role of the dopaminergic system in chronic pain—a fluorodopa-PET study. Pain 2001;90(3):257–260
18. Jääskeläinen SK. Clinical neurophysiology and quantitative sensory testing in the investigation of orofacial pain and sensory function. J Orofac Pain 2004;18(2):85–107
19. Hagelberg N, Forssell H, Aalto S, et al. Altered dopamine D2 receptor binding in atypical facial pain. Pain 2003;106(1–2):43–48
20. Forssell H, Jääskeläinen S, Tenovuo O, Hinkka S. Sensory dysfunction in burning mouth syndrome. Pain 2002;99(1–2):41–47
21. Heckmann SM, Heckmann JG, Hilz MJ, et al. Oral mucosal blood flow in patients with burning mouth syndrome. Pain 2001;90(3):281–286
22. Formaker BK, Mott AE, Frank ME. The effects of topical anesthesia on oral burning in burning mouth syndrome. Ann N Y Acad Sci 1998;855:776–780
23. Nagler RM, Hershkovich O. Sialochemical and gustatory analysis in patients with oral sensory complaints. J Pain 2004;5(1):56–63
24. Lim J, Green BG. The psychophysical relationship between bitter taste and burning sensation: evidence of qualitative similarity. Chem Senses 2007; 32(1):31–39
25. Linden RW. Taste. Br Dent J 1993;175(7):243–253
26. Suarez P, Clark GT. Burning mouth syndrome: an update on diagnosis and treatment methods. J Calif Dent Assoc 2006;34(8):611–622
27. Birnbaum J. Peripheral nervous system manifestations of Sjögren syndrome: clinical patterns, diagnostic paradigms, etiopathogenesis, and therapeutic strategies. Neurologist 2010;16(5):287–297
28. Gøransson LG, Brun JG, Harboe E, Mellgren SI, Omdal R. Intraepidermal nerve fiber densities in chronic inflammatory autoimmune diseases. Arch Neurol 2006;63(10):1410–1413
29. Afrin LB. Burning mouth syndrome and mast cell activation disorder. Oral Surg Oral Med Oral Pathol Oral Radiol Endod 2011;111(4):465–472
30. Cho GS, Han MW, Lee B, et al. Zinc deficiency may be a cause of burning mouth syndrome as zinc replacement therapy has therapeutic effects. J Oral Pathol Med 2010;39(9):722–727
31. Bartoshuk LM, Snyder DJ, Grushka M, Berger AM, Duffy VB, Kveton JF. Taste damage: previously unsuspected consequences. Chem Senses 2005; 30(Suppl 1):i218–i219
32. Grushka M, Bartoshuk L. Burning mouth syndrome and oral dysesthesias. Can J Diagnosis 2000;99–109
33. Lehman CD, Bartoshuk LM, Catalanotto FC, Kveton JF, Lowlicht RA. Effect of anesthesia of the chorda tympani nerve on taste perception in humans. Physiol Behav 1995;57(5):943–951
34. Yanagisawa K, Bartoshuk LM, Catalanotto FA, Karrer TA, Kveton JF. Anesthesia of the chorda tympani nerve and taste phantoms. Physiol Behav 1998;63(3):329–335
35. Tie K, Fast K, Kveton J, et al. Anesthesia of chorda tympani nerve and effect on oral pain. Chem Senses 1999;24:609
36. Bartoshuk LM, Duffy VB, Miller IJ. PTC/PROP tasting: anatomy, psychophysics, and sex effects. Physiol Behav 1994;56(6):1165–1171
37. Eliav E, Kamran B, Schaham R, Czerninski R, Gracely RH, Benoliel R. Evidence of chorda tympani dysfunction in patients with burning mouth syndrome. J Am Dent Assoc 2007;138(5):628–633
38. Snyder DJ, Prescott J, Bartoshuk LM. Modern psychophysics and the assessment of human oral sensation. Adv Otorhinolaryngol 2006;63:221–241
39. Bartoshuk LM, Duffy VB, Green BG, et al. Valid across-group comparisons with labeled scales: the

gLMS versus magnitude matching. Physiol Behav 2004;82(1):109–114

40. White TL, Kent PF, Kurtz DB, Emko P. Effectiveness of gabapentin for treatment of burning mouth syndrome. Arch Otolaryngol Head Neck Surg 2004; 130(6):786–788

41. Yamazaki Y, Hata H, Kitamori S, Onodera M, Kitagawa Y. An open-label, noncomparative, dose escalation pilot study of the effect of paroxetine in treatment of burning mouth syndrome. Oral Surg Oral Med Oral Pathol Oral Radiol Endod 2009;107(1):e6–e11

42. Grushka M, Epstein J, Mott A. An open-label, dose escalation pilot study of the effect of clonazepam in burning mouth syndrome. Oral Surg Oral Med Oral Pathol Oral Radiol Endod 1998;86(5):557–561

43. Gremeau-Richard C, Woda A, Navez ML, et al. Topical clonazepam in stomatodynia: a randomised placebo-controlled study. Pain 2004;108(1–2):51–57

44. Petruzzi M, Lauritano D, De Benedittis M, Baldoni M, Serpico R. Systemic capsaicin for burning mouth syndrome: short-term results of a pilot study. J Oral Pathol Med 2004;33(2):111–114

45. Femiano F, Lanza A, Buonaiuto C, et al. Burning mouth syndrome and burning mouth in hypothyroidism: proposal for a diagnostic and therapeutic protocol. Oral Surg Oral Med Oral Pathol Oral Radiol Endod 2008;105(1):e22–e27

46. Cowart B, Klock CV, Pribitkin E, Breslin P. Relative impact of taste versus smell dysfunctions on quality of life. Chem Senses 2007;32:A16

47. Panayiotou H, Small SC, Hunter JH, Culpepper RM. Sweet taste (dysgeusia). The first symptom of hyponatremia in small cell carcinoma of the lung. Arch Intern Med 1995;155(12):1325–1328

48. Nakazato Y, Ito Y, Naito S, Tamura N, Shimazu K. Dysgeusia limited to sweet taste in myasthenia gravis. Intern Med 2008;47(9):877–878

49. Schiffman SS. Taste and smell in disease (first of two parts). N Engl J Med 1983;308(21):1275–1279

50. Ackerman BH, Kasbekar N. Disturbances of taste and smell induced by drugs. Pharmacotherapy 1997;17(3):482–496

51. Avoni P, Contin M, Riva R, Albani F, Liguori R, Baruzzi A. Dysgeusia in epileptic patients treated with lamotrigine: report of three cases. Neurology 2001;57(8):1521

52. Ohkoshi N, Shoji S. Reversible ageusia induced by losartan: a case report. Eur J Neurol 2002;9(3):315

53. Roob G, Fazekas F, Hartung HP. Peripheral facial palsy: etiology, diagnosis and treatment. Eur Neurol 1999;41(1):3–9

54. Taillibert S, Bazin B, Pierrot-Deseilligny C. Dysgeusia resulting from internal carotid dissection. A limited glossopharyngeal nerve palsy. J Neurol Neurosurg Psychiatry 1998;64(5):691–692

55. Lee BC, Hwang SH, Rison R, Chang GY. Central pathway of taste: clinical and MRI study. Eur Neurol 1998;39(4):200–203

56. Adler A. Zur Topik des Verlaufes der Geschmacks-sinnsfasern und anderer afferenter Bahnen im Thalamus. [Article in German] Z Gesamte Neurol Psychiatr 1934;149:208–220

57. Hausser-Hauw C, Bancaud J. Gustatory hallucinations in epileptic seizures. Electrophysiological, clinical and anatomical correlates. Brain 1987;110 (Pt 2):339–359

58. Cho GS, Han MW, Lee B, et al. Zinc deficiency may be a cause of burning mouth syndrome as zinc replacement therapy has therapeutic effects. J Oral Pathol Med 2010;39(9):722–727

59. Heckmann SM, Hujoel P, Habiger S, et al. Zinc gluconate in the treatment of dysgeusia—a randomized clinical trial. J Dent Res 2005;84(1):35–38

60. Halyard MY, Jatoi A, Sloan JA, et al. Does zinc sulfate prevent therapy-induced taste alterations in head and neck cancer patients? Results of phase III double-blind, placebo-controlled trial from the North Central Cancer Treatment Group (N01C4). Int J Radiat Oncol Biol Phys 2007;67(5):1318–1322

61. Leopold D. Distortion of olfactory perception: diagnosis and treatment. Chem Senses 2002;27(7): 611–615

62. Zarinko K. Über Kakosmia subjectiva. In: Festschrift zur Feier des 80-jährigen Stiftungsfestes des ärztlichen Vereins zu Hamburg. Leipzig: Langkammer; 1896: 339–342

63. Zilstorff K. Parosmia. J Laryngol Otol 1966;80:(11) 1102–1104

64. Reden J, Maroldt H, Fritz A, Zahnert T, Hummel T. A study on the prognostic significance of qualitative olfactory dysfunction. Eur Arch Otorhinolaryngol 2007;264(2):139–144

65. Deems DA, Doty RL, Settle RG, et al. Smell and taste disorders, a study of 750 patients from the University of Pennsylvania Smell and Taste Center. Arch Otolaryngol Head Neck Surg 1991;117(5):519–528

66. Holbrook EH, Leopold DA, Schwob JE. Abnormalities of axon growth in human olfactory mucosa. Laryngoscope 2005;115(12):2144–2154

67. Begum M, McKenna PJ. Olfactory reference syndrome: a systematic review of the world literature. Psychol Med 2011;41(3):453–461

68. Frasnelli J, Landis BN, Heilmann S, et al. Clinical presentation of qualitative olfactory dysfunction. Eur Arch Otorhinolaryngol 2004;261(7):411–415

69. Bitter T, Siegert F, Gudziol H, et al. Gray matter alterations in parosmia. Neuroscience 2011;177: 177–182

70. Muller A, Rodewald A, Reden J, Gerber J, von Kummer R, Hummel T. Reduced olfactory bulb volume in post-traumatic and post-infectious olfactory dysfunction. Neuroreport 2005;16(5): 475–478

71. Leopold DA, Loehrl TA, Schwob JE. Long-term follow-up of surgically treated phantosmia. Arch Otolaryngol Head Neck Surg 2002;128(6):642–647

17 Structural Imaging in Chemosensory Dysfunction

Nasreddin Abolmaali

Summary

Structural imaging in chemosensory dysfunction can visualize the morphological anatomy and pathology of the entire chemosensory pathway, from the oral and nasal mucosa and adjacent structures (e.g., paranasal sinuses), along the particular cranial nerves, and through the respective ganglia to the brain. While some of these structures display only subtle and mainly size-related changes during life, the olfactory system contains highly plastic structures. For example, research indicates that smell deficits leading to a reduced sensory input result in structural changes at the level of the olfactory bulb. Therefore, certain cases require highly specific and optimized imaging with quantitative image analysis. However, in most patients, structural imaging in chemosensory dysfunction is a comparatively nonspecific diagnostic tool used mainly to exclude malignancy in the brain and the head and neck region. Clinical symptoms prompting imaging of the chemosensory system typically occur only if both sides of the respective structures are affected, which is more frequent in olfaction than in gustation. If only one side is affected, most patients will neither experience any chemosensory dysfunction nor be able to lateralize the loss of chemosensory input.

This chapter discusses some of the radiological basics for the assessment of chemosensory structures, results of quantitative imaging, and major pathologies in which imaging is clinically relevant.

Imaging Technique

> Magnetic resonance imaging is the modality of choice for imaging chemosensory dysfunction.

Technical Considerations: Magnetic Resonance Imaging

Field Strength

Magnetic resonance imaging (MRI) is the major imaging modality used to visualize the anatomy and pathology of chemosensory dysfunction, mainly because of its inherent high soft tissue contrast. It relies on signals from hydrogen atoms. The number of hydrogen atoms contributing to the MRI signal is increased at higher field strengths. Therefore, it may seem that small structures, such as the olfactory bulb (OB) (**Fig. 17.1**) and the olfactory tract (OT), are best visualized at 3 to 7 T. However, certain artifacts that increase with field strength reduce the applicability of these systems. For example, the main parts of the OT are not easily visualized at a field strength at or above 3 T, as so-called susceptibility artifacts, occurring at

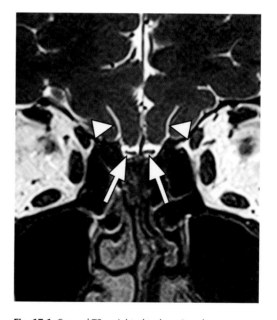

Fig. 17.1 Coronal T2-weighted turbo spin-echo magnetic resonance imaging. The olfactory bulbs (arrows) are surrounded by cerebrospinal fluid and located above the cribriform plate and below the olfactory sulci (arrowheads) of the frontal lobes.

the posterior frontobasis between cerebrospinal fluid (CSF) and the air-filled paranasal sinuses, may deteriorate signal (**Fig. 17.2**). Furthermore, these systems are still not available everywhere. Therefore, the imaging technique was optimized at 1.5 T, using advanced receiver-coil techniques or selected imaging sequences. The techniques discussed herein were performed at 1.5 T, which remains the reference standard for many applications. Most of the images in this chapter were acquired at 1.5 T.

Receiver Coils

When MRI was first used to visualize the OB, mostly small-loop coils were employed, which were placed on the nasion, and enabled comparatively high-resolution images of the OB to be obtained.[1] Owing to the limited field of view ("depth penetration") of these coils, the OT and posterior parts of the olfactory system could not be visualized, and standard head coils were applied, allowing imaging of the whole brain at somewhat lower spatial resolution. New head coils (e.g., multichannel head array coils) allow similar or even better spatial

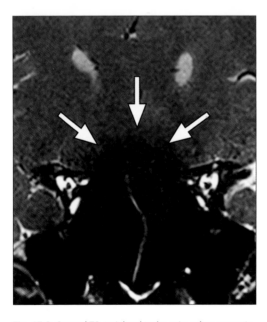

Fig. 17.2 Coronal T2-weighted turbo spin-echo magnetic resonance imaging at 3 T. The olfactory tracts (posterior to the olfactory bulbs) are not visible as a large susceptibility artifact has destroyed the image dataset (arrows). These artifacts do not limit visualization of this region at 1.5 T.

resolution than small-loop coils and provide information from the entire brain.

Sequence Techniques

Basically, two different tissue characteristics may be assessed: the T1 time, using T1-weighted sequences; and the T2 time, using T2-weighted sequences. Different sequence types (mainly turbo spin echo [TSE], constructive interference in steady-state precession [CISS], turbo fast low-angle shot) are capable of generating different contrasts between tissues. Additionally, and independent of the desired tissue contrast, sequences may be optimized for three-dimensional (3D) imaging or two-dimensional (2D) imaging.

For high-resolution imaging, 2D data acquisition is preferably performed using TSE techniques, which generate a voxel size of 0.405 mm³. A voxel is a 3D picture element (volume element) consisting of the slice thickness (mm) multiplied by the in-plane resolution (mm × mm). With such small voxels, accurate volumetry of the OB is feasible. To accurately assess this, 2D TSE sequences should be acquired in coronal slice orientation (perpendicular to the frontobasis; maximum slice thickness 2 mm) covering the entire frontal skull base and the pituitary gland. To visualize pathology along the OB or within the Meckel cave, a sequence with stronger T2-weighting (e.g., CISS[2]) appears to be advantageous. This technique generates bright signals from CSF and very low signal intensities from all other tissues and structures (i.e., high contrast for the sensitive visualization of structures surrounded by CSF [**Fig. 17.3**]). The disadvantage of this sequence is the poor contrast among nerves, brain, air, and bone.

If the entire afferent olfactory or gustatory system, including nasal and oral cavity and posterior structures, needs to be investigated, 3D imaging with isotropic voxels (which reveal identical lengths of the margins of every voxel in all three spatial orientations) covering the entire cranium is preferred. The acquired datasets allow for multiplanar reformation in any orientation and may be acquired before and after intravenous administration of contrast material. For such large volume acquisitions, imaging is preferably performed at 3 T to keep the acquisition time short whilst providing adequate spatial resolution.

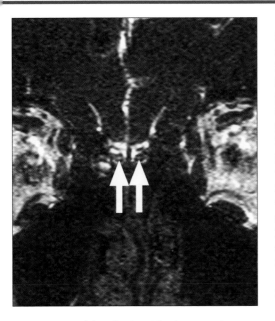

Fig. 17.3 Coronal, heavily T2-weighted, constructive interference in steady-state precession (CISS) magnetic resonance imaging. High contrast is provided between cerebrospinal fluid and other structures. Therefore, subtle liquid structures, e.g., small fluid-filled spaces within the olfactory bulbs (arrows), can be appreciated, while the contrast between other structures is too low for detailed analysis.

For clinical purposes, and mainly to exclude frontal, prepontine, or intra-axial tumors or infections, the imaging protocol includes T1-weighted 2D imaging before and after intravenous administration of contrast material. Imaging should be performed using axial, coronal, and sagittal planes to provide sufficient information for preoperative planning. The use of fat suppression techniques improves the delineation of extracranial tumors growing along cranial nerves and invading subcutaneous fat. For tumor detection in the head and neck region, so-called TIRM (turbo inversion recovery magnitude) sequences with strong fat suppression (inversion time above 160 milliseconds) are preferably performed, as these imaging techniques are highly sensitive at detecting pathologies surrounded by normal soft tissues, especially fat.

Table 17.1 shows important technical parameters of recommended sequence designs.

New Developments

As the signal in MRI relies on hydrogen, the contrast between cortical bone and air is low. New techniques, such as sequences delivering ultrashort echo times, allow for enhanced contrast between air and bone, and may be applied to MRI of the paranasal sinuses in the near future.

Table 17.1 Useful features of magnetic resonance imaging sequences for application in chemosensory imaging

	T1 TSE (2D)	T1 TSE w&w/o FS (2D)	T1 TFL (3D) (MP-RAGE)	T2 TSE (2D)	T2 TSE (3D)	CISS (3D)	TIRM (2D)
TR (ms)	400	450	2180	4800	2500	12.2	6000
TE (ms)	14	11	3.2	148	354	6.1	80
TI (ms)	–		1100	–	–	–	170
Bandwidth (Hz / pixel)	70	130	160	130	930	130	130
Slice thickness (mm)	2	3	0.8	2	0.8	0.7	3
In-plane resolution (mm²)	0.45 × 0.45	0.8 × 0.8	0.8 × 0.8	0.45 × 0.45	0.8 × 0.8	0.7 × 0.7	0.8 × 0.8
Voxel size (mm³ = nL)	0.41	1.92	0.51	0.41	0.51	0.34	1.92
Approximate acquisition time (min)	14	4	6 (PAT factor 2)	8	11	6	4

TR, repetition time; TE, echo time; TI, inversion time; PAT, parallel acquisition technique; TSE, turbo spin echo; TFL, turbo FLASH (FLASH, fast low-angle shot); CISS, constructive interference in steady-state precession; MP RAGE, magnetization prepared rapid acquisition gradient echo; 2D, two dimensional; 3D, three dimensional; TIRM, turbo inversion recovery magnitude; FS, fat suppression; w&w/o, with and without.

Limitations

Current limitations of MRI in structural imaging of chemosensory dysfunction are related to the size of the object and the contrast of the object in relation to its surroundings. Higher field strengths are pushing the limits, but cellular imaging, for example, is only possible using labeled cells. Imaging of single neurons or even groups of cells is currently not possible with MRI without labeling.

Patient-related contraindications of MRI are continuously decreasing. While cardiac pacemakers have been an absolute contraindication, some institutes are now performing MRI in patients with such devices under dedicated surveillance. Continuing contraindications are ferromagnetic foreign bodies in regions where their movement may destroy structures, especially vessels or neural structures.

The use of gadolinium-based contrast agents continues to be considered very safe, even in patients suffering from severe renal insufficiency (glomerular filtration rate < 30 mL/min/1.73 m²).

Technical Considerations: Computed Tomography

Image Acquisition

Computed tomography (CT) imaging contrast is dependent on the electron density of the visualized tissues. Therefore, soft tissue contrast is low compared with MRI, and some structures are not easily visualized (e.g., the OB). However, CT imaging of bone- and air-filled structures reveals a high difference in electron density and can provide sufficient diagnostic information in some cases of chemosensory dysfunction. Destruction of bones related to trauma or infiltration and replacement of air in cranial cavities are the main pathologies visualized by CT (**Fig. 17.4**). Additionally, the visualization of the foramina where the cranial nerves penetrate the skull base is a major indication for CT in chemosensory imaging. For this indication, CT is only limited by spatial resolution (e.g., the foramina of the cribriform plate are not visualized in standard CT imaging). Typically, a 3D dataset of the skull is acquired and reformatted in three orthogonal imaging planes. Data acquisition is mainly performed in an axial imaging plane, but also may be performed or supplemented in a coronal imaging plane. This depends on the clinical question:

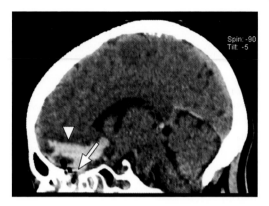

Fig. 17.4 Sagittal reformation of computed tomography of the head of a polytrauma patient in soft tissue window. Displaced fracture of the frontal skull base (arrow) indicating possible later problems with olfaction due to olfactory nerve and bulb injury. The dark areas resemble intracranial air collections. Additionally, intracranial frontal lobe bleeding is detected (bright, arrowhead).

while trauma and tumor questions are most often answered with axial imaging, pathology of the paranasal sinuses is mainly assessed using coronal imaging. Additionally, artifacts related to metal-based dental implants, which may impair image quality, have to be taken into consideration when planning image acquisition.

Nowadays, CT is acquired as a true (isotropic) 3D dataset revealing a voxel size between 0.6 mm × 0.6 mm × 0.6 mm (voxel size: 0.216 mm³) and 1 mm × 1 mm × 1 mm (voxel size: 1 mm³), and the desired imaging planes are reformatted out of this dataset.

Considerations on Dose Exposure

Unlike MRI, CT is always associated with radiation exposure. In most regions of many countries, the natural annual radiation exposure of the human body reaches ~2 to 3 mSv (millisievert) and is mainly related to the inhalation of[222] radon, terrestrial radiation, and to the ingestion of radioactive isotopes such as[40] potassium. One CT of the head delivers about the same radiation dose in a few seconds. In most cases, this may not be relevant for the individual patient, but it is related to a dose risk in adults of ~5% per sievert for the induction of lethal cancer.[3] In other words: if 1,000,000 people receive a CT of the head with a dose exposure of 2.5 mSv, 125 of them may die from cancer induced by this diagnostic procedure. Other risks of radiation exposure may be higher, for example, the risk of developing a cataract. For reasons of radiation protection, the risk factor of 5% per sievert was estimated in a pessimistic fashion. The risk factor is expected to be lower, as the relation between dose and risk is not linear, especially at low radiation exposure, but data for a more valid risk approximation are not available. The risk of dose exposure must be considered before a CT of the head is carried out, but must not prevent the patient from receiving an adequate diagnosis prior to therapy. Radiologists are able to reduce CT-related radiation burden, conserving high sensitivity and specificity of images, if the clinical question is precisely specified.

Projection Radiography

In the clinical setting, projection radiography (PRG) is mainly used for the visualization of the paranasal sinuses in sinusitis, but many standardized projections exist for the evaluation of the cranial nerves as they pass through the foramina penetrating the base of the skull (**Fig. 17.5**). The aim of PRG is either to visualize an enlarged or destroyed foramen that indicates tumor extent along the respective cranial nerve or to demonstrate bony pathologies in trauma or inborn osteochondral diseases. With MRI and CT available, PRG nowadays is a second-line diagnostic tool for certain infrequent indications. In the diagnostic workup of the paranasal sinuses, PRG is frequently of no value.

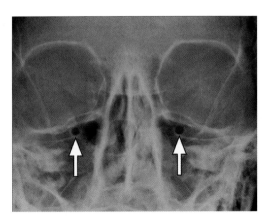

Fig. 17.5 Projection radiography of the skull with optimal visualization of the round foramina (arrows) letting the second branch of the trigeminal nerve (cranial nerve V/II) pass through the base of the skull.

Ultrasound and FDG-PET/CT

Ultrasound and [18F]-fluorodeoxyglucose positron emission tomography–computed tomography (FDG-PET/CT) may only supplement MRI and CT and play a minor role in chemosensory imaging. In oncological imaging, on the other hand, both modalities are of considerable importance.

Olfactory Imaging

> Dedicated imaging, mainly using specific MRI techniques, is needed to optimize therapeutic decisions.

Introduction

The olfactory nerve (ON) is the sum of the axons of all olfactory receptor neurons, which are located in the nasal mucosa on both sides of the nasal cavity. The ganglion of the ON collects all these sensory afferents and constitutes the primary olfactory cortex. It is called the olfactory bulb. The ON passes through the perforations of the cribriform plate to make contact with the OB. The OB is aligned in a strict ventrodorsal orientation and has an average volume of 125 ± 17 mm^3 (mean $\pm$ standard deviation).[4] The olfactory sulcus (OS) of the frontal lobe is located above the OB and the OT, and its morphology appears to be dependent on the presence of the OB.[4] The OT runs from anteromedial to posterolateral (perforate substance) and its cross-sectional area is ~1/10 of the cross-sectional area of the OB. Adding up the volumes of OB and OT results in an average of up to 160 mm^3, but this volume shows considerable variation depending on age.[5]

Evaluation of the nasal mucosa containing the ON (which is invisible in humans in vivo) is preferably performed by MRI using T2-weighted sequences in a coronal image orientation.[6] In many centers, the nasal mucosa is investigated by CT, but MRI should be considered in every patient to reduce radiation exposure.[7]

Adequate visualization of the human OB and OT in vivo is only possible using MRI (see **Fig. 17.1**). However, owing to the size and orientation of these structures, they are often not visible on standard clinical MRIs of the brain and skull used to exclude malignant disease. Pathologies affecting the olfactory system include inborn diseases such as Kallmann syndrome, tumors such as meningiomas, and metastatic disease.

Imaging of the Nasal Mucosa Containing the Olfactory Nerves

In the nasal cavity, the most frequent causes of olfactory loss are inflammatory disorders such as sinonasal disease with and without polyposis.[8] In addition, respiratory problems may prevent airflow to the olfactory cleft and thus produce olfactory loss. More recently, localized inflammation of the olfactory cleft with consecutive thickening of the mucosa has been described as a possible cause of olfactory loss.[9]

Imaging of the Olfactory Bulb

Congenital Anosmia

Largely based on work by Yousem and colleagues[10] magnetic resonance–based imaging of the OB has found its way into clinical practice (**Fig. 17.6**).

Interestingly, flattening of the OS in the plane of the posterior tangent through the eyeballs can be used as an additional criterion to separate patients with isolated congenital anosmia from normosmic

controls.[4] This might be important when the OBs are difficult to identify (e.g., for technical reasons).

Tumors Affecting Olfactory Bulb Function

Tumors of the frontal skull base commonly induce alterations of the olfactory sense, such as hyposmia, anosmia, or parosmia. Such distortions of olfaction only occur in bilateral damage. Most commonly meningiomas (**Fig. 17.7**) affect the OB and OT.[11] Esthesioneuroblastomas typically involve the frontal skull base and grow along the cranial nerves into and out of the skull base. Therefore, the ON, OB, and OT are commonly affected by such tumors (**Fig. 17.8**). In rare cases, other tumors, such as olfactory-ensheathing cell tumors[12] or primitive neuroectodermal tumors in children (**Fig. 17.9**), affect the olfactory system.

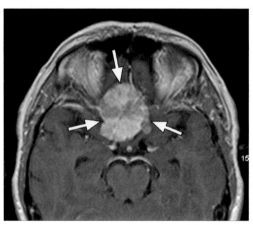

Fig. 17.7 Axial T1-weighted turbo spin-echo magnetic resonance imaging after intravenous administration of contrast agent. As frequently seen, this meningioma (arrows) shows a marked contrast enhancement. Neither olfactory bulbs nor olfactory tracts are visible. Typically, meningiomas show a shallow contrast enhancement in the adjacent meninges, referred to as a dural tail.

The Volume of the Olfactory Bulb may be Modified

Morphological imaging in healthy, normosmic subjects showed that OB volume is highly variable.[5,13] Importantly, the reliability of measures of OB volume does not contribute to this variability, as a

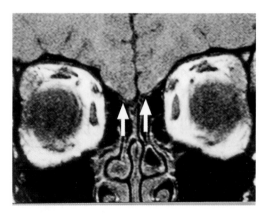

Fig. 17.6 Coronal T1-weighted turbo spin-echo magnetic resonance imaging in a patient with congenital anosmia. Neither the olfactory bulbs (OBs) (arrows) nor the olfactory tracts are visible and the olfactory sulci are developed, which are frequent findings in aplastic OBs.

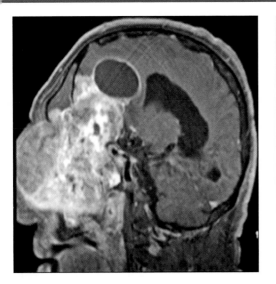

Fig. 17.8 Axial T1-weighted turbo spin-echo magnetic resonance imaging after intravenous administration of a contrast agent. This massive frontobasal tumor (esthesioneuroblastoma) shows inhomogeneous, partly septated enhancement, cystic regions, and a severe mass effect.

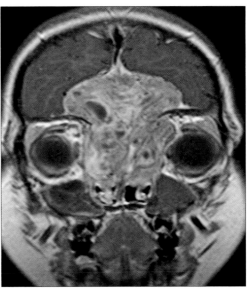

Fig. 17.9 Coronal contrast-enhanced T1-weighted turbo spin-echo magnetic resonance imaging in a child suffering from a primitive neuroectodermal tumor with cystic components. The olfactory nerve, olfactory bulb, olfactory tract, and parts of the frontal lobes are destroyed.

high interobserver reliability has been reported in numerous studies.[4,14] It seems likely that, on an individual level, changes of the OB provide a measure of the prognosis of olfactory dysfunction.

The reason for the high plasticity of the OB volume can be found in the continuing synaptogenesis in the OB, which remains highly plastic throughout adult life, reflecting, to some degree, the level of afferent neural activity.[15,16] In patients with olfactory loss, OB volume correlates with decreased olfactory sensitivity regardless of the cause of olfactory loss.[17] It varies with regard to olfactory function, and decreases with duration of olfactory loss.[18]

Imaging of the Olfactory Tract

The OT has a comparatively small cross-sectional area and an oblique course along the frontobasis. Imaging is therefore demanding and only MRI can successfully visualize the OT. As with the OB, tumors (e.g., meningiomas and metastases) and trauma are the main causes of damage to the OT. In rare cases, large aneurysms of the anterior cerebral artery may also compress the OT (**Fig. 17.10**).

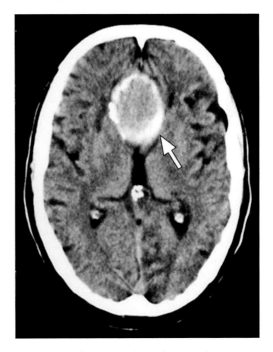

Fig. 17.10 Axial contrast-enhanced computed tomography of the brain. Emanating from the anterior cerebral artery, a large contrast-enhancing aneurysm (arrow) with a partly calcified margin has compressed both olfactory tracts, leading to anosmia as a first symptom in this patient.

Imaging of Olfactory Eloquent Brain Structures

Several brain structures are highly significant in processing olfactory information. These are divided into the primary olfactory cortex and secondary or tertiary olfactory projection areas.[19] Among other processes, tumors, infarctions, hemorrhage, superficial siderosis, or changes in blood perfusion may affect olfactory function.

Mesial tumors (e.g., of the amygdala) seem to play an important role in the genesis of olfactory auras.[20] Furthermore, in patients who have undergone brain surgery it has been shown that the temporal lobe and the orbitofrontal cortex play a role in the execution of various olfactory functions and odor memory.[21,22]

Conclusions

In conclusion, olfactory dysfunction may be caused at various levels during the processing of olfactory information.[23] Interestingly, olfactory function appears to be assessable through measurement of the volume of the OB. It can be expected that techniques with higher resolution will provide even better insights into the structural and functional organization of the olfactory system.

As with the entire chemosensory system, olfactory function can be affected by brain lesions even when they are not directly associated with the OB or OT. In turn, when using MRI as a diagnostic tool, the whole brain of patients with olfactory dysfunction needs to be thoroughly investigated.

Trigeminal Imaging

The sensory parts of the trigeminal nerve (TN, cranial nerve V) transfer sensations of pain, temperature differences, and chemical stimulation in the nasal and oral mucosa to central processing, and thereby modify and enhance olfactory and gustatory chemosensation.[24] The most prominent chemical compound stimulating trigeminal receptors in the mouth and nose is probably capsaicin, which can be found, for example, in pepperoni. The three branches of the TN leave the skull through three different peripheral foramina (branch I [NV/I], supraorbital foramen; branch II [NV/II], infraorbital foramen; branch III [NV/III], mental foramen—touch these trigeminal trigger

points synchronously for *mind melding*) and three different central canals (NV/I, superior orbital fissure; NV/II, round foramen [see **Fig. 17.5**]; NV/III, oval foramen). All these canals can be visualized by PRG, but destruction of bony structures surrounding the nerves is better visualized on CT (**Fig. 17.11**). Axial, T1-weighted, fat-suppressed, contrast-enhanced MRI sequences allow direct visualization and superior detection of schwannomas or metastatic or direct tumor spread along the nerves. These are supplemented by axial TIRM imaging (CSF is bright and fat is dark), especially for extracranial lesion detection. Squamous cell carcinomas of the head and neck region may induce damage of the peripheral branches of the TN, but only in rare cases can olfaction or gustation be altered by such tumors. The major ganglion of the trigeminal nerve that collects all sensory and most motor afferents constitutes the primary trigeminal cortex, and is called the ganglion of Gasser (GG). The GG is located bilaterally within the Meckel cave and is best visualized by heavily T2-weighted MRI (CISS, **Fig. 17.12**). These sequences provide high contrast between the bright CSF and the dark nerves, and are also used to investigate the

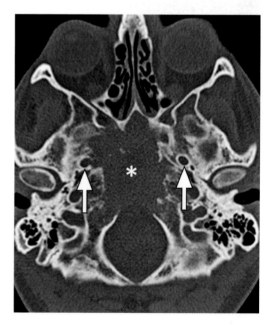

Fig. 17.11 Axial computed tomography of the skull base, bone window. The bony medial skull base is destroyed by a large, squamous cell carcinoma of the nasopharynx (asterisk). The right and left oval foramina are also depicted (arrows).

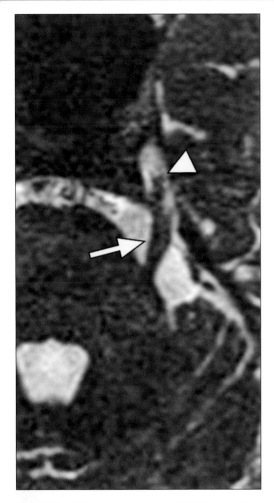

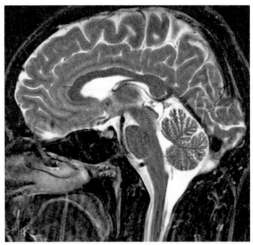

Fig. 17.13 Sagittal T2-weighted turbo-gradient spin-echo of the brain and brainstem. The red line shows the position of the nuclei involved in trigeminal signal processing (sensory: nucleus pontinus, nucleus spinalis; motor: nucleus mesencephalicus, nucleus motorius).

Fig. 17.12 Axial image from isotropic 3D CISS magnetic resonance imaging. Within the cerebrospinal fluid–filled (bright) Meckel cave (arrowhead), the ganglion of Gasser (dark) is visualized. More posteriorly, the cisternal segment of the trigeminal nerve root is visualized (arrow).

cisternal segment of the nerve roots of the TN between the GG and the brainstem (**Fig. 17.13**). In this region, the major pathologies affecting the trigeminal system are tumors (vestibular schwannomas compressing the cisternal segment of the TN, meningiomas, epidermoid cysts, and, less commonly, trigeminal schwannomas, neurofibromatosis type II, and meningeal carcinomatosis), congenital (arachnoid cysts, aplasia), inflammatory or infectious (multiple sclerosis, sarcoidosis, tuberculosis, bacterial and viral infections), and vascular (contact or compression of the TN root causing focal demyelination, which is the most

frequent detectable cause of classic trigeminal neuralgia). The sensory (major) nerve root is far larger than the motor nerve root, but separation on imaging is frequently difficult. Sensory input from the nasal and oral mucosa is processed in two (nucleus pontinus and nucleus spinalis) of the four nuclei located in the brainstem (**Fig. 17.14**) and connected to the TN. These nuclei are connected to the reticular formation, the olfactory and gustatory centers, and other deep structures (especially the nucleus accumbens) for information analysis. Imaging of the brain and brainstem is preferably performed using sagittal T2-weighted and axial T1-weighted sequences after intravenous injection of contrast material or, with higher sensitivity, by applying fluid-attenuated inversion recovery (FLAIR) imaging after contrast enhancement. Major pathologies of the brainstem are again divisible into vascular lesions (stroke caused by occlusion of the posterior inferior cerebellar artery or the basilar artery; hemorrhage caused by hypertension, arteriovenous malformations or cavernous angiomas; trauma), inflammation or infection (multiple sclerosis, acute demyelinating encephalomyelitis, human immunodeficiency virus encephalitis, and others), and tumors (especially pontine gliomas, lymphomas, hemangioblastomas, and metastases).

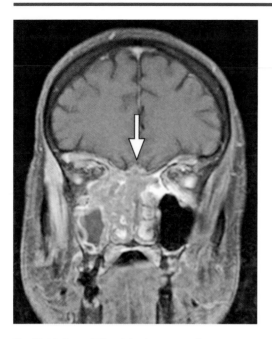

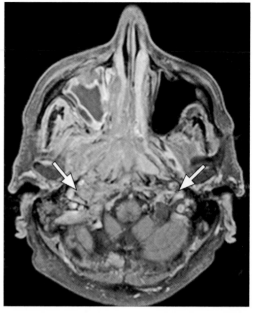

Fig. 17.14 Coronal T1-weighted sequence after intravenous administration of contrast material with fat suppression. This patient suffers from a massive tumor (squamous cell cancer) destroying large areas of the skull base and infiltrating the cranium. Both the olfactory bulb and the olfactory tract are destroyed by the anterior parts of the large mass (arrow).

Fig. 17.15 Axial T1-weighted sequence after intravenous application of contrast material with fat suppression. Same patient as in **Fig. 17.14**. Both jugular foramina are infiltrated by tumor masses; cranial nerves IX and X on both sides are destroyed (arrows).

Gustatory Imaging

Gustation is the sum of afferents collected from the taste buds along the outer edge of the tongue and delivered via the TN, the chorda tympani (facial nerve, cranial nerve VII), the glossopharyngeal nerve (cranial nerve IX), and the vagus nerve (cranial nerve X) to ganglia and brain. Single-sided conditions affecting the chorda tympani are one of the unusual exceptions from the fact that chemosensation is not usually lateralized. Hence, in certain rare (and typically very sensitive) patients, unilateral conditions of the chorda tympani may be perceived as disturbance of gustatory sensation. Gustation is far less frequently affected by specific pathologies than olfaction, and research into gustation has not been as detailed as it has been in the olfactory system. In fact, disturbance of the gustatory system is a quite rare clinical symptom and mainly occurs in patients with very large tumors destroying most parts of the peripheral gustatory system of the head and neck region (**Figs. 17.14 and 17.15**). Many of these patients are frequently and continuously exposed to certain toxins (e.g., alcohol, cigarette smoke), which themselves reduce gustatory sensations. As a result, even with extensive tumors destroying large (typically more peripheral) parts of the gustatory system, these patients commonly do not experience modifications or restrictions in gustation. Tumors and metastases affecting the respective cranial nerves traveling through the head and neck region and entering the skull should be considered and imaged. Tumors and infections affecting the ganglia and nerve roots (mainly meningeal carcinomatosis, meningiomas, and infectious diseases of the posterior skull base) should also be visualized. Lastly, the brainstem and the brain have to be evaluated, mainly to exclude primary brain tumors and metastases. Activation and deactivation of the primary gustatory cortex is dependent on the sensory input: sweet and salty tastes activate, while bitter stimuli lead to deactivation.[25]

A fast and sensitive imaging protocol visualizing the entire gustatory system would include axial TIRM sequences of the head and neck region, T2-weighted and T1-weighted sequences of the brain before and after intravenous administration of contrast material (probably supplemented by FLAIR imaging), and contrast-enhanced T1-weighted sequences of the brain and head and neck region with fat suppression.

Conclusion

> Close communication between ear, nose, and throat doctors and radiologists assures best imaging quality for the patient's symptoms—identify the question you want imaging to answer as precisely as possible.

In the clinical context, structural imaging in chemosensory dysfunction in the first instance requires nonspecific exclusion of malignancy and inflammation affecting the brain, the base of the skull, and the head and neck region. Especially in the context of olfaction, research has confirmed that more specific visualization techniques, requiring highly adapted and optimized imaging and quantification of chemosensory structures, are mandatory. MRI is the modality of choice for both fields and only very few questions may be preferentially assessed by CT. Adequate selection of imaging techniques takes account of the fact that chemosensory input is not lateralized; therefore, in general, anosmia or ageusia will only develop if the peripheral input of both the right and the left side is impaired, or if a central lesion has evolved. For optimal results in chemosensory imaging, details of the clinical question for the specific patient should be discussed with the involved radiologist.

Acknowledgments

The authors thank Professor Dr. Rüdiger von Kummer, Chairman of the Department for Neuroradiology, PD Dr. Volker Hietschold, Institute and Policlinics for Diagnostic Radiology, and Dr. Gabriele Hahn, Pediatric Radiology, from the University Clinics and Medical Faculty Carl Gustav Carus, Dresden University of Technology, for their support with some of the images presented in the chapter.

References

1. Suzuki M, Takashima T, Kadoya M, Takahashi S, Miyayama S, Taira S. MR imaging of olfactory bulbs and tracts. AJNR Am J Neuroradiol 1989; 10(5):955–957

2. Casselman JW, Kuhweide R, Deimling M, Ampe W, Dehaene I, Meeus L. Constructive interference in steady state-3DFT MR imaging of the inner ear and cerebellopontine angle. AJNR Am J Neuroradiol 1993;14(1):47–57

3. ICRP. The 2007 Recommendations of the International Commission on Radiological Protection. ICRP publication 103. Ann ICRP 2007;37(2–4):1–332

4. Abolmaali ND, Hietschold V, Vogl TJ, Hüttenbrink KB, Hummel T. MR evaluation in patients with isolated anosmia since birth or early childhood. AJNR Am J Neuroradiol 2002;23(1):157–164

5. Yousem DM, Geckle RJ, Bilker WB, Doty RL. Olfactory bulb and tract and temporal lobe volumes. Normative data across decades. Ann N Y Acad Sci 1998;855:546–555

6. Abolmaali N, Kantchew A, Vogl TJ, Hummel T. Evaluation of the "nasal cycle" using MR-imaging. XVI International Congress of Head and Neck Radiology 4–6 September 2003, Frankfurt/Main, Germany. Eur Radiol 2003;13:C2

7. Abolmaali N, Hummel T, Damm M. Two- and three-dimensional, morphologic and functional MR-imaging in smelling disorders. [Article in German] Laryngorhinootologie 2009;88(1):10–16

8. Kern RC. Chronic sinusitis and anosmia: pathologic changes in the olfactory mucosa. Laryngoscope 2000;110(7):1071–1077

9. Trotier D, Bensimon JL, Herman P, Tran Ba Huy P, Døving KB, Eloit C. Inflammatory obstruction of the olfactory clefts and olfactory loss in humans: a new syndrome? Chem Senses 2007;32(3):285–292

10. Yousem DM, Turner WJ, Li C, Snyder PJ, Doty RL. Kallmann syndrome: MR evaluation of olfactory system. AJNR Am J Neuroradiol 1993;14(4):839–843

11. Welge-Luessen A, Temmel A, Quint C, Moll B, Wolf S, Hummel T. Olfactory function in patients with olfactory groove meningioma. J Neurol Neurosurg Psychiatry 2001;70(2):218–221

12. Yasuda M, Higuchi O, Takano S, Matsumura A. Olfactory ensheathing cell tumor: a case report. J Neurooncol 2006;76(2):111–113

13. Azoulay R, Fallet-Bianco C, Garel C, Grabar S, Kalifa G, Adamsbaum C. MRI of the olfactory bulbs and sulci in human fetuses. Pediatr Radiol 2006;36(2):97–107

14. Yousem DM, Geckle RJ, Doty RL, Bilker WB. Reproducibility and reliability of volumetric measurements of olfactory eloquent structures. Acad Radiol 1997;4(4):264–269

15. Baker H, Kawano T, Albert V, Joh TH, Reis DJ, Margolis FL. Olfactory bulb dopamine neurons survive deafferentation-induced loss of tyrosine hydroxylase. Neuroscience 1984;11(3):605–615

16. Margolis FL, Roberts N, Ferriero D, Feldman J. Denervation in the primary olfactory pathway of mice: biochemical and morphological effects. Brain Res 1974;81(3):469–483

17. Mueller A, Rodewald A, Reden J, Gerber J, von Kummer R, Hummel T. Reduced olfactory bulb volume in post-traumatic and post-infectious olfactory dysfunction. Neuroreport 2005;16(5): 475–478

18. Rombaux P, Mouraux A, Bertrand B, Nicolas G, Duprez T, Hummel T. Olfactory function and olfactory bulb volume in patients with postinfectious olfactory loss. Laryngoscope 2006;116(3):436–439

19. Gottfried JA. Smell: central nervous processing. Adv Otorhinolaryngol 2006;63:44–69

20. Chen C, Shih YH, Yen DJ, et al. Olfactory auras in patients with temporal lobe epilepsy. Epilepsia 2003;44(2):257–260

21. Frasnelli J, Lundström JN, Boyle JA, Djordjevic J, Zatorre RJ, Jones-Gotman M. Neuroanatomical correlates of olfactory performance. Exp Brain Res 2010;201(1):1–11

22. Jones-Gotman M, Zatorre RJ, Cendes F, et al. Contribution of medial versus lateral temporal-lobe structures to human odour identification. Brain 1997;120(Pt 10):1845–1856

23. Abolmaali N, Gudziol V, Hummel T. Pathology of the olfactory nerve. Neuroimaging Clin N Am 2008;18(2):233–242, preceding x

24. Bensafi M, Iannilli E, Gerber J, Hummel T. Neural coding of stimulus concentration in the human olfactory and intranasal trigeminal systems. Neuroscience 2008;154(2):832–838

25. Savic-Berglund I. Imaging of olfaction and gustation. Nutr Rev 2004;62(11 Pt 2):S205–S207; discussion S224–S241

18 Providing Expert Opinion on Olfactory and Gustatory Disorders

Boris A. Stuck, Axel Muttray, Terence M. Davidson

Summary

In discussing olfactory and gustatory disorders, it is often necessary to provide an expert legal opinion—a task that differs greatly from everyday clinical work. A series of factors makes a legal assessment difficult, particularly missing initial examinations and the limited possibilities to obtain objective examination results. The question of work-related causes of olfactory and gustatory disorders is of particular interest, despite the fact that these disorders are often not cited in lists of occupational diseases (e.g., in Germany). Presenting complaints depend greatly on their cause. In general, the patient reports a limited capability of smell as well as of taste. It is important to distinguish between a subjective gustatory dysfunction (generally an olfactory dysfunction) and a real dysfunction in terms of hypogeusia or ageusia.

A thorough medical history is the basis of every assessment, supplemented by clinical examinations, and completed by specific tests of olfactory and gustatory capabilities. For German-speaking countries, the Olfactology and Gustology Task Force of the German Society of Otolaryngology (Deutsche Gesellschaft für Hals-Nasen-Ohrenheilkunde) has published recommendations regarding the provision of expert opinion on olfactory disorders, which facilitate the assessment in practice.

Introduction

It is often necessary to provide an expert assessment on presumed or confirmed olfactory and gustatory disorders. In total, olfactory disorders outnumber gustatory disorders. A series of factors complicates the assessment of olfactory and gustatory disorders. Aside from missing initial examinations in almost all cases (convincing examinations of smelling and tasting capabilities are rarely conducted and are usually not among the screening examinations of the Employers' Liabilities Insurance Association), this is mainly due to the lack of results from olfactory or gustatory examinations. In this chapter, we will demonstrate the assessor's principal tasks as well as the obligatory examinations and basics of assessment in the authors' view. Also, we will present recommendations for providing an expert opinion. Furthermore, this complex problem will be illustrated with two case studies from everyday practice.

Providing Expert Opinion

The task of providing an expert opinion is complex and differs greatly from the everyday activities of clinical practice. Within the framework of social legislation, a physician is often asked to function as an expert assessor for the Employers' Liabilities Insurance Association, as well as for cases concerning compensation and the Severely Handicapped Persons Act. Private insurers have regulations of their own, which will not be discussed here. Finally, it might be necessary to take a stand in a liability suit if there are allegations of treatment errors and compensation claims (e.g., after nasal or sinus surgery). Iatrogenic olfactory disorders, for example, may be due to overzealous nasal surgery, most commonly polypectomy. These may be litigated as malpractice. Experts are required to testify that the nasal surgery was overzealous and so a departure from the standard of care. Defense experts testify the opposite.

Regarding the Employers' Liabilities Insurance Association's legislation, the question of work-related causes of olfactory and gustatory disorders is of utmost significance. **Table 18.1** gives an overview, without claiming to be complete, of substances that are able to cause toxic olfactory disorders. In each case, an evaluation of the particular workplace is mandatory. Mixed exposures are numerous (e.g., chromates, bases and acids in electroplating). The precondition for toxic olfactory disorders is a *substantial* overstepping of critical values defined by occupational medicine. Most

Table 18.1 Selected working materials that can cause olfactory disorders in humans

Metals and their compounds	Organic solvents
Lead	Inter alia several alloys, including benzenes
Chromium	Esters (acetates)
Cadmium	Carbon disulfide
Nickel	Trichloroethylene
Mercury	
	Aldehydes
Dust and smoke	
Welding fumes	**Acids and bases**
Cement	
	Hydrogen sulfide
Irritant gases	
Inter alia ammonia	**Carbon monoxide**
Nitrous gases	
Sulfur dioxide	**Cyanide**

Reproduced from Stuck and Muttray (2008)[36]; not all original papers were verified.

of today's toxin exposures are therefore the result of an acute, intense injury. In the case of exposure to caustic or irritant agents in very high concentrations, the possibility of a toxic olfactory disorder and rhinitis must be considered.

An overview of toxin-induced anosmia may be found in Smith et al 2009.[1] This review points out that in the past, and prior to **Occupational Safety and Health Administration** protection, anosmia was seen as a result of chronic exposure to toxins such as formaldehyde and photo developing chemicals (see also Chapter 9: Miscellaneous Causes of Olfactory Dysfunction).

In addition, zinc gluconate nasal sprays, touted as a homoeopathic treatment for the common cold, are reported to cause anosmia based on numerous patient complaints to the Food and Drug Administration. Zinc gluconate nasal sprays have been removed from the market and presumably the flurry of current lawsuits will soon be resolved. Several scientific publications support the diagnosis of zinc-induced anosmia.[2,3]

In the case of a well-founded suspicion of an occupational disorder, it is usually mandatory (e.g., in Germany, Switzerland, or Austria) to report this to the Employers' Liabilities Insurance Association, even if a reduction in earning capacity that may lead to retirement is not expected. The insured

patient must be informed of this report by his physician. A comprehensive comment on the legal basis of assessment cannot be given here, as it differs substantially among different countries and social systems.

Expert Opinion in Olfactory Disorders

The symptoms involved in the assessment of olfactory disorders depend greatly on their cause. Persons who have lost their capacity to smell in an accident can normally define the circumstances and moment of the damage very clearly. They often experience the symptoms very vividly, as in the majority of these cases, an uninhibited ability to smell existed previously. If an olfactory disorder has evolved through the years because of occupational exposure to toxins or is claimed as a result of a medical intervention with a possibly preexisting impairment of smell, the situation clearly becomes more difficult for the assessor.

In general, not only an impairment of smell but also an impairment of taste is reported. The differentiation between a concomitant disorder of taste that occurs as a result of an olfactory disorder and a real gustatory dysfunction in terms of hypogeusia or ageusia is of substantial importance for an adequate assessment. This differentiation is often difficult to explain to the parties concerned. Factual gustatory disorders are relatively rare and will be discussed later. An appropriate medical history and a diligent gustatory examination ought to be part of every assessment of olfactory disorders. It must be pointed out, however, that disorders of the factual gustatory capabilities and subjective impairment of taste can both occur with a pre-existing olfactory disorder. Impaired sensitivity to flavors, as well as reduced trigeminal sensitivity in olfactory disorders,[4-7] is ascribed to the loss of reinforcing neuronal interaction, and not to damage to receptive structures. A reduced reaction to trigeminal stimuli can be assessed as an indication, but not as proof, of an amplification of existing symptoms, or of malingering.

Medical History

At the beginning of the medical history, the nature and extent of the olfactory disorder must be established, and the origin and course must be ascertained. Qualitative olfactory disorders (e.g., parosmias and phantosmias) without an associated decline of olfactory capabilities (hyposmia or anosmia) are rare and not typically assessed for medicolegal purposes. For isolated qualitative olfactory disorders, concrete directives for action do not exist; compensation is, therefore, usually not provided.

In olfactory disorders that have developed over the years, a precise date of onset cannot be given quite frequently. Owing to their gradual onset, the symptoms often are not experienced or described as vividly as sudden onset disorders, and quite often olfactory disorders are noted as a secondary complaint to other disorders that are to be assessed. Questions regarding the accidental consumption of spoiled food, or occasions when smoke or hazardous materials that can be smelled were not recognized in time, can be helpful in chronological determination, as such occurrences are often remembered. This can be vital for the assessment of correlation, as toxic olfactory disorders develop in close chronological correlation with the causative exposure. Quite often, patients complain of a loss of appetite in association with the perceived taste disorders. However, some gain weight as a result of overeating to seek some taste. Change in body weight should be ascertained.

Additionally, special attention should be paid if the patient has previously seen a doctor for olfactory disorders or if appropriate examinations have already been performed. Generally, however, relevant examination results are not available. Patients are often assessed initially for other occupational disorders (e.g., hardness of hearing due to noise and disorders of the lung and the musculoskeletal system) and work-related olfactory disorders are not described until later in the process.

As a rule, traumatic damage resulting from accidents leads to an immediate defect in the fila olfactoria themselves, or in the brain areas responsible for processing olfactory stimuli. The majority of cases of post-traumatic anosmia are a result of frontal or occipital trauma, but are occasionally the result of temporal or parietal trauma. The generally accepted mechanism of injury is that the trauma results in an abrupt anterior or posterior movement of the brain. The thin olfactory fila of the cranial nerve are presumably stretched or torn as they exit the cribriform plate. If the fila are stretched, olfaction may recover; if torn, the olfactory disorder will usually persist. Some such patients will develop phantosmia, which may dissipate after several months. Loss of consciousness is not a prerequisite for post-traumatic anosmia. Isolated intracranial injury is uncommon.[8] Although the onset is usually immediate, patients with severe cranial injuries or multiple trauma may not perceive the disorder until the acute phase of the injury has resolved, which can take up to several months depending on the severity of the injury. A gradual decrease in olfactory function in this period is not impossible, though very unlikely.

Obviously, a comprehensive review of the course of events and the resulting injuries must be attained and, if indicated, examination findings (e.g., magnetic resonance imaging [MRI] or paranasal sinus computed tomography [CT]) should be requested.

In cases of suspected occupational olfactory disorder due to exposure to toxic matter, the character, duration, and extent of the exposure must be evaluated thoroughly, including use of any protective measures. For example, mobile vacuum devices for welding outside the workshop are often not used, and paper screens do not protect from organic solvent fumes. Questions regarding work-related symptoms are also important. Such symptoms could be due to irritation of mucous membranes by irritant substances. Organic solvent fumes acutely affect the central nervous system depending on dosage. Typical symptoms are loss of appetite, nausea, dizziness, headaches, and intoxication (see Case Study 2). Older patients, in particular, have been "used" to such symptoms for many years and do not mention them spontaneously, so it is important that the assessor asks about them directly. Investigations into occupational disorders normally do not register these symptoms. An inquiry with the company medical officer could be helpful.

As with any assessment, other possible causes for the disorder (e.g., inflammatory or structural sinonasal causes, or nonsinonasal or neurodegenerative causes) must be excluded. If the patient suffers from acute inflammatory disorders (such as acute rhinitis or rhinosinusitis) at the time of examination, the required olfactory tests should be postponed until the acute inflammation has resolved. The existence of chronic paranasal sinus inflammation can impede the assessment significantly, as recovery often is either not possible or prolonged, and this must always be considered as a differential diagnosis. On the other hand, there is the possibility that toxin exposure could also be responsible for the development of chronic inflammation of the nose or the paranasal sinus.[9,10] If this is definitely the case, then the olfactory disorder would rank as a direct result of an occupational disorder.

When taking the medical history of a patient presenting with an olfactory disorder, it is important to ask about previous surgical interventions on the nose or the cranium. Olfactory disorders can exist that are not primarily reported, particularly in patients with chronic inflammation of the paranasal sinuses.[11] After surgical intervention, these patients often ascribe their (quite frequently persisting) olfactory disorder to the surgery. In view of subsequent legal claims based on an assumed malpractice on the part of the surgeon (which normally entails an expert opinion), the authors recommend performing olfactory testing before surgery (e.g., before septal surgery or surgery of the paranasal sinuses), and explaining to the patient the possible (potentially permanent) disorders associated with the intervention. Postinfectious anosmia is also a common cause of olfactory dysfunction.

Examination

Clinical and Technical Examinations

During the clinical examination of the nose, special attention must be paid to inflammatory changes, chronic inflammatory or atrophic changes of the mucous membranes, relevant structural abnormalities (obstructing deviations of the septum, significant hyperplasia of the nasal concha), and signs of acute or chronic inflammation of the paranasal sinuses, including nasal polyposis. As well as anterior rhinoscopy, endoscopy should be included in the examination; special attention should be paid to the fossa olfactoria. Furthermore, signs of previous surgical interventions (e.g., synechias or perforations of the septum) should be sought. However, the latter can also be attributed to chronic damage of the mucous membranes due to occupational exposure to toxic substances such as chromates or acids.

Purely structural changes with reduced nasal airflow are very rarely the sole cause for a relevant olfactory disorder, and rhinomanometric findings do not show any causal relationship with olfactory capability. (Here, the previously mentioned inspection of the fossa olfactoria using angular optics is the most significant test.) However, owing to its minimal invasiveness and its widespread use, rhinomanometry is used frequently to determine nasal airflow. If, in the course of the medical history or clinical examination, signs of a chronic disorder (e.g., chronic rhinosinusitis) are discovered, additional tests might be necessary, such as CT of the paranasal sinuses. These, however, should be discussed beforehand with the commissioning party. Additional images of the cranium (CT or MRI) are required to rule out a space-occupying intracranial process or tumor of the skull base if there are no relevant radiological findings.

If there are complaints of disorders of taste (which usually exist), the clinical examination and assessment of gustatory disorders should also be applied as described on p. 168–178.

Olfactory Testing

Quantitative validated tests of olfactory function are mandatory in all cases. In Europe, the authors recommend the extended "Sniffin' Sticks" test battery.[12] Other test systems that are recommended (especially for the USA) are the University of

Pennsylvania Smell Identification Test (UPSIT) or the test of the Connecticut Chemosensory Clinical Research Center (for further details see Chapter 6: Smell Testing).

A test of retronasal olfactory capability can also be performed if the relevant resources are available. Qualitative olfactory disorders cannot be tested to date. They must be specified in detail, in particular the frequency of their occurrence. Testing with mainly trigeminal substances such as acetic acid or ammonia can give clues regarding an amplification of existing symptoms, or simulation of such symptoms.

In this context, we would like to point out that even a patient with anosmia can score a minimal number of points in the Sniffin' Sticks test because of the probability of guessing correctly in the "forced choice" test. Conspicuously low results, or a TDI (threshold, discrimination, and identification score) of 0, points to simulation of symptoms (malingering). The probability for a TDI score of 0 is 0.002%; a TDI score of 1 has a probability of 0.02%. The UPSIT is a 40-item multiple-choice test. Malingering in this test is defined as a score of 5 correct, as it is statistically extremely improbable for a patient with anosmia to score 5. Nevertheless, malingering is still possible for both tests.

In all cases of doubt and to rule out simulation, in the authors' opinion, the assessment of olfactory disorders should also include an objective examination, primarily using olfactory and trigeminal event-related potentials (ERPs). The assessment may need to be performed by a specialized institution if essential technical equipment is not available. Lack of ERPs with preserved responses to trigeminal stimuli substantiates the diagnosis of anosmia (even if it does not answer the question of its cause). The persistence of olfactory potentials, however, clearly speaks against the presence of anosmia. Despite the publication of standard parameters for latencies and amplitudes,[13] a reliable verification of hyposmia is not possible at the time.[14]

Special Aspects of Assessment

Germany

Expert opinions for the Statutory Pension Insurance and within the Severely Handicapped Persons Act are merely assessments of the present state. In the case of occupational accidents and poten-

tial occupational diseases, however, the assessor must also comment on their causes. As quantitative baseline physical examination results are not usually available, the assessor must analyze the plausibility of the stated causative mechanisms. Legislation demands that the exposure (or the occupational accident) is *secured*. At least, the work-related exposure must be a major cause of the olfactory disorder. The causative correlation must be *probable*. If there are several competing causes, possible interactions must also be considered. It is useful in such cases if an experienced occupational physician comments on the causative mechanisms. If the given disorder is not cited in the list of occupational diseases and new medical findings exist, compensation might be granted according to § 9, clause 2, of the Code of Social Law VII (CSL VII).[15] In addition, we would like to mention § 9, Chapter 3, of CSL VII: "If the insurant who, due to specific conditions of his insured occupation, was exposed to increased danger of falling ill with an occupational disorder cited in the regulations according to Chapter 1 (i.e., the disease is quoted in the list of occupational diseases) comes down with such a disorder, and if indications for a cause outside the insured occupation cannot be found, it is assumed that this disorder was caused by the occupation insured." This can be significant if the extent of the exposure cannot be ascertained accurately in retrospect.

Regarding the level of reduction in earning capacity, different recommendations exist, which amount to 10 to 20% in the case of complete anosmia without particular occupational impact.[16,17] These amounts are significantly lower than those normally given for the loss of vision (one-sided blindness, 25%; two-sided blindness, 100%) or the loss of hearing (one-sided deafness, 20%; two-sided deafness, 70%). This applies to compensation law as well as the laws regarding accident insurance. The regulations regarding the task of medical assessment within the social compensation laws and the Severely Handicapped Persons Act state 15% for complete loss of olfactory capability and resulting impairment of taste perception (see textbox on the recommendations of the German Task Force, p. 213). Within the regulations of accident insurance, the level of reduction in earning capacity is based on "the extent—resulting from the impairment of the physical and intellectual capacities—of reduced possibilities for occupation in the entire domain of professional life" (CSL

VII, § 56, Chapter 2). However, the literal implementation of this is problematic. In practice, the assessor normally refers to tables or to figures based on experience. A 15% level of reduction in earning capacity is quoted—according to scientific doctrine—for an anosmia with resulting subjective impairment of taste. Figures for hyposmia are accordingly lower.[17–19] If, beyond that, a relevant disorder of gustatory capability (ageusia) is found (which rarely happens, however), a 20% reduction in earning capacity may be considered according the Olfactology and Gustology Task Force of the German Society of Otolaryngology (Deutsche Gesellschaft für Hals-Nasen-Ohrenheilkunde),[19] even if a level of only 15% is stated in relevant literature.[18]

The particular circumstances of the individual case must be taken into account. For example, a direct eating disorder with substantial weight loss can result in an increased level of reduction in earning capacity. With olfactory disorders, any work-related impact has to be investigated. For some occupations (e.g., bakers, confectioners, cooks, etc.), faultless olfactory capabilities are essential. The level of reduction in earning capacity might have to be raised. The criteria, however, are defined rather narrowly.[17] Also, in other specialized trades, such as perfumers, anosmia might make continuation of the occupation impossible. This might result in occupational disability. In other occupations where the olfactory sense is essential for recognizing hazardous situations in time (e.g., chemical industry, fire brigade, plumbers dealing with gas, etc.) the particular work situation has to be considered. Technical devices (e.g., gas alarm units) might enable the continuation of these occupations.

Switzerland

Complete loss of olfactory capability (anosmia) caused by an accident and still persisting after 2 years leads to a disbursement of a one-time compensation of 15% for loss of integrity. Hyposmia leads to a compensation of 7.5%. Such damage events must be reported to the Suva (the Swiss National Accident Insurance Fund). If the person affected by the olfactory loss works in a field where olfactory function is essential (e.g., cook, perfumer), an enactment of nonsuitability can be initiated and occupational re-training started. Recognition and declaration of occupation-related toxic olfactory disorders are also handled by the Suva in Switzerland.

Austria

Complete loss of olfactory capability (anosmia) caused by an accident and still persisting after 2 years is considered to amount to a reduction in earning capacity of 10% and is compensated accordingly. A complete anosmia amounts to 10%, and hyposmia to 5%.

Qualitative olfactory disorders (parosmia) as a sole symptom are not recognized in the German assessment regulations based on the lack of quantification, or the impossibility for a clear diagnosis. However, if a quantifiable limitation of olfactory or gustatory capability exists and symptoms of parosmia are characterized, this fact can be integrated into the assessment. The decisive question is, however, whether the parosmia has a relevant adverse effect on the person at issue (e.g., loss of appetite, weight loss, etc.).

Owing to the special regenerative ability of the olfactory senses, a spontaneous remission or an improvement should always be taken into consideration. If the onset of the symptoms is recent, the possibility of remission should be mentioned in the expert opinion, and reassessment suggested in due course (e.g., after 2 years). This hardly ever arises in cases of work-related olfactory disorder that have developed over a number of years, but a spontaneous remission must always be considered in the case of a sudden occurrence such as an accident. Though the possibility of a remission decreases with time, a fixed period of time after which a spontaneous remission is impossible cannot be defined.

In advisory issues, certain questions regarding olfactory and gustatory disorders come up quite frequently. These include assessments for the supposed existence of an occupational disease caused mainly by chronic exposure to toxic substances such as organic solvents or smokes (e.g., welding smokes). A set of documented cases already exists where a work-related olfactory disorder was acknowledged outside the list of occupational disorders, formerly § 551, Chapter 2, Federal Insurance Code (RVO), at present § 9, Chapter 2, CSL.

Furthermore, expert opinions may be provided within civil law, particularly for traumatic olfactory disorders caused by accidents due to an outside source (e.g., traffic accidents resulting in traumatic anosmia). Expert opinions may also be required in liability suits regarding olfactory disorders supposedly caused during medical interventions (usually surgical interventions on the nasal cavity or the paranasal sinuses).

United States of America

While awards for loss of vision, loss of hearing, and loss of limbs seem to be relatively standard in the courts, the awards for loss of smell vary widely. Awards in California vary between $250,000 and $750,000.

Recommendation of the German Task Force

The Olfactology and Gustology Task Force of the German Society of Otolaryngology (Deutsche Gesellschaft für Hals-Nasen-Ohrenheilkunde) has published recommendations regarding the assessment of olfactory disorders,[19] although these recommendations are in part very specific for Germany. A more general modification of these recommendations is given in the following textbox.

Information of the Olfactology and Gustology Task Force for Providing Expert Opinion for Olfactory and Gustatory Disorders within the Statutory Accident Insurance (modified version for this book)

According to the criteria for providing medical expert opinion in social compensation legislation and according to the German Severely Handicapped Persons Act of 2004 and its amendments, a 15% reduction in earning capacity for the complete loss of olfactory capabilities and the associated impairment of taste, and a 10% reduction for the complete loss of taste, is usually recommended.[18] With partial damage, the reduction in earning capacity is lower. Hyposmia, for example, with a TDI score between 15 and 20 can absolutely justify a reduction in earning capacity of 10%. That the gustatory perception of food or drink is always affected in anosmia is explained by the discontinuation of the olfactory input. The taste of food is a complex experience of olfactory, gustatory, trigeminal, visual, and also sonic perception and their central processing. A complete loss of olfactory or gustatory perception means the complete loss of the perception of sweet, sour, salty, or bitter tastes.

An important point in assessing the level of reduction in earning capacity—when the function of chemical senses in working life is lost—is a more precise assessment that takes into account the increased importance of chemical senses (e.g., the ability to detect hazardous situations). This also reflects the increased esteem of the olfactory and gustatory senses in the health consciousness of the general population. The reduction in earning capacity must be seen here as an abstract parameter of loss of health.

In general, a loss of olfactory capacity is associated with a decline—but not complete loss—in gustatory capability and the trigeminal sensitivity of the nasal mucosa. In providing expert opinion, this combined effect of damage must always be verified individually and acknowledged where appropriate. Obviously, in providing expert opinion, the total olfactory and gustatory abilities are at issue, and not the verification of a regional loss of function.

The rare (0.5% of all craniocerebral traumas) post-traumatic anosmia/ageusia syndrome represents the most severe form of this combined effect of damage. In this syndrome, the Task Force recommends an integrated reduction in earning capacity of 20%. The combined effect of damages should be rated higher than the sole anosmia.

According to the Task Force, a parosmia or parageusia associated with an impairment of olfactory or gustatory capabilities with a simultaneous psychovegetative aftereffect such as loss of appetite, dysphagia, or malnutrition should be rated with an integrated level of 0 to 10% of reduction in earning capacity. If the parosmia or parageusia is not caused by damage to the chemical senses, a neuropsychiatric expert opinion should be obtained. If the symptoms of parosmia or parageusia are not primarily and spontaneously reported by the patient, they are not rated as relevant.

If an olfactory disorder caused by occupational pollutants is suspected, this should be reported to the proper Employers' Liabilities Insurance Association. Work-related olfactory disorders are not cited in the list of occupational diseases. Patients with anosmia with a particular occupational impact (e.g., those employed in the food industry) are awarded a level of 20% reduction in earning capacity according to current ruling. In the case of highly specialized occupations (i.e., perfumers, or food supervision and control), the courts or administrative authorities can declare the individual incapable to practise his profession.

Expert Opinion in Gustatory Disorders

Disorders of perception of the basic tastes sweet, sour, salty, bitter, and umami—as they are relayed by the gustatory system—require expert opinion substantially less frequently than olfactory disorders, not least because of the sensory innervation of the tongue. Gustatory disorders, however, are almost always reported by patients being assessed for olfactory and gustatory disorders. Primarily, patients report gustatory impairment due to olfactory disorders (see assessment of olfactory disorders, p. 63). Examination of olfactory capability is, therefore, essential in patients with gustatory disorders, and vice versa.

Medical History

In the assessment of gustatory disorders, the medical history is vital to distinguish between a gustatory disorder itself and a primarily olfactory disorder. Furthermore, gustatory function before the onset of the disorder should be ascertained, as well as the course of its development. The medical history should also reveal if a quantitative dysfunction (hypogeusia or ageusia) or a qualitative dysfunction (parageusia, where taste sensations are altered, e.g., perceived as bitter or metallic) of the gustatory system exists. Also, clear gustatory disorders, in particular dysgeusia, are often accompanied by loss of appetite. In all cases, a history of food intake and any resulting weight loss must be taken.

Another aspect of the medical history is a systematic interrogation into well-known triggers for gustatory disorders. This particularly applies to medical conditions that can often cause gustatory disorders (e.g., diseases of the liver and kidneys, vitamin B12 deficiency with consecutive glossitis, diabetes, Sjögren syndrome, hypothyroidism, or Cushing syndrome) as well as the intake of medications that have been documented to cause gustatory disorders (e.g., chlorhexidine, penicillamine, cytostatics, or a metallic taste caused by carboanhydrase inhibitors).[20]

Work-related disorders of gustatory function are rare. A report by the German Statutory Accident Insurance showed that a total of five gustatory disorders ("reduced gustatory sense") were recorded as occupational disease between 1999 and 2006. "Aromatic halogenated carbon hydride," trichloroethylene, "chrome and its compounds," "phosphorus, inorganic," and hydrogen sulfide were cited once each as the cause; more specific data are not available. According to current scientific knowledge, relatively few working materials cause hypogeusia or ageusia. Reduced gustatory function was also reported after occupational exposure to antimony, cadmium, chromates, cyanides, hydrogen sulfide, selenium, and vanadium[21-24]; a few more substances are under suspicion.[25,26] A metallic taste was experienced after intoxication with, for example, arsenic, lead (sweetish metallic taste), inorganic mercury, and tellurium. It was also found with metal fume fever and in deep-sea welders.[23,27-29] A detailed medical history of the occupational environment can be helpful for the evaluation of gustatory disorders as well as impairment of olfactory senses. Work-related gustatory disorders can only be expected if there has been a significant breach of industrial safety regulations, or in occupational accidents.

Disorders of salivation as an undesirable side effect of medication or as a result of radiotherapy must also be mentioned here. Traumatic or surgical damage to relevant neural structures (e.g., due to interventions in the upper aerodigestive tract, the neck, or the skull base) should be asked about, if not already stated as possible triggers for gustatory disorders. Central nervous causes of gustatory disorders are rare (e.g., brain tumors, neurodegenerative diseases, lesions of the brainstem, or epileptoid disorders) but should nevertheless be included in the medical history. It is essential to ask about previous tonsillectomy or surgery of the middle ear. Transient changes in gustatory function are often reported in the immediate postoperative period, but longer lasting impairment after tonsillectomy is not infrequent (especially dysgeusia).[30] This is important in terms of expert opinion in a compensation trial. Direct damage to the glossopharyngeal nerve in the spatium parapharyngeum, as well as damage to neural or receptive structures due to the pressure from the surgical spatula, are discussed as possible causative factors.[31-33] Gustatory disorders following surgery of the middle ear can be a consequence of a lesion of the chorda tympani, although such lesions may have pre-existed with relevant conditions of the middle ear. It cannot always be avoided, and one-sided impairment often is not even noticed by the patient and generally lessens with time. In addition, damage to the lingual nerve can occur during oral surgery or dental procedures, resulting in unilateral ageusia. Potential taste disorders as a complication of such interventions should be included in the informed consent, especially before tonsillectomy and middle ear surgery.

If a gustatory disorder is reported after an intracranial injury (generally associated with olfactory dysfunction), then comprehensive information should be obtained regarding the extent of the damage (e.g., CT or MRI of the cranium, or reports on diagnostic findings and progression), as already outlined above. Combined failure of both sensory systems is rare and is, in general, associated with severe trauma (e.g., contusion, prolonged unconsciousness). Isolated bilateral ageusia, as a direct result of an accident, occurs even less frequently, if at all.

Examination

Clinical and Technical Examination

The clinical examination can help detect insufficient oral hygiene, faulty prosthetic materials (fillings, inlays, etc.), or morphological changes on the surface of the tongue that must be taken into consideration in a differential diagnosis. Even though congenital or acquired morphological mutations of the surface of the tongue (e.g., lingua geographica, or hairy tongue) are not associated with a gustatory dysfunction, such aberrations should be documented. Particularly in the case of unclear or suspicious changes, a biopsy might be beneficial, not least to exclude neoplastic changes. Furthermore, clinical examination might reveal possible effects of surgical intervention or trauma, or the presence of acute inflammation or tumors of the oral cavity or oropharynx. A clinical examination of the upper respiratory tract, the nose and its mucous membranes should be conducted, as described on pp. 49–57. Examination of the middle ear should also be included so inflammatory changes and previous surgery are not overlooked.

If there is any suggestion of unilateral dysfunction or local trauma of the chorda tympani, the sensitivity of the buccal mucosa should be examined to detect involvement of the lingual nerve, which runs adjacent to the chorda tympani in the oral cavity.

Gustatory Testing

Apart from extensive olfactory testing, as described on p. 58–75, gustatory function should be tested as follows. This can be done in the form of a full mouth test, but, in patients complaining of unilateral symptoms, a separate test should be performed on each side of the tongue. Initially, an orienting identification test with supraliminal testing substances can be conducted for each side separately. This tests identification of sweet, sour, salty, and bitter tastes. In advisory issues, a quantitative test should also be used, for example, using the "three drop method" or "taste strips" (see Chapter 14). It is important, however, that standard parameters are available for the chosen methods that allow classification of normogeusia, hypogeusia, or ageusia. If tests of the gustatory ability of particular areas of the tongue are required (e.g., if a damage of distinct neural structures is suspected), "taste strip" testing or electrogustometry can be performed (see Chapter 14). Not least because of the limited availability and poor compliance of this method, the authors feel that neither electrogustometry nor gustatory-evoked potentials or functional MRI should be routine clinical investigations for advisory issues. In advisory issues in western Europe and the USA, the quality umami is not tested, as patients and examiners are usually unfamiliar with it.

Special Aspects of Assessment

A common problem in the assessment of gustatory disorders is the lack of availability of quantitative—or even qualitative—gustatory testing before the onset of the disorder. Therefore, as a rule, the advisor has to rely on the patient's subjective report. An objective test of gustatory function has recently been developed based on gustatory ERPs; nevertheless, this technique is so far only available in a very limited number of centers.[34] As a consequence, directed simulations are hard to detect. Usually, the advisor will have to rely on the plausibility of the symptoms in the context of an adequate comprehensible cause. Overall, isolated gustatory disorders are extremely rare in advisory issues. From their own experience, the authors have been involved in the assessment of gustatory disorders (ageusia) after tonsillectomy or decimation of gustatory function (hypogeusia) after middle ear surgery. Additionally, the authors know of a case of hemiageusia with ipsilateral dysfunction of sensitivity, combined with a lesion of the chorda tympani and the lingual nerve, after dental surgery.

In terms of assessment of a possible impairment of earning capacity within the regulations of the Statutory Accident Insurance, a reduction of 10% is suggested in Germany for an isolated ageusia.[14] A particular occupational impact can occur in the case of cooks and comparable work situations where gustatory function plays a major role in the occupation analogous to olfactory dysfunction. Here, the specific requirements for gustatory function must be evaluated in the particular work situation. Additionally, a gustatory disorder associated with a documented olfactory disorder (anosmia) can necessitate an increase of the anosmia-induced impairment of earning capacity up to 20%.

Case Studies

Case Study 1: Post-traumatic Anosmia

A 45-year-old school teacher was hit by a car that had taken her right of way while she was riding her bicycle to the market. She was flung onto the street and struck her head on the surface. Owing to loss of consciousness and subsequent amnesia, she was not able to make a statement concerning the immediate period after the accident. She was taken to a nearby hospital by the emergency medical service. Her medical files state that a closed craniocerebral trauma was diagnosed, which had led to several minor frontoparietal hemorrhages due to contusion. An initial rhinoliquorrhea resolved after a few days. Neurosurgical intervention was not required. A series of small, superficial injuries of the facial soft tissues was initially treated surgically, and a distal radius fracture was treated conservatively with a forearm plaster splint.

The patient reported noticing a complete loss of olfactory function and a clear impairment of gustatory function after a few days in the hospital. She was no longer able to smell the flowers in her room, or her breakfast coffee. Her meals had tasted bland, so she had not been able to regain her appetite and had lost several kilograms in the course of a few weeks. Her olfactory and gustatory function have not improved since. She did not report any other complaints of the nose or paranasal sinuses.

Apart from occasional analgesics that she takes for intermittent pain in the lumbar spine, no drugs are taken. The patient had a tonsillectomy as a child; an appendectomy was performed 4 years ago. Additional interventions in the ear, nose, and throat region were not specified. There are no other relevant pre-existing conditions.

Expert opinion was requested 8 months after the accident. The woman had sued the party responsible for the accident for damages and compensation; the adversary's liability insurance doubted the olfactory disorder was caused by the accident and requested an expert opinion.

Clinical examination did not reveal any visible injuries of the neurocranium or viscerocranium that could have been caused by the accident. Rhinoscopy was normal, without relevant impairment of nasal airflow. Endoscopy of the main nasal cavity showed normal nasal mucosa; the fossa olfactoria was unobstructed and clearly visible. Intraoral examination was unremarkable and bilateral ear microscopy normal.

Rhinomanometry confirmed sufficient nasal airflow. Subjective olfactory testing with Sniffin' Sticks revealed a TDI score of 12 (threshold, 1; discrimination, 5; identification, 6), accordant with a functional anosmia. Results of the taste strips test were normal for the qualities sweet, sour, and bitter, but salty taste was not recognized until the concentration had been increased. Subsequent objective olfactometry showed residual potentials of 40 and 60% v/v CO_2 on trigeminal stimulation; accordant potentials on olfactory stimulation with H_2S (2 and 4 ppm) could not be evoked. Previous findings of olfactory and gustatory function were not available. MRI carried out days after the accident showed the described contusions. An initial CT did not show any discernible fractures. The paranasal sinuses were inconspicuous in both examinations.

The patient was diagnosed with anosmia. It was stated that the anosmia was caused by the accident "with the utmost probability" (post-traumatic anosmia) and a re-evaluation in 12 months was suggested.

Case Study 2: Anosmia as an Occupational Disorder

In 2004, a 44-year-old German plumber was examined for an expert opinion to determine if his anosmia was work related. He had been welding on and off from 1975 to 1993, mainly without vacuum devices or respiratory protection. During a major contract from late 1993 to early 1996, he laid polyvinyl chloride pipes for taps in poorly ventilated rooms. First, he cleaned the pipes with paper towels soaked in solvent mixtures. Then, he applied the adhesive with a brush, and fitted the pipes together. The basic solvents were tetrahydrofuran, cycloheranone, acetone, and further ketones. These operations often lasted several hours per day. Respiratory protection was not available. When cleaning and bonding, the plumber always felt a stinging sensation in his eyes and nose. In the course of 1 or 2 hours, nasal secretions turned from watery to bloody. Less frequently, he also had headaches and a feeling of slight tipsiness without having consumed alcohol earlier. All these symptoms appeared strictly work related. From 1996 to today the patient has rarely conducted bonding. In late 1995, he first noticed an impairment of his olfactory function. However, he continued to install gas lines. In March 1996, he was examined as an outpatient by an ear, nose, and throat specialist, and a deviated septum and reddened nasal mucosa were found. Rhinomanometry showed slightly impaired nasal airflow on both sides. Gustatory testing and radiography results of the paranasal sinuses were normal. The company physician reported these results as an occupational disease as late as 2001. The patient smoked one packet of cigarettes per day. The medical history gave no indication of other causes of olfactory dysfunction. On the occasion of the expert opinion examination in March 2004, the nasal mucosa was dry with some crusts. The lower nasal conchae were slightly enlarged; the fossa olfactoria was not visualized. Anterior rhinomanometry and acoustic rhinometry were normal. Olfactory examination with Sniffin' Sticks showed a TDI score of 10 (threshold, 1; discrimination, 5; identification, 4), which suggests functional anosmia. The diagnosis was secured by means of objective olfactometry.

On subjective gustatory testing (full mouth test), the qualities sweet, bitter, and salty were identified in contrast to sour. The result was assessed as non-impaired gustatory function. The medical history, skin prick test, and intracutaneous test with the most frequent seasonal and perennial allergens did not suggest allergic rhinitis. CT of the paranasal sinuses showed a minimal shadow in the area of the ethmoid cells. The basic cause of the disorder was the very high exposure

to solvents. The Employers' Liabilities Insurance Association followed the expert advisor's recommendation to acknowledge a toxic anosmia and rhinitis, with a reduction in earning capacity of 20%. Part of the plumber's job included laying gas lines and connecting appliances operating on gas. Hence the Employers' Liabilities Insurance Association initiated the purchase of a gas detector, so that the patient was able to stay in his workplace. Without this technical solution, an increased level of reduction in earning capacity would have been possible because of the particular work-related impact.[35]

References

1. Smith WM, Davidson TM, Murphy C. Toxin-induced chemosensory dysfunction: a case series and review. Am J Rhinol Allergy 2009;23(6):578–581

2. Alexander TH, Davidson TM. Intranasal zinc and anosmia: the zinc-induced anosmia syndrome. Laryngoscope 2006;116(2):217–220

3. Davidson TM, Smith WM. The Bradford Hill criteria and zinc-induced anosmia: a causality analysis. Arch Otolaryngol Head Neck Surg 2010;136(7):673–676

4. Gudziol H, Rahneberg K, Burkert S. Anosmics are more poorly able to taste than normal persons. [Article in German] Laryngorhinootologie 2007;86(9):640–643

5. Frasnelli J, Hummel T. Interactions between the chemical senses: trigeminal function in patients with olfactory loss. Int J Psychophysiol 2007;65(3):177–181

6. Frasnelli J, Schuster B, Zahnert T, Hummel T. Chemosensory specific reduction of trigeminal sensitivity in subjects with olfactory dysfunction. Neuroscience 2006;142(2):541–546

7. Hummel C, Frasnelli J, Gerber J, Hummel T. Cerebral processing of gustatory stimuli in patients with taste loss. Behav Brain Res 2007;185(1):59–64

8. Wu AP, Davidson T. Posttraumatic anosmia secondary to central nervous system injury. Am J Rhinol 2008;22(6):606–607

9. Samet JM. Adverse effects of smoke exposure on the upper airway. Tob Control 2004;13(Suppl 1):i57–i60

10. Shusterman D. Toxicology of nasal irritants. Curr Allergy Asthma Rep 2003;3(3):258–265

11. Delank KW, Stoll W. Olfactory function after functional endoscopic sinus surgery for chronic sinusitis. Rhinology 1998;36(1):15–19

12. Kobal G, Klimek L, Wolfensberger M, et al. Multicenter investigation of 1,036 subjects using a standardized method for the assessment of olfactory function combining tests of odor identification, odor discrimination, and olfactory thresholds. Eur Arch Otorhinolaryngol 2000;257(4):205–211

13. Stuck BA, Frey S, Freiburg C, Hörmann K, Zahnert T, Hummel T. Chemosensory event-related

potentials in relation to side of stimulation, age, sex, and stimulus concentration. Clin Neurophysiol 2006;117(6):1367–1375

14. Lötsch J, Hummel T. The clinical significance of electrophysiological measures of olfactory function. Behav Brain Res 2006;170(1):78–83

15. Muttray A, Klimek L, Jung D, Rose DM, Mann W, Konietzko J. Die toxische Hyp- und Anosmie—eine "vergessene" Berufskrankheit? Zbl Arbeitsmed 1998;48:66–71

16. Muttray A, Moll B, Letzel S. Die sozialmedizinische Bedeutung von Riechstörungen am Beispiel einer Kasuistik. Arbeitsmed Sozialmed Umweltmed 2003; 38:428–434

17. Schönberger A, Mehrtens G, Valentin H. Arbeitsunfall und Berufskrankheit. Rechtliche und medizinische Grundlagen für Gutachter, Sozialverwaltung, Berater und Gerichte. Erich Schmidt Verlag; 2009: 261–264

18. Feldmann H. Das Gutachten des Hals-Nasen-Ohren-Arztes. 6th ed. Stuttgart, New York: Thieme; 2006

19. Gudziol H. Mitteilung der Arbeitsgemeinschaft Olfaktologie und Gustologie zur Begutachtung von Riech- und Schmeckstörungen in der gesetzlichen Unfallversicherung. 2007. http://www.uniklinikum-dresden.de/das-klinikum/kliniken-polikliniken-institute/hno/forschung/interdisziplinares-zentrum-fur-riechen-und-schmecken/downloads/kongresse/prot_muenchen_06.pdf

20. Reiter ER, DiNardo LJ, Costanzo RM. Toxic effects on gustatory function. Adv Otorhinolaryngol 2006; 63:265–277

21. Hirsch AR, Zavala G. Long-term effects on the olfactory system of exposure to hydrogen sulphide. Occup Environ Med 1999;56(4):284–287

22. Seeber H, Fikentscher R, Roseburg B. Smell and taste disturbances in chromium dye workers. [Article in German] Z Gesamte Hyg 1976;22(11):820–822

23. Shusterman DJ, Sheedy JE. Occupational and environmental disorders of the special senses. Occup Med 1992;7(3):515–542

24. Seeber H, Fikentscher R. Taste disorders in chromium exposed workers. [Article in German] Z Gesamte Hyg 1990;36(1):33–34

25. Rossberg G, Schaupp H, Schmidt W. Geruchs- und Geschmacksvermögen bei Arbeitern der Chemischen und Metallverarbeitenden Industrie (Olfaktometrische und Elgustometrische Schwellenuntersuchungen). Z Laryngol Rhinol Otol 1966;45:571–590

26. Seeber H, Hanson J, Happrich F. Änderung der chemischen Sinne unter täglicher Karbidstaubexposition. Zbl HNO 1993;143:775–776

27. Hall AH. Chronic arsenic poisoning. Toxicol Lett 2002;128(1–3):69–72

28. Kachru DN, Tandon SK, Misra UK, Nag D. Occupational lead poisoning among silver jewellery workers. Indian J Med Sci 1989;43(4):89–91

29. Müller R, Zschiesche W, Steffen HM, Schaller KH. Tellurium-intoxication. Klin Wochenschr 1989; 67(22):1152–1155

30. Heiser C, Landis BN, Giger R, et al. Taste disturbance following tonsillectomy—a prospective study. Laryngoscope 2010;120(10):2119–2124

31. Tomita H, Ohtuka K. Taste disturbance after tonsillectomy. Acta Otolaryngol Suppl 2002; (546): 164–172

32. Collet S, Eloy P, Rombaux P, Bertrand B. Taste disorders after tonsillectomy: case report and literature review. Ann Otol Rhinol Laryngol 2005;114(3): 233–236

33. Tomofuji S, Sakagami M, Kushida K, Terada T, Mori H, Kakibuchi M. Taste disturbance after tonsillectomy and laryngomicrosurgery. Auris Nasus Larynx 2005;32(4):381–386

34. Hummel T, Genow A, Landis BN. Clinical assessment of human gustatory function using event related potentials. J Neurol Neurosurg Psychiatry 2010;81(4):459–464

35. Muttray A, Haxel B, Mann W, Letzel S. Toxic anosmia and rhinitis due to occupational solvent exposure. [Article in German] HNO 2006;54(11):883–887

36. Stuck BA, Muttray A. Begutachtung von Riech- und Schmeckstörungen. In: Hummel T, Welge-Lüssen A, eds. Riech- und Schmeckstörungen. Stuttgart: Georg Thieme Verlag; 2008: 123–136, 157–158

19 Flavor: Interaction Between the Chemical Senses

Antje Welge-Luessen, Dana M. Small, Thomas Hummel

Summary

Both chemical senses, smell and taste, contribute enormously to flavor perception, but it has been shown that visual and trigeminal inputs also influence olfactory and gustatory perception. In terms of olfaction, orthonasal and retronasal perception differ: Retronasal thresholds are higher and perceived intensity of identical stimuli is reduced, suggesting different central processing, which has been confirmed on functional magnetic resonance imaging studies. Application of congruent olfactory and gustatory stimuli has been shown to produce superadditive central responses compared with unimodal stimulation alone. Moreover, simultaneous application of congruent odorants can increase the perceived intensity of tastants. Trigeminal and olfactory stimuli, both perceived intranasally, interact; and the trigeminal threshold is increased in patients with anosmia. Visual stimuli, if present as congruent visual cues while presenting odorants, can also enhance odorant processing. These interactions explain the complaints of patients suffering from an isolated olfactory loss who nevertheless complain about changes in the perception of trigeminal and gustatory stimuli as well.

Introduction

The chemical senses of taste and smell interact with each other during eating and drinking to produce flavor perceptions. In everyday life, it is very rare to sense taste without also sensing smell. This contrasts with how taste and smell are generally studied in the laboratory as independent modalities. It is also recognized that other factors influence flavor perception.[1] This is illustrated by imagining a dinner in a nice restaurant with music and candlelight: Not only is the flavor of the food perceived, but also the visual and acoustic sensory inputs. These additional sensations contribute not only to the atmosphere, but also to the perception of flavor. However, although there is general agreement that many modalities contribute to flavor perception, there continues to be significant debate over just how many modalities should be included. Here, the core flavor modalities are defined as those sensations that arise, or appear to arise, from the mouth.[2] These sensations include olfaction, gustation, and oral somatosensation. The goal of this chapter is to provide an overview of chemosensory integration in healthy subjects, and then in subjects with known chemosensory deficits.

Flavor Perception

Olfactory and gustatory inputs are the main contributors to flavor perception, alongside trigeminal inputs such as temperature and texture of the given food.[3] Before looking at further details, one has to keep in mind that odorants are perceived in two ways: Orthonasally, before they enter the mouth; and retronasally, when odorants traverse the nasopharynx. To understand interactions in flavor perception and the important role of retronasal odorant perception in flavor perception, the main differences between orthonasal and retronasal perception will be briefly discussed.

Orthonasal versus Retronasal Olfactory Perception

The olfactory components of food are first sensed orthonasally, before the food is placed inside the mouth, and then retronasally, when the food enters the mouth (**Fig. 19.1**). In both cases the odor molecules bind to receptors in the olfactory epithelium.[4] In 1982, Rozin noted that olfaction is the only dual sense modality, in that it provides information about objects distal and proximal to the observer.[5] He therefore suggested that olfaction should be considered as two distinct senses. It is nowadays known that odorants of the same concentration are perceived less intensely when

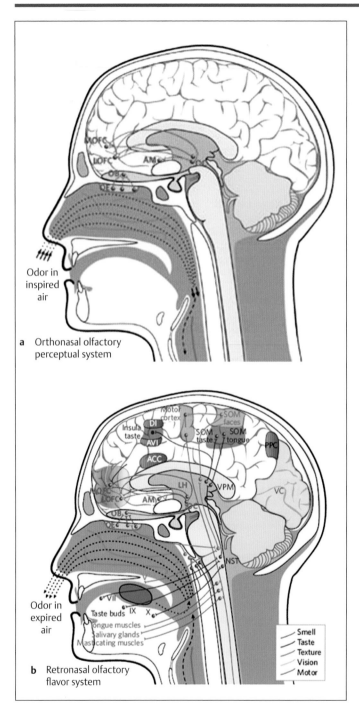

Fig. 19.1a, b The dual olfactory system. (Reproduced with kind permission of Nature Publishing Group from Shepherd G. Smell images and the flavour system in the human brain. Nature 2006;444:316–321.)

a Brain systems involved in smell perception during orthonasal olfaction (sniffing in).

b Brain systems involved in smell perception during retronasal olfaction (breathing out), with food in the oral cavity. Air flows indicated by dashed and dotted lines; dotted lines indicate air carrying odor molecules.

ACC, accumbens; AM, amygdala; AVI, anterior ventral insular cortex; DI, dorsal insular cortex; LH, lateral hypothalamus; LOFC, lateral orbitofrontal cortex; MOFC, medial orbitofrontal cortex; NST, nucleus of the solitary tract; OB, olfactory bulb; OC, olfactory cortex; OE, olfactory epithelium; PPC, posterior parietal cortex; SOM, somatosensory cortex; V, VII, IX, X, cranial nerves; VC, primary visual cortex; VPM, ventral posteromedial thalamic nucleus.

applied retroansally.[6] Moreover, retronasal thresholds are higher than orthonasal thresholds even in odorants identical in hedonics and concentration, thus supporting the idea that orthonasal and retronasal odorants are processed differently.[7,8] Using functional magnetic resonance imaging (fMRI), Small and colleagues showed that the brain responds differently to the same food odor sensed orthonasally than retronasally.[9] In a subsequent study using olfactory event-related potentials (OERPs), Hummel and Heilmann[10] were able to demonstrate that OERP responses were larger when an odor unrelated to food was presented in an unusual site (i.e., retronasally) than when the same odor was presented at an orthonasal site. The result was the other way around for a food-related odor. Odorants were presented using an olfactometer and a tube close to the epipharynx, mimicking molecules coming from the epipharynx (see **Fig. 19.2**). In patients with endonasal polyps, retronasal function was found to be significantly better than orthonasal olfactory function compared with controls.[11] Retronasal olfactory function was also found to be better than orthonasal function in patients with olfactory disorders because of other reasons, further supporting the different processing of orthonasal and retronasal stimuli.[12] Performing an interesting experiment involving mechanical blocking of the anterior part of the olfactory cleft, Pfaar et al were able to demonstrate

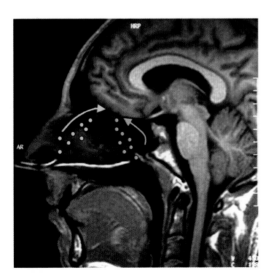

Fig. 19.2 Magnetic resonance image labeled to show orthonasal and retronasal odorant stimulation via tubes located in the vestibulum nasi (yellow odorant stimulation) and at the choana (blue odorant stimulation).

that orthonasal and retronasal perception differ.[13] Further findings regarding orthonasal and retronasal olfaction will be discussed below within the flavor perception section.

Interaction Between Olfactory–Gustatory and Gustatory–Olfactory Systems

Almost two decades ago in monkeys, single-cell recording techniques identified single cells responding to both taste and smell in the orbitofrontal cortex,[14] as well as in the insula/operculum.[15] Interestingly, these bimodal cells in the orbitofrontal cortex of the macaque were selective for congruent stimuli: For example, a cell responding optimally to a sweet taste such as glucose also responded optimally to sweet-like odors rather than to odors related to salty food. Also in primates, bimodal cells have been identified that react to both gustatory and visual stimuli. As such techniques are not applicable in humans, it took the implementation of functional imaging techniques to gain further insight into multimodal processing in humans. Initial functional imaging work focused on the identification of primary and secondary olfactory and gustatory cortices. The piriform cortex and medial orbitofrontal cortex,[16] caudal orbitofrontal cortex,[17] and the anterior insula/frontal operculum[18] have been identified. In all these studies, however, the brain's reaction to isolated olfactory or gustatory stimuli was recorded. Using positron emission tomography, Small et al[19] were the first to examine the brain's reaction to simultaneous olfactory and gustatory stimuli. They were able to show that the evoked cerebral blood flow in primary gustatory and secondary gustatory and olfactory cortices decreased during simultaneous presentation of olfactory and gustatory stimuli compared with independent presentation of these stimuli alone. This decrease in response was later interpreted to reflect competition between the taste and smell systems, arising from the fact that the odors were delivered orthonasally by asking subjects to sniff, rather than retronasally, as would naturally occur during bimodal taste and odor stimulation during eating or drinking.[8] In this study, olfactory or gustatory stimuli were not only applied "alone" but also in a "matched" and "mismatched" flavor condition (for example, sour taste and grapefruit smell as a matched condition; sweet taste and soy sauce odorant as a "mismatched" condition). In the "mismatched" condition, an increase in blood flow was observed in the left amygdaloid region and in the left and right basal forebrain. These results have been interpreted as confirmation of the function of the amygdala and basal forebrain in processing novel or unpleasant stimuli.[19]

This study was followed by others using fMRI techniques. Cerf-Ducastel et al[20] tested the interaction of gustatory and lingual somatosensory perception at a cortical level in humans. Stimulating subjects with either pure gustatory stimuli or stimuli containing both gustatory and somatosensory qualities, they were able to demonstrate that gustatory and somatosensory lingual representation fields overlap hugely, as similar cortical areas (namely the insula, the Rolandic operculum [base of the pre- and post-central gyri], the frontal operculum, and the temporal operculum) were activated by both kinds of stimuli. Moreover, in 2001, Cerf-Ducastel and Murphy[21] applied aqueous solutions of odorant intraorally, thus mimicking retronasal odorant perception. The observed activation pattern included all the brain regions usually activated when odorants were applied orthonasally, such as the piriform and orbitofrontal cortex, the hippocampal region, the amygdala, the insular lobe, the cingulate gyrus, and the cerebellum. In this study, however, no comparison with orthonasally applied odorants was made. A region in the lateral anterior part of the orbitofrontal cortex was identified in 2003 by de Araujo et al as the region activated by combined olfactory and taste stimuli, but not by unimodal stimuli alone.[22] Odorants in this study were delivered in aqueous form, again to mimic retronasal stimulation in combination with taste stimuli, just as they were in another study by Small et al in 2004.[23] Using familiar/congruent taste odor pairs and unfamiliar/incongruent taste odor pairs, as well as unimodal stimuli, the authors were able to show superadditive responses in the anterior cingulate cortex, the insula, the orbitofrontal cortex, and the posterior parietal cortex following stimulation with the congruent pair compared with unimodal stimulation alone.

In summary, these initial studies using intraorally applied aqueous stimuli in combination with taste stimuli to examine flavor perception were able to identify the orbitofrontal cortex, the insula, and the cingulate cortex as the main areas where odorants and tastants integrate. Moreover,

it became obvious that the experimental set-up (namely the route of delivery of the stimuli) was of great relevance.

The form of stimulation used in these studies (namely, the application of odorants in aqueous form), however, is not always comparable with food consumption and flavor perception in our everyday life. Small et al[9] therefore conducted a study examining brain activation in response to identical orthonasal and retronasal stimuli applied in gaseous form with an olfactometer. As shown in **Fig. 19.2**, stimuli were applied twice, orthonasally and then retronasally. Using a food odor (chocolate) and other, nonfood odors, Small et al were able to show that brain activation differed depending on the route of delivery of the food odor but not of the nonfood odors.[9] These findings prove that food odorants perceived retronasally—which happens during food intake normally—are processed in different central networks from nonfood odors perceived retronasally. In combination with gustatory stimuli, retronasal olfactory stimulation, but not orthonasal olfactory stimulation, has been shown to accelerate swallowing activity.[24] This is not surprising considering that retronasal olfactory stimulation activates a region of the Rolandic operculum at the base of the central sulcus,[9] and that this area corresponds to a primary representation of the oral cavity.[25] Looking at interactions the other way around, Bult et al[26] were able to show that a simultaneous odor stimulus was able to influence perceived oral texture (in this case, thickness and creaminess) of food, but only when it was presented retronasally. The effect was most pronounced when odor presentation coincided with swallowing.

Simultaneous odor perception (if the odorants are perceptually similar) can enhance the perceived intensity of tastants; however, blocking the nose severely diminishes this effect.[27] This phenomenon was shown by Sakai et al, who were able to demonstrate taste enhancement caused by simultaneously presented odors and, moreover, confirm that the effect observed was really due to simultaneous olfactory perception and not to taste stimulation.[28] It has also been shown that the pure presence of an oral stimulus increases odor intensity, irrespective of whether the odorant is perceived orthonasally or retronasally.[29] In a psychological experiment, Dalton et al were able to demonstrate that subthreshold concentrations of olfactory and gustatory stimuli integrate.[30]

However, there is more recent evidence that taste stimulation influences odor intensity perception[31] and is important for localizing retronasally sensed odorants to the oral cavity.[32] Interestingly, the localization effect occurs only for congruent taste-odor pairs. A sweet but not salty taste sensation causes subjects to report a vanilla odor appearing to come from the mouth, whereas a salty but not sweet taste sensation produces the appearance of a soy sauce odor.

In summary, all these data confirm that (1) odorants are processed differently when they are perceived orthonasally versus retronasally; and (2) they interact and influence taste perception differently.

Clinical Implications

So far, there has been a limited number of studies explicitly examining patients with isolated lesions. However, as previously mentioned, it has been shown that in patients with mainly orthonasal mechanical obstructions, such as polyps or chronic rhinosinusitis, retronasal olfactory perception is better than orthonasal olfactory perception.[11] However, it has also been shown that in cases of olfactory loss for other reasons, retronasal olfactory perception can remain, at least partly.[12] In cases of reduced orthonasal airflow (e.g., post-laryngectomy patients), retronasal olfaction is reduced as well.[33] The exact underlying pathophysiology that might explain why orthonasal and retronasal olfactory perception differ is currently unknown.

There are also studies examining the effect of gustatory stimulation on olfactory perception. In a study by Welge-Luessen et al, it was shown that congruent paired stimuli, such as a sweet tastant in combination with a sweet odorant, modulate OERPs of the odorant and enlarge them, while a concomitant sour tastant enlarges the event-related potentials (ERPs) of simultaneously applied gaseous carbon dioxide.[34] Olfactory stimulation, however, was only performed in an orthonasal way. Applying odorants not only orthonasally but also retronasally, it has been shown that food-like retronasally applied odors are processed significantly faster, resulting in shorter OERP latencies, in congruent odor–taste situations (food-like odor vanillin, plus sweet taste) than in incongruent smell–taste combinations (food-like odor vanillin, plus sour taste). Incongruent simultaneous gustatory stimulation applied during orthonasal olfaction seemed to induce conflict priming, also resulting in faster processing.[35]

To examine the influence of the vagal nerve on gustatory and olfactory processing, a small group of patients with vagal nerve stimulators (VNSs) was examined. It has long been suggested that interruption of a laryngeal–vagal feedback mechanism[36] might contribute to olfactory dysfunction after laryngectomy,[37] which might be considered to be consistent with findings from the early 1980s.[38] On the other hand, it has also been shown that part of the hyposmia in post-laryngectomy patients is due to reduced airflow.[39,40] Examining olfactory function in subjects with vagal stimulators, it was shown that vagal nerve stimulation prolonged P2 latencies of OERPs. In patients receiving a therapeutic benefit from VNSs in terms of seizure control, larger amplitudes during the "on" period than during the "off" period were observed.[41] Even though the number of studies examining vagal–olfactory interaction is limited, there seems to be growing evidence that vagal–olfactory interaction does occur. It has also been shown that patients with olfactory disorders exhibit higher gustatory thresholds.[42]

Visual–Olfactory and Flavor Interactions

As discussed in the introduction, visual inputs influence olfactory and, in particular, flavor perceptions. In a study by DuBose et al in 1980, participants often misidentified flavors of drink because their answers were misled by inappropriate coloring of the tested drink, providing evidence that visual cues influence flavor perception.[43] Consistent with this result is the fact that white wine that has been colored red has been described as featuring typical "red wine characteristics" by students in an experimental set-up in 2001.[44] Anatomically possible sites of integration are the orbitofrontal cortex,[14] the hippocampus,[45] or the intraparietal sulcus and the superior temporal sulcus.[46] Even though the latter are known to be regions processing multimodal interactions, direct inputs from olfactory regions such as the piriform cortex have not yet been identified. Indirect olfactory projections via the amygdala or orbitofrontal cortex might serve as a route of information transfer to these regions. Using fMRI and combining an olfactory detection task with visual presentation, Gottfried and Dolan were the first to show olfactory–visual integration in humans.[47] Olfactory detection was accelerated when odorants were presented in the context of semantically congruent visual cues (congruent odor–picture pairs) compared with incongruent combinations. Enhanced activity was observed in the anterior hippocampus and the orbitofrontal cortex, proving their participation in the crossmodal facilitation of olfactory and visual perception. Besides pure visual perception, subjects' belief also interacts with olfactory and flavor perception. If subjects believe that different colors are associated with different flavors, subjects are more likely to judge a flavor as different even if the offered samples differ only in color and not in flavor.[48] Further evidence that "believing" modulates olfactory perception comes from an interesting experiment by de Araujo et al in 2005.[49] Subjects had to rate the valence of either clean air or one odor, which, however, was labeled once as "cheddar cheese" and once as "body odor." Using fMRI, it could be shown that the rostral anterior cingulate cortex, the medial orbitofrontal cortex, and the amygdala were significantly more activated when the odor was labeled "cheddar cheese" than when it was labeled "body odor." Even labeling the clean air "cheddar cheese" showed more activation in the cingulate cortex and the orbitofrontal cortex than labeling it "body odor." These data show that pure semantic and cognitive inputs modulate sensory perception and processing.

Clinical Implications

To date, there is a limited number of studies examining small numbers of patients with reduced visual function (mainly completely blind people). Some of these behavioral studies have yielded contradictory results. While some studies did not show any difference between odor detection thresholds in blind subjects compared with sighted people,[50,51] others, using olfactory identification tasks, did show better results in blind subjects.[52–54] Rombaux et al were able to show increased olfactory bulb (OB) volume in blind subjects compared with sighted controls as well as increased olfactory function in the blind subjects.[55]

Olfactory–Trigeminal and Trigeminal–Olfactory Interaction

Inside the nose, olfactory receptor neurons and trigeminal nerves are not only located very close to each other, but also often stimulated simultaneously. Several odorants are known not only to be so-called pure olfactory odorants, but also to contain characteristics enabling them to elicit simultaneous trigeminal stimulation. Most odorants, if applied in higher concentrations, have olfactory and trigeminal properties. It is therefore not surprising that interactions have been postulated to occur peripherally at the level of the olfactory epithelium, as well as centrally. In mammals, it has been shown that trigeminal ganglion cells with sensory endings in the respiratory epithelium also get input from the OB or the spinal trigeminal complex.[56] Experimental approaches to selectively induce temporary anosmia or trigeminal anesthesia intranasally have been performed,[57] but have not been reproduced to study interactions between the two systems, as selective temporary elimination of only one system intranasally is almost impossible to achieve.

Eliciting chemosensory ERPs (CSERPs) with increasing concentrations of intranasally applied nicotine, Hummel et al[58] were able to show that, with increasing concentration, the perceived quality of nicotine changed from an olfactory perception to a stinging sensation, suggesting trigeminal stimulation. At the highest concentration, the trigeminal system seemed to "suppress" the olfactory perception. Moreover, the pattern of the recorded CSERPs changed to a "trigeminal pattern," meaning that the largest amplitude using the higher concentration was observed at Cz position, while, at olfactory concentrations, the largest amplitude was observed at Pz.[58] This confirmed former data.[59] On a psychophysical level using a behavioral paradigm, the suppression of olfactory perception caused by a simultaneous trigeminal stimulus had been previously shown.[60] Using fMRI, central regions of interaction have been identified and it has been shown that the combination of both trigeminal and olfactory stimuli elicit higher cortical activation than the sum of each part.[61]

Clinical Implications

It has been shown that the trigeminal sensitivity in patients with anosmia is reduced.[62,63] Interestingly, only intranasal trigeminal threshold changes, while cutaneous trigeminal threshold seems not to be influenced by the loss of olfactory function. Moreover, the etiology of the olfactory loss (post-traumatic versus postinfectious), as well as the degree of the olfactory disturbance, seems to have an influence on trigeminal threshold: In patients with anosmia there seems to be no difference in trigeminal threshold between post-traumatic and postinfectious olfactory disorders; in patients with hyposmia, however, those with post-traumatic disorders had higher trigeminal

thresholds than those with postinfectious disorders.[64] As well as the etiology of the olfactory disorder, age and olfactory status affect trigeminal sensitivity.[65] Recording electrophysiological responses from the intranasal mucosa and ERPs in subjects with congenital anomia[66] and acquired anosmia,[67] Frasnelli et al were able to reveal different interaction levels, both peripherally and centrally, compared with healthy controls. A negative correlation between threshold, discrimination, and identification score and the components of the CSERP typically occurred after trigeminal stimulation has also been shown.[68] Olfactory–trigeminal interaction can also be observed in patients suffering from reduced trigeminal sensitivity, a rare, but sometimes observed, entity. In a patient with

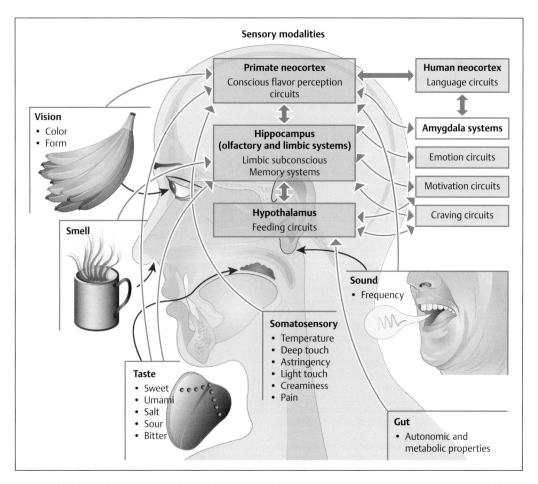

Fig. 19.3 The different sensory modalities (smell, taste, vision, hearing, somatosensory) that, together with the information provided from the gut, contribute to flavor perception. Moreover, different brain systems participating in food intake regulation and evaluation and its

interaction are depicted. (Modified with kind permission of Nature Publishing Group from Shepherd G. Smell images and the flavour system in the human brain. Nature 2006;444:316–321.)

225

unilateral loss of trigeminal sensitivity due to a meningioma, olfactory threshold was severely elevated on the affected side,[69] just as it was in patients following balloon compression for cases of trigeminal neuralgia.[70]

In summary, in patients with olfactory deficits, trigeminal thresholds are elevated. It is especially important to keep this in mind in medicolegal cases in order not to misinterpret such results as signs of malingering.

Conclusions

There is growing evidence that the olfactory, gustatory, and trigeminal systems interact. Flavor perception can also be influenced by visual inputs and beliefs and expectations (**Fig. 19.3**).[71] This is of great importance for the clinician examining patients with lesions previously considered "isolated," as this knowledge helps to better understand deficits and impairments reported by patients. Until now, many of these complaints have not been taken seriously or even considered possible, as the underlying pathophysiology has not yet been identified.

References

1. Auvray M, Spence C. The multisensory perception of flavor. Conscious Cogn 2008;17(3):1016–1031
2. Small DM. Flavor is in the brain. Physiol Behav 2012;107(4):540–552
3. Bartoshuk LM, Beauchamp GK. Chemical senses. Annu Rev Psychol 1994;45:419–449
4. Pierce J, Halpern BP. Orthonasal and retronasal odorant identification based upon vapor phase input from common substances. Chem Senses 1996; 21(5):529–543
5. Rozin P. "Taste–smell confusions" and the duality of the olfactory sense. Percept Psychophys 1982; 31(4):397–401
6. Heilmann S, Hummel T. A new method for comparing orthonasal and retronasal olfaction. Behav Neurosci 2004;118(2):412–419
7. Hummel T, Heilmann S, Landis BN, et al. Perceptual differences between chemical stimuli presented through the ortho- or retronasal route. Flavour Frag J 2006;21:42–47
8. Small DM, Prescott J. Odor/taste integration and the perception of flavor. Exp Brain Res 2005; 166(3–4):345–357
9. Small DM, Gerber JC, Mak YE, Hummel T. Differential neural responses evoked by orthonasal versus retronasal odorant perception in humans. Neuron 2005;47(4):593–605
10. Hummel T, Heilmann S. Olfactory event-related potentials in response to ortho- and retronasal stimulation with odors related or unrelated with food. Int Dairy J 2008;18:874–878
11. Landis BN, Giger R, Ricchetti A, et al. Retronasal olfactory function in nasal polyposis. Laryngoscope 2003;113(11):1993–1997
12. Landis BN, Frasnelli J, Reden J, Lacroix JS, Hummel T. Differences between orthonasal and retronasal olfactory functions in patients with loss of the sense of smell. Arch Otolaryngol Head Neck Surg 2005; 131(11):977–981
13. Pfaar O, Landis BN, Frasnelli J, Hüttenbrink K-B, Hummel T. Mechanical obstruction of the olfactory cleft reveals differences between orthonasal and retronasal olfactory functions. Chem Senses 2006; 31(1):27–31
14. Rolls ET, Baylis LL. Gustatory, olfactory, and visual convergence within the primate orbitofrontal cortex. J Neurosci 1994;14(9):5437–5452
15. Scott TR, Plata-Salamán CR. Taste in the monkey cortex. Physiol Behav 1999;67(4):489–511
16. Zatorre RJ, Jones-Gotman M, Evans AC, Meyer E. Functional localization and lateralization of human olfactory cortex. Nature 1992;360(6402):339–340
17. Small DM, Jones-Gotman M, Zatorre RJ, Petrides M, Evans AC. A role for the right anterior temporal lobe in taste quality recognition. J Neurosci 1997; 17(13):5136–5142
18. Faurion A, Cerf B, Le Bihan D, Pillias A-M. fMRI study of taste cortical areas in humans. Ann N Y Acad Sci 1998;855:535–545
19. Small DM, Jones-Gotman M, Zatorre RJ, Petrides M, Evans AC. Flavor processing: more than the sum of its parts. Neuroreport 1997;8(18):3913–3917
20. Cerf-Ducastel B, Van de Moortele P-F, MacLeod P, Le Bihan D, Faurion A. Interaction of gustatory and lingual somatosensory perceptions at the cortical level in the human: a functional magnetic resonance imaging study. Chem Senses 2001; 26(4):371–383
21. Cerf-Ducastel B, Murphy C. fMRI activation in response to odorants orally delivered in aqueous solutions. Chem Senses 2001;26(6):625–637
22. de Araujo IED, Rolls ET, Kringelbach ML, McGlone FP, Phillips N. Taste-olfactory convergence, and the representation of the pleasantness of flavour, in the human brain. Eur J Neurosci 2003;18(7): 2059–2068
23. Small DM, Voss J, Mak YE, Simmons KB, Parrish T, Gitelman D. Experience-dependent neural integration of taste and smell in the human brain. J Neurophysiol 2004;92(3):1892–1903
24. Welge-Lüssen A, Ebnöther M, Wolfensberger M, Hummel T. Swallowing is differentially influenced by retronasal compared with orthonasal stimulation in combination with gustatory stimuli. Chem Senses 2009;34(6):499–502
25. Boling W, Reutens DC, Olivier A. Functional topography of the low postcentral area. J Neurosurg 2002;97(2):388–395
26. Bult JHF, de Wijk RA, Hummel T. Investigations on multimodal sensory integration: texture, taste, and ortho- and retronasal olfactory stimuli in concert. Neurosci Lett 2007;411(1):6–10

27. Schifferstein HNJ, Verlegh PWJ. The role of congruency and pleasantness in odor-induced taste enhancement. Acta Psychol (Amst) 1996;94(1): 87–105

28. Sakai N, Kobayakawa T, Gotow N, Saito S, Imada S. Enhancement of sweetness ratings of aspartame by a vanilla odor presented either by orthonasal or retronasal routes. Percept Mot Skills 2001;92(3 Pt 2):1002–1008

29. Roudnitzky N, Bult JHF, de Wijk RA, Reden J, Schuster B, Hummel T. Investigation of interactions between texture and ortho- and retronasal olfactory stimuli using psychophysical and electrophysiological approaches. Behav Brain Res 2011; 216(1):109–115

30. Dalton P, Doolittle N, Nagata H, Breslin PA. The merging of the senses: integration of subthreshold taste and smell. Nat Neurosci 2000;3(5):431–432

31. Green BG, Nachtigal D, Hammond S, Lim J. Enhancement of retronasal odors by taste. Chem Senses 2012;37(1):77–86

32. Lim J, Johnson MB. The role of congruency in retronasal odor referral to the mouth. Chem Senses 2012;37(6):515–522

33. Leon EA, Catalanotto FA, Werning JW. Retronasal and orthonasal olfactory ability after laryngectomy. Arch Otolaryngol Head Neck Surg 2007; 133(1):32–36

34. Welge-Lüssen A, Drago J, Wolfensberger M, Hummel T. Gustatory stimulation influences the processing of intranasal stimuli. Brain Res 2005;1038(1): 69–75

35. Welge-Lüssen A, Husner A, Wolfensberger M, Hummel T. Influence of simultaneous gustatory stimuli on orthonasal and retronasal olfaction. Neurosci Lett 2009;454(2):124–128

36. Henkin RI, Larson AL. On the mechanism of hyposmia following laryngectomy in man. Laryngoscope 1972;82(5):836–843

37. Henkin RI, Hoye RC, Ketcham AS, Gould WJ. Hyposmia following laryngectomy. Lancet 1968;2 (7566):479–481

38. García-Díaz DE, Aguilar-Baturoni HU, Guevara-Aguilar R, Wayner MJ. Vagus nerve stimulation modifies the electrical activity of the olfactory bulb. Brain Res Bull 1984;12(5):529–537

39. Mozell MM, Schwartz DN, Youngentob SL, Leopold DA, Hornung DE, Sheehe PR. Reversal of hyposmia in laryngectomized patients. Chem Senses 1986;11:397–410

40. Welge-Luessen A, Kobal G, Wolfensberger M. Assessing olfactory function in laryngectomees using the Sniffin' Sticks test battery and chemosensory evoked potentials. Laryngoscope 2000;110(2 Pt 1):303–307

41. Kirchner A, Landis BN, Haslbeck M, Stefan H, Renner B, Hummel T. Chemosensory function in patients with vagal nerve stimulators. J Clin Neurophysiol 2004;21(6):418–425

42. Landis BN, Scheibe M, Weber C, et al. Chemosensory interaction: acquired olfactory impairment is associated with decreased taste function. J Neurol 2010;257(8):1303–1308

43. DuBose CN, Cardello AV, Maller O. Effects of colorants and flavorants on identification, perceived flavor intensity, and hedonic quality of fruit-flavored beverages and cake. J Food Sci 1980;45: 1393–1399

44. Morrot G, Brochet F, Dubourdieu D. The color of odors. Brain Lang 2001;79(2):309–320

45. Kreiman G, Koch C, Fried I. Category-specific visual responses of single neurons in the human medial temporal lobe. Nat Neurosci 2000;3(9):946–953

46. Bruce C, Desimone R, Gross CG. Visual properties of neurons in a polysensory area in superior temporal sulcus of the macaque. J Neurophysiol 1981;46(2):369–384

47. Gottfried JA, Dolan RJ. The nose smells what the eye sees: crossmodal visual facilitation of human olfactory perception. Neuron 2003;39(2):375–386

48. Levitan CA, Zampini M, Li R, Spence C. Assessing the role of color cues and people's beliefs about color–flavor associations on the discrimination of the flavor of sugar-coated chocolates. Chem Senses 2008;33(5):415–423

49. de Araujo IED, Rolls ET, Velazco MI, Margot C, Cayeux I. Cognitive modulation of olfactory processing. Neuron 2005;46(4):671–679

50. Smith RS, Doty RL, Burlingame GK, McKeown DA. Smell and taste function in the visually impaired. Percept Psychophys 1993;54(5):649–655

51. Schwenn O, Hundorf I, Moll B, Pitz S, Mann WJ. Do blind persons have a better sense of smell than normal sighted people? [Article in German] Klin Monatsbl Augenheilkd 2002;219(9):649–654

52. Murphy C, Cain WS. Odor identification: the blind are better. Physiol Behav 1986;37(1):177–180

53. Rosenbluth R, Grossman ES, Kaitz M. Performance of early-blind and sighted children on olfactory tasks. Perception 2000;29(1):101–110

54. Cuevas I, Plaza P, Rombaux P, De Volder AG, Renier L. Odour discrimination and identification are improved in early blindness. Neuropsychologia 2009;47(14):3079–3083

55. Rombaux P, Huart C, De Volder AG, et al. Increased olfactory bulb volume and olfactory function in early blind subjects. Neuroreport 2010;21(17): 1069–1073

56. Schaefer ML, Böttger B, Silver WL, Finger TE. Trigeminal collaterals in the nasal epithelium and olfactory bulb: a potential route for direct modulation of olfactory information by trigeminal stimuli. J Comp Neurol 2002;444(3):221–226

57. Welge-Lüssen A, Wille C, Renner B, Kobal G. Anesthesia affects olfaction and chemosensory event-related potentials. Clin Neurophysiol 2004; 115(6):1384–1391

58. Hummel T, Livermore A, Hummel C, Kobal G. Chemosensory event-related potentials in man: relation to olfactory and painful sensations elicited by nicotine. Electroencephalogr Clin Neurophysiol 1992;84(2):192–195

59. Kobal G, Hummel C. Cerebral chemosensory evoked potentials elicited by chemical stimulation of the human olfactory and respiratory nasal mucosa. Electroencephalogr Clin Neurophysiol 1988;71(4): 241–250

60. Cain WS, Murphy CL. Interaction between chemoreceptive modalities of odour and irritation. Nature 1980;284(5753):255–257

61. Boyle JA, Frasnelli J, Gerber J, Heinke M, Hummel T. Cross-modal integration of intranasal stimuli: a functional magnetic resonance imaging study. Neuroscience 2007;149(1):223–231

62. Hummel T, Barz S, Lötsch J, Roscher S, Kettenmann B, Kobal G. Loss of olfactory function leads to a decrease of trigeminal sensitivity. Chem Senses 1996; 21(1):75–79

63. Gudziol H, Schubert M, Hummel T. Decreased trigeminal sensitivity in anosmia. ORL J Otorhinolaryngol Relat Spec 2001;63(2):72–75

64. Frasnelli J, Schuster B, Zahnert T, Hummel T. Chemosensory specific reduction of trigeminal sensitivity in subjects with olfactory dysfunction. Neuroscience 2006;142(2):541–546

65. Frasnelli J, Schuster B, Hummel T. Olfactory dysfunction affects thresholds to trigeminal chemosensory sensations. Neurosci Lett 2010;468(3): 259–263

66. Frasnelli J, Schuster B, Hummel T. Subjects with congenital anosmia have larger peripheral but similar central trigeminal responses. Cereb Cortex 2007;17(2):370–377

67. Frasnelli J, Schuster B, Hummel T. Interactions between olfaction and the trigeminal system: what can be learned from olfactory loss. Cereb Cortex 2007;17(10):2268–2275

68. Rombaux P, Mouraux A, Keller T, Hummel T. Trigeminal event-related potentials in patients with olfactory dysfunction. Rhinology 2008;46(3):170–174

69. Husner A, Frasnelli J, Welge-Lüssen A, Reiss G, Zahnert T, Hummel T. Loss of trigeminal sensitivity reduces olfactory function. Laryngoscope 2006;116(8):1520–1522

70. Siqueira SRDT, Nóbrega JCM, Teixeira MJ, Siqueira JTT. Olfactory threshold increase in trigeminal neuralgia after balloon compression. Clin Neurol Neurosurg 2006;108(8):721–725

71. Seo H-S, Hummel T. Auditory–olfactory integration: congruent or pleasant sounds amplify odor pleasantness. Chem Senses 2011;36(3):301–309

Index

Page numbers in **bold** refer to material in tables and page numbers in *italics* refer to material in figures.

A

Aachen "rhinotest" 63
acupuncture 100
adaptation 36
adenosine monophosphate, cyclic 22, 26, 46
adrenergic fibers 18
afferent connections
  gustatory cortex, primates 158–159
  parvicellular part of ventral posteromedial nucleus 157–158
age-related loss (older/elderly persons)
  nasal trigeminal system function 143–144
  smell 1, 3–4, 102
  taste 1, 4–5
ageusia 180
  definition 1, 68, **180**
air conditioning, nasal 10–11
air passages, nasal 10
airborne particles, nasal response to 144
airways *see* respiratory tract
Alcohol-Sniff-Test 59
  children 121
allergy, nasal (allergic rhinitis) 81–83
  trigeminal system and 143–144, 145
alliesthesia 119
  negative 119
Alzheimer dementia 132, 183
ambient odorants, impact on behavior and health 6
AMP, cyclic 22, 26, 46
amygdala 33–34
  gustation and 160, 165
  olfaction and 27, 33–34
anatomy (functional)
  gustatory system *see* gustatory system
  olfactory system *see* olfactory system
  trigeminal system 138–139

aneurysm, anterior cerebral artery 201
anosmia 141, 216–217
  case study 216–217
  congenital *see* congenital olfactory disorders
  definition 1
  expert opinion 209, 210, 211, 216–217
    Austria 212
    Switzerland 212
  occupational cause 216–217
  post-traumatic (PTA), 92, 209, 212, 216
  prognosis 101–102
  treatment 100
  postviral/postinfectious 67, 211
  specific compounds 2
  trigeminal system and 141, 225
antibiotics
  acute bacterial rhinosinusitis 81
  chronic rhinosinusitis 85
  gustatory dysfunction induced by **185**
  olfactory dysfunction induced by **108**
antidepressants
  olfactory dysfunction called by **108**
  tricyclic, in burning mouth syndrome 191
antihistamines, chronic rhinosinusitis 85
antineoplastic (cytostatic) drug-induced dysfunction
  gustation **185**
  olfaction **108**
antipsychotic-induced olfactory dysfunction **108**
antithyroid drugs
  gustatory dysfunction induced by **185**
  olfactory dysfunction induced by **108**

area 1 (primate primary gustatory cortex) 159
area 2 (primate primary gustatory cortex) 159
area 3 (primate primary gustatory cortex) 159, 162
area 12 (primate primary gustatory cortex) 159, 160, 161
area 13 (primate higher order gustatory cortex) 159
area 43 (human primary gustatory cortex) 161, 162
area G (human primary gustatory cortex) 162
arousal, infant/child 118
asthma and asthma-like mimics 146
ataxia, Friedreich 133
atrophic rhinitis 77, 83
aura
  epilepsy 134
  migraine 135
Austria, expert opinion on olfactory disorders 212–213
autonomic functions, trigeminal system 139
autonomic syndromes triggered by olfactory or trigeminal stimulation 145

B

bacterial acute rhinosinusitis 78–81
balloon dilatation, chronic rhinosinusitis 86
basal cells
  horizontal 19–20
  taste buds 150
basal ganglia and parkinsonism 128, 129
bed nuclei of stria terminalis 28
behavior, olfactory cues influencing
  ambient odorant 6
  amygdala and 33
  sexual behavior and *see*

sexual behavior
benzene 106
bimodal (taste/smell) cells,
   orbitofrontal cortex 221
biopsies
   olfactory epithelium/
      mucosa 20, 22, 67
   olfactory neuroepithelium 22
bipolar cells
   olfactory receptor neurons
      as 18
   vomeronasal 24
bitterness 150
   gustatory cortex,
      primate 159
   inability to detect specific
      bitter compounds 2
   nerve fibers 154
   receptors 152
   transduction 153
brain
   contusions or hemorrhage 94
   gustation and 155–165
      disorders of 183
      interaction between
         olfaction and 221–222
   imaging see imaging
   olfaction and 27–38
      imaging 202
      interaction between
         gustation and 221–222
      orthonasal 220, 221
      retrononasal 220, 221
      vision and 223–224
   in Parkinson's disease,
      pathology 128, 130
   trigeminal system anatomy
      relating to 138–139
   see also neurological disease
brainstem lesions
   gustatory disorders 183
   imaging 203
brainstem reflexes and trigeminal system 139
breathing and trigeminal
   system 139
bulbofugal fibers 27–29
burning mouth syndrome 169,
   189–191
   therapy 186, 191
butanol detection test 60, 62

butyl acetate 106

C
cacosmia, investigations 97
cadmium 106
calcium ions
   olfactory receptor neurons
      and 22
   sensorineural olfactory
      disorders and 99
   taste transduction and 153
cancer see antineoplastic
   drug-induced dysfunction;
   malignant tumors
Candy Smell Test 121, 122
capsaicin
   in burning mouth
      syndrome 191
   threshold test 173
cardiovascular drug-induced
   disorders
   gustation 185
   olfaction 108
carotid gustatory
   syndrome 183
caroverine, postinfectious
   hyposmia 99–100
central nervous system
   gustatory 155–165, 181
      disorders 180, 183
   olfactory 27–38
   see also brain; neurological
      diseases
cerebrovascular disease
   aneurysm 201
   ischemic 135
   taste disorders 193
chemical senses
   (chemosensation/
   chemoreception)
   flavor and interactions
      between 219–228
   insula and 34
   pediatric 116–126
   rationales for assessment 58
   role/function 1
   vomeronasal
      system-independent 45–46
chemoreceptor cells, solitary
   (SCCs) 19, 141
chemosensory event-related
   potentials

acute rhinitis/rhinosinusitis
   and 80
epilepsy and 134
olfactory–trigeminal interactions and 224
chemosensory imaging
   see imaging
children,
   chemosensation 116–126
Children's Olfactory
   Behaviors in Everyday Life
   questionnaire 122
cholinergic fibers 18
chorda tympani (CTN) 152,
   153, 154, 157, 159, 204
   assessment 172, 176
   lesions/damage 123, 171,
      204, 214, 215, 216
      burning mouth syndrome
         and 190
      case report 174
   taste changes and anesthesia
      of 190
circumvallate papillae 151, 152,
   154, 172, 191
clinical examination 53–54
   expert opinion
      gustation 215
      olfaction 210
clonazepam in burning mouth
   syndrome 191
cold, common 78–81, 91
common cold 78–81, 91
Compu-Sniff test 65
computational fluid
   dynamics 16
computed tomography
   (CT) 198–199
   chronic rhinosinusitis (with/
      without polyps) 78, 88
   PET combined with 199
   postinfectious or
      post-traumatic olfactory
      disorders 96
   technical
      considerations 198–199
   trigeminal nerve 202
conchae, nasal 10
conduction problems (olfaction), nasal 10–11
confocal laser scanning
   microscope, taste buds 174

congenital olfactory disorders
(incl. anosmia) 109–110, 114,
200
definition 1
diagnosis incl. imaging 55,
200
conjunctiva, trigeminal
innervation 142
Connecticut Chemosensory
Clinical Research Center
Test 62, 211
contingent negative
variation 65
contusions, olfactory bulb or
brain 94
cornea, trigeminal
innervation 142
cortical areas
gustatory 158–165
disorders 183
non-human
primates 158–160
olfactory 27, 29–34
see also specific cortices
corticobasal degeneration
(CBD) 128–129
corticofugal fibers 29
corticosteroids (referred to as
steroids sometimes)
postinfectious hyposmia 97,
100
post-traumatic anosmia 100
in sinonasal pathology 55
acute bacterial
rhinosinusitis 81
allergic rhinitis 82
chronic rhinosinusitis 85,
86, 87
coughing 139
chronic 139
cranial nerves and their
disorders see neuropathies
and specific nerves
craniomaxillofacial injury see
post-traumatic disorders
Cross-Cultural Smell
Identification Test 59
cyclic AMP 22, 26, 46
cytostatic drugs see antineoplastic drug-induced
dysfunction

D
dark cells 150
data acquisition (image
acquisition)
CT 198
MRI 196
decongestants, acute bacterial
rhinosinusitis 81
degenerin/epithelial sodium
channel family 152
dementia
Alzheimer's 132, 183
Lewy body 129
depression 135
see also antidepressant
Deutsche Gesellschaft für Hals-
Nasen-Ohrenheilkunde 213
development
chemosensory
function 116–118
vomeronasal system 39–42
directional responses to smell,
infants 118
dopamine and Parkinson's
disease 128, 133
dorsomedial nucleus of
thalamus 28
dose exposure (CT) 198–199
drug-induced dysfunction
gustatory 168, 184
olfactory 108
perioperative 112
drug therapy
acute viral/bacterial
rhinosinusitis 80–81
allergic rhinitis 82, 83
burning mouth
syndrome 186
chronic rhinosinusitis 85–86
parosmia 101
postinfectious
hyposmia 97–100
taste disorders 185–186
qualitative 191
dusts **107**, **208**
dysgeusia 68, 180, 191–192
definition **180**, 192
therapy 186
dysosmia, postinfectious or
post-traumatic 91, 101
investigation 96–97
dyspnea, episodic 146

E
education, food 101
EEG see electroencephalography
efferent connections
parvicellular part of ventral
posteromedial nucleus 158
solitary tract nucleus 156
elderly see age-related loss
electroencephalography (EEG)
gustation 161
olfaction 64, 65
newborns/infants 120
trigeminal system 142
electrogustometry (EGM) 69,
70, 171–173
children 124
filter paper disc method
compared with 171
electro-olfactograms 65
electrophysiological (neurophysiological) tests 64–65
trigeminal system 142–143
endocrine disorders 109, 114
endoscopy
diagnostic endonasal 53
vomeronasal duct 46
interventional
sinonasal 86–87
olfactory dysfunction
following 112
see also rhinoscopy
entorhinal cortex 27–28, 34
environmental odorants, impact
on behavior and health 6
eosinophilia syndrome, non-allergic rhinitis with 83
epidemiology 2–3
sinonasal disorders 76–78
epilepsy 134–135
episodic dyspnea 146
epithelial sodium channels
(ENACs) 152, 153
epithelium
olfactory see olfactory
epithelium
vomeronasal 39, 42
erosive pattern in chronic
rhinosinusitis 85
esthesioneuroblastoma **111**,
200
European Position Paper

on Rhinosinusitis and Nasal Polyps (EPOS) guidelines 76–78
European Test of Olfactory Capabilities 59
event-related potentials
chemosensory see chemosensory event-related potentials
olfactory 64, 211, 221, 223
trigeminal 65, 72, 142–143, 211
see also evoked potentials
evoked potentials, gustatory 69, 70, 173, 215
see also event-related potentials
examination (of patient) 50–54
expert opinion
gustation 215
olfaction 210–211
expert opinion 207–218
gustatory disorders 214–216
olfactory disorders 208–213

F
facial injury see post-traumatic disorders
facial nerve (VIIth cranial nerve) 2, 68, 139, 153, 154, 156, 191, 204
branches see chorda tympani; petrosal nerve, greater
facial palsy 182
familial parkinsonism 129
fat suppression in MRI, 197
FDG-PET/CT 199
fetal (prenatal) development
chemosensory function 116
vomeronasal system 39–42
field strength (MRI) 195–196
filter paper disc method 70, **170**, 170–171
flavor (and its perception) 219–228
factors contributing to 3, 219–220
fluid dynamics, computational 16
fluorodeoxyglucose (F-18)-PET/CT 199

FN model 15–16
foliate papillae 151, 152, 154, 168, 172
food education 101
formaldehyde 106
fractures, craniomaxillofacial see post-traumatic disorders
Friedreich ataxia 133
frontal lobe contusions 94, 95
functional anatomy see anatomy
functional neuroimaging
flavor perception 221
gustatory stimuli and structures 70, 161, 162, **163**, 165, 173, 221, 222
olfactory stimuli and structures 21, 65, 221
amygdala 34
insula 34
non-specific olfactory brain regions 35
piriform cortex 33
visual perception and 223–224
fungiform papillae 151, 152, 168, 174, 189, 190

G
G-protein coupled receptors
gustatory 152, 153
olfactory 21, 22
GABAergic periglomerular cells 31
gabapentin in burning mouth syndrome 191
gases, toxic/irritant 106, **208**
Gasserian ganglion 138
imaging 202, 203
gemmae see taste buds
German Task Force recommendations on olfactory disorders 213
Germany, expert opinion on olfactory disorders 211–212
ginkgo biloba 100
glomeruli, olfactory 31
glossopharyngeal nerve (GLN; IXth cranial nerve) 2, 68, 154, 155, 156, 159
lingual branch see lingual

nerve
goblet cell hyperplasia 84
gonadotrophin-releasing hormone (GnRH) and the vomeronasal system 39–42
granular cells 31
gustatory cortex 158–165
humans 161–165
lesions 183
non-human primates 158–160
gustatory evoked potentials/event-related potentials *69*, 70, 173, 215
gustatory sensation see taste
gustatory system 150–167
functional anatomy 150–165
central 155–165
peripheral 150–155, 181
olfactory system interactions with 221–223

H
habituation 36
head injury see post-traumatic disorders
health
impact of ambient odorants 6
nasal trigeminal function affected by 143–144
hemorrhage, brain 94
herpes zoster
ophthalmicus 145
higher order gustatory cortices
humans 165
primates 159–160
hippocampus 28
histamine antagonists, chronic rhinosinusitis 85
history taking
gustation 50, 168–169, 180, 214–215
olfaction 50, 209–210
HLAs and pheromones 43
horizontal basal cells 19–20
human lymphocyte antigens and pheromones 43
humidification 13
Huntington disease 132
hypergeusia, definition 1, 68, **180**

hypogeusia, definition 1, 68, **180**
hyposmia
  definition 1
  postinfectious,
    treatment 97–100
  trigeminal system and 225
hypothalamus 28, 33
  sexual behavior and 32, 42, 43

I

iatrogenic damage see surgery
image acquisition see data
  acquisition
imaging (incl.
  neuroimaging) 195–206
  functional see functional
    neuroimaging
  postinfectious or
    post-traumatic olfactory
    disorders 96
  structural
    gustatory 204–205
    olfactory 199–202
  in vivo, gustatory
    structures 174
  see also specific imaging
    modalities
immune system and allergic
  rhinitis 81
immunotherapy, allergic
  rhinitis 82
imposed mucosal activity
  patterns 13–15
industrial chemicals 106–107, 144
  gustatory disorders 184
  olfactory disorders 106–107
  see also occupational
    disorders; toxicants
infant chemosensory
  function 117–118
  evaluation 119–120
  importance 118–119
  premature infant 116
  see also newborns
infection, rhinitis caused by **77**
  see also postinfectious
    disorders
  inflammatory causes of

rhinitis **77**
inflammatory phase of acute
  viral rhinitis 79–80
inherent mucosal activity
  patterns 13–15
injury, disorders following see
  post-traumatic disorders;
  surgery
innervation see nerve supply
inorganic compounds
  metallic **107, 208**
  non-metallic **107**
insula 28, 34, 162, 173, 192, 221, 222
intermediate nerve of Wrisberg
  (IMN) 153–154, 156, 156
intracranial tumors 110, **111**, 135
  skull base 113, 200
intranasal drug-induced
  olfactory dysfunction **108**
intranasal trigeminal system see
  trigeminal nerve/system
intranasal tumors (extracranial) 110, **111**
intravenous odorant tests 63
irritant (toxic) gases 106, **208**
ischemic lesions 135

K

Kallmann syndrome 42, 109

L

lamina propria 17–18
lateralization
  gustatory 165
  olfactory 27, 36
    trigeminal system test-
    ing 71, 123, 141–142
leukotriene receptor
  antagonists 82
  chronic rhinosinusitis with
    polyps 85
Lewy body 128
Lewy body disease/
  dementia 129
"lie detector test" 65
light cells 150
lingual nerve (branch of
  glossopharyngeal nerve) 152, 153, 159

damage 182
α-lipoic acid, postinfectious
  hyposmia 97–98
liquid solutions **170**, 171
local/regional/spatial taste
  tests 69–70
  burning mouth
    syndrome 170–171
  children 124
Lund–Mackay scores 78

M

magnetic resonance imaging
  (MRI) 195–198
  functional
    gustation 70, 161, 162, **163**, 165, 173, 221, 222
    olfaction 65, 221
  structural 195–198
    congenital olfactory
      disorders 55, 200
    gustatory 204–205
    postinfectious or
      post-traumatic olfactory
      disorders 96
    technical
      considerations 195–198
    trigeminal system 202, 203
    visual perception
      and 223–224
  tumors 110, *111, 112*
magnetoencephalography
  (MEG), gustation 161, 162, **163**
malignant tumors **111**
  see also antineoplastic
    drug-induced dysfunction
mandibular nerve 138
manufacturing processes **107**
mast cells and burning mouth
  syndrome 190
Match-to-Sample Odor
  Identification test (MTST) 121
maxillary nerve 138
maxillofacial injury see
  post-traumatic disorders
mechanoreceptors,
  trigeminal 141
medioposterior nucleus of
  thalamus 35
meningioma *112*, 135, 200, 226

menthol 144
metallic compounds **107**, **208**
metallurgical processes **107**
microvilli, taste bud 150
microvillous cells 19
migraine 135, 144
mitral (tufted) cells 27, 28, 31, 32, 35, 36
molecules, odorant *see* odorant
monosodium glutamate use 101
morphological changes in peripheral taste structures, assessment 70
motor neuron disease 133
mouth *see* burning mouth syndrome; local/regional/ spatial taste tests; taste; whole-mouth taste tests
mucosa
  olfactory/nasal respiratory biopsy 20, 22, 67
    imaging 199, 200
    imposed and inherent activity patterns 13–15
    trigeminal system and 139, 143
mucosal potentials (peripheral) 65
  negative 143
mucus, nasal, partitioning of odorant molecules in 13
multiple sclerosis 134, 183
multiple system atrophy (MSA) 128–129
muscle relaxant-induced olfactory dysfunction **108**

N
nasal cavity
  chemoreception *see* olfaction
  functional anatomy 10–23
  mucosa *see* mucosa
  polyps *see* polyps
  reflex airflow obstruction 139
  surgery, olfactory dysfunction following 112, **113**
  see also entries under intranasal
nasal cycle 11

nasal dilators 16
nasal fractures 93, 96
nasal hyper-reactivity and challenge tests 145
nasal response to airborne particles 144
nasal secretory reflexes 139
nasoincisor duct 157
nasopalatine duct, persistent, vomeronasal duct orifice misinterpreted as 46
negative alliesthesia 119
negative mucosal potentials 143
neocortical areas, olfactory 28, 33, 35
neonates *see* newborns
neoplasms *see* antineoplastic drug-induced dysfunction; tumors
nerve supply (gustation) 153–154
  electrogustometry in assessment of *see* electrogustometry
  lesions 182–183
  taste papillae 152
neuralgia, trigeminal 144
neurodegenerative disease
  gustatory 183
  olfactory disorders 102, 126–134
neuroepithelium
  olfactory 17, 20, 22
    biopsy 22
    in postinfectious olfactory disorders 92
    toxicant agent exposure 106, 107
  vomeronasal, degeneration 42
neurological diseases
  degenerative *see* neurodegenerative disease
  gustatory disorders 183
  imaging 203
  olfactory disorders 126–147
    non-degenerative 134–135
neurological drug-induced taste disorders **185**
neuropathies (sensorineural/

cranial nerve)
  burning mouth syndrome and 189–190
  gustation 182–183
  olfaction (SNODs)
    postinfectious disorders as 92, 97
    treatment 97–98, 99–100
neurophysiological
  function 17–23
  tests *see* electrophysiological tests
newborns, chemosensation/ chemoreception 116–117
  evaluation 119
nose *see entries under* nasal
nucleus accumbens 28, 32, 203
nucleus dorsomedialis thalamus 28
nucleus medialis posterior thalami (medioposterior thalamic nucleus) 35
nucleus olfactorius anterior *see* olfactory nucleus, anterior
nucleus tractus solitarius (solitary tract nucleus; NTS) 153, 154, 155–157
nucleus ventralis posteromedialis (VPM) 156, 157–158
NVT model 15

O
objective tests, taste 173–174, 215
occupational (work-related) disorders 107
  expert opinion 207, 208, 209, 210, 211, 212
    case study 217–218
    German Task Force recommendations 213
    Germany 211
    gustatory 214, 216
    olfactory 208, 209, 210, 211, 212
  see also industrial chemicals; toxicants
odorants
  ambient, impact on behavior and health 6
  behavior influenced by *see*

behavior
detection *see* olfaction
molecules
  olfactory response and
    number of 15
  partitioning in nasal
    mucus 13
  panic attacks triggered
    by 146
  task-specific odor
    processing 35–36
older people *see* age-related loss
olfaction (smell; odor detection; nasal chemoreception)
  assessment 49, 49–50, 50,
    53–54, 58–68
    newborns/infants 119–120
    rationale 58
    school-age
      children 120–123
  development
    fetal/premature infant 116
    infants and
      children 117–118
    neonatal 116
  disorders/dysfunction (basic/
    major refs only)
    in acute rhinitis/
      rhinosinusitis 80
    in allergic rhinitis 82
    diagnosis 49, 49–50, 50,
      53–54
    expert opinion 208–213
    idiopathic 108–109, 114
    miscellaneous
      causes 106–115
    neurological *see* neurologi-
      cal diseases
    postinfectious *see* postin-
      fectious (postviral upper
      respiratory tract infection)
      disorders
    post-traumatic *see*
      post-traumatic disorders
    qualitative 53–54, **68**, 92,
      97, 191–192
    quantitative *see* loss
      (*subheading below*)
  endonasal regions influencing
    performance *80*

flavor and 223–224
history taking 50, 209–210
imaging *see* imaging
loss (quantitative disorders)
  age-related 1, 3–4, 102–103
  epidemiology *see*
    epidemiology
  orthonasal vs. retronasal
    perception and 223
  QoL impact 5–6
  quantification 53–54
  orthonasal *see* orthonasal
    olfaction
  retronasal *see* retronasal
    olfaction
  role 1
  see also entries under
    olfactory
Olfactology and Gustology Task
  Force of the German Society of
  Otolaryngology 213
olfactory bulb 22, 27, 29–31,
  200–201
  absence/aplasia 109–110
  contralateral information
    and 32
  contusions 94
  imaging 195, 199, 200–201
  intracranial tumors
    affecting 110
  mitral/tufted cells 27, 28, 31,
    32, 35, 36
  Parkinson's disease and 128,
    131
  parosmia and 92
  specialness in humans 31
  tumors 200
  volume
    assessment 65–67
    blind subjects 223
    modification/plas-
      ticity 65–67, 200–201
olfactory cleft
  syndrome 113–114
olfactory cortex 27, 28, 32
  primary 27, 199, 202
  secondary and tertiary 27,
    202
olfactory epithelium (OE) 13,
  17–20
  biopsies 20, 22, 67

  see also mucosa
  vomeronasal receptors 44–45
olfactory event-related potentials 64, 211, 221, 223
olfactory fila 27, 28
  stretched or torn 209
olfactory intolerance 54
olfactory lateralization 27, 36
olfactory marker protein
  (OMP) 19, 39
olfactory nerve (1st cranial) 28
  imaging 199, 200
olfactory neuroepithelium *see*
  neuroepithelium
olfactory nucleus, anterior 27,
  28, 31, 32
  Parkinson Disease and 128
olfactory peduncle 32
olfactory receptor(s) (ORs;
  odorant receptors) 10, 21
  steroid-derived odors 46
olfactory receptor neurons
  (ORNs) 13, 17, 18–19, 21, 27
  convergence in olfactory
    bulb 31
  parosmia and phantosmia
    and 192
  vomeronasal system and 44
olfactory system
  dual *see* orthonasal olfaction;
    retronasal olfaction
  flavor and 223–224
  functional anatomy
    central pathways/
      events 27–38
    peripheral pathways/
      events 10–26, 39–42
  gustatory system interactions
    with 221–223
  subset vs. main 45–46
  trigeminal system relation-
    ship with 143, 224–226
olfactory tests (smell tests) 53,
  59–62
  expert opinion 210–211
    case study of post-traumatic
      anosmia 216
olfactory tract 27
  absence 109, 110
  imaging 195, 199
  intracranial tumors

affecting 110
lateral 27
medial 29
operculum
orbitofrontal (OFO) 159, 162
Rolandic 161, 162, 222
ophthalmic nerve 138
oral cavity/mouth
chemoreception see taste
taste tests see local/regional/
spatial taste tests; whole-
mouth taste tests
see also burning mouth
syndrome
orbitofrontal cortex 34, 165
gustatory–olfactory interactions 221, 222
visual–olfactory and flavor
interactions 223, 224
orbitofrontal gyri 28, 34
orbitofrontal operculum
(OFO) 159, 162
organic compounds **107**
solvents 106, **208**, 217
orthonasal olfaction 219–223
clinical implications 223
psychophysical
assessment 59–63

P
paint solvent 106
palate 150, 157, 172
soft 151, 152, 157, 168
panic attacks,
odor-triggered 146
papillae, taste see taste papillae
parageusia, definition 1, 68,
180
paranasal sinus pathology see
sinonasal pathology
parkinsonian syndromes (incl.
Parkinson's disease) 126–132
case study 133–134
gustatory disorders 183
olfactory disorders 126–132,
133–134
parosmia 54, 101, 192
evaluation 67–68
expert opinion in Austria 212
investigations 97
pathophysiology 92
postinfectious 92, 95, 97

post-traumatic (PTA) 92–93,
96, 97
treatment 101
parvicellular part of ventral
posteromedial nucleus 156,
157–158
pathological loss of smell,
definition 1
pediatric
chemosensation 116–126
pentoxifylline, postinfectious
hyposmia 98–99
perforated substance, anterior 32, 35
periamygdaloid cortex/com-
plex 27, 33
periglomerular cells 31
peripheral gustatory system
disorders 180, 182–183
functional anatomy 150–155,
181
peripheral mucosal potentials
see mucosal potentials
petrosal nerve, greater/superfi-
cial (SGP) 152, 153–154, 155,
171, 172
testing 176
phantageusia 180
definition 1, 68, **180**
phantosmia 54, 192
evaluation 67–68
Parkinson's disease 128
phenylethyl alcohol (PEA) odor
detection
olfactory ERPs elicited by 64,
64
tests 60, 62, 100
pheromones 39, 42–44
piriform cortex 27, 33
adaptation and 36
habituation and 36
Pocket-Smell-Test 59
polyneuropathy, taste
disorders 182
polyps, nasal
chronic rhinosinusitis with
(CRSwNP), distinction
from without polyps
(CRSsNP) 84
computed tomography 88
medical treatment 85–86
surgical treatment 87

positron emission tomography
(PET), gustation 161, 162
positron emission tomography/
CT (PET/CT) 199
postinfectious (postviral upper
respiratory tract infection)
disorders
gustation 168–169, 184–185
olfaction 2, 76
anosmia 67, 211
clinical findings 95–96
diagnosis 55
etiology/prevalence/
pathophysiology 91–92
history taking 209
investigations 96–97
prognosis 101
treatment 97–100
post-traumatic disorders
(following head/skull/
craniomaxillofacial injury or
fracture)
gustatory 174–176
olfactory 92–94, 96
biopsies 67
case study 216
clinical findings 96
diagnosis 55
etiology/prevalence/
pathophysiology 92–94
expert opinion 209, 212
investigations 96–97
prognosis 101–102
treatment 100
pregabalin in burning mouth
syndrome 191
premature infant, chemosensory function 116
prenatal development see fetal
development
primary gustatory cortex
(PGA) 158
human 161–165
primates
(non-human) 158–159
primates (non-human),
gustatory cortex 158–160
primitive neuroectodermal
tumors 200, **201**
progressive supranuclear palsy
(PSP) 128–129

projection radiography 199
pseudosmia 54
pseudotumors, rhinitis caused by **77**
psychiatric diseases 135
psychiatric drug-induced taste disorders **185**
psychogalvanic skin reaction 65
psychological impact of ambient odorants 6
psychophysical (subjective) assessment
  gustation, children 123–124
  olfaction 58
    children 121–123
    orthonasal olfaction 59–63
    postinfectious or post-traumatic disorders 97
    retronasal olfaction 63–64
    trigeminal system 141–142
puberty 118
public health, impact of smells 6
pupillary reflexes 65

Q
qualitative smell/olfaction assessment/diagnosis 67–68, 97
  children 122–123
  disorders 53–54, 92, 97, 192
  expert opinion 212
qualitative taste disorders **68**, 180, 191–192
quality of life (QoL) 1
  smell loss 5–6
  taste loss 6
quantitative disorders *see* olfaction, loss; taste, loss
quantitative tests
  smell 64, 210–211
  taste 50, 170, 171, 215

R
radiation dose exposure (CT) 198–199
radiography (projection/plain film) 199
reactive upper airways dysfunction syndrome 145
receiver coils (MRI) 196

reflexes and trigeminal system 139
  reflex rhinorrhea 139, 145
regional taste tests *see* local/regional/spatial taste tests
respiratory changes after olfactory stimulation 65
respiratory syndromes triggered by olfactory pr trigeminal stimulation 145
respiratory tract/airways, upper reactive upper airways dysfunction syndrome 145
  reflexes 139
  viral infection *see* postinfectious disorders
retronasal olfaction 3, 219–223
  assessment 64–65
    children 121–122
    expert opinion 211
  clinical implications 223
rhinorrhea, reflex 139, 145
rhinoscopy, anterior 53
rhinosinusitis (rhinitis and/or sinusitis) 76–88
  acute (ARS) 76
    bacterial 78–81
    recurrent 76
    viral (common cold) 78–81, 91
  allergic *see* allergy
  atrophic 77, 83
  chronic (CRS) 76, 84–87
    computed tomography 78, 88
  definition 76–78
  differential diagnosis **77**
  epidemiology 76–78
  idiopathic/noninfectious/nonallergic/vasomotor 145
Rolandic operculum 161, 162, 222

S
salivation disorders 214
saltiness 150
  gustatory cortex, primate 159
  nerve fibers 154
  receptors 152
San Diego Odor Identification

test (SDOIT) 121
schizophrenia 135
school-age children, chemosensory function
  measurement 120
  puberty and 118
screening tests
  gustation 50
  olfaction 50, 59
self-assessment of olfactory function 49
senses *see* chemical senses
sensorineural neuropathies *see* neuropathies
septal nuclei 28
septum, nasal 10
  traumatic deviation *93*
sequence techniques (MRI) 196
sex steroids/hormones, vomeronasal 45
sexual behavior, olfactory cues 32–33
  GnRH and 42
  pheromones and 42, 43
  vomeronasal system and 42, 43, 45
sick building syndrome 144
signal transduction pathways
  gustatory 153
  olfactory 20–21, 46
sinonasal pathology 76–90
  differentiation 54–55, 55
  endoscopic surgery *see* endoscopic sinonasal surgery
  examination/assessment for 53, 54–55
    biopsy 56
  steroid therapy 55, 85, 86, 87
  see also rhinosinusitis
Sjögren syndrome 189–190
skull base tumors 113, 200
skull injury *see* post-traumatic disorders
smell *see* olfaction
sneezing 139
Sniff Magnitude test (SMT) 121
sniff variables and olfactory response 15
Sniffin' Sticks test 53, 60–62
  children 121, 122
  expert opinion 210
  in postinfectious or

post-traumatic disorders 97
screening 59
TDI score *see* Threshold
+ Discrimination +
Identification score
sodium channels, epithelial
(ENACs) 152, 153
sodium citrate, postinfectious
disorders as 99
soft palate 151, 152, 157, 168
solitary chemoreceptor cells
(SCCs) 19, 141
solitary tract nucleus
(NTS) 153, 154, 155–157
solvents 106, **208**, 217
somatic functions, trigeminal
system 139
somatosensory perception of
taste 222
testing 173
sourness 150
gustatory cortex,
primate 159
nerve fibers 154
receptors 152, 153
spatial taste tests *see* local/
regional/spatial taste tests
spinocerebellar ataxias (SCA)
type 2 and 3, 133
squamous metaplasia 84–85
steroids
endogenous
olfactory receptors 36
vomeronasal 45
exogenous administration *see*
corticosteroids
stria terminalis, bed nuclei
of 28
striatum, ventral 28, 32
stroke, taste disorders 193
subjective assessment *see*
psychophysical assessment
supporting cells
olfactory epithelium 19
taste buds 150
supralaryngeal nerve 152, 154,
155
surgery
chronic rhinosinusitis 86–87
endoscopic sinonasal *see*
endoscopy
iatrogenic damage

gustation 168, 214–215
olfaction 112–113, 114
sustentacular cells (olfactory
epithelium) 19
sweetness 150
gustatory cortex
(primate) 159
nerve fibers 154, 155
receptors 152
transduction 153
Switzerland, expert opinion on
olfactory disorders 212
Sydney Children's Hospital
Gustatory Test 123
Sydney Children's Hospital Odor
Identification Test 120–121
systemic diseases
acute rhinosinusitis associated with 76
burning mouth syndrome
associated with 189
endocrinological 109, 114
gustatory dysfunction 50,
169, 184

T
T&T Test 62
T1- vs. T2-weighted MRI, 196
task-specific odor
processing 35–36
taste (gustation; oral
chemoreception)
assessment 49, 50, 53, 68–71,
168–178
newborns/infants 119, 120
school-age
children 123–124
see also taste tests
development
fetal/premature infant 116
neonatal 117
older children 118
disorders (basic/major refs
only) 179–188
case reports 174–176
clinical findings 179
definition/types/classifica-
tion 68, 180
diagnosis 49, 50, 53, 185
etiology 181, 182
expert opinion 214–216

idiopathic 184–185
pathophysiology 182
qualitative **68**, 180,
191–192
quantitative *see* loss
(*subheading below*)
therapy 185–186
five basic types 150
functional anatomy 150–167
history taking 50, 168–169,
180, 214–215
imaging 173–174, 204–205
loss (quantitative disor-
ders) **68**, 169, 180
age-related 1, 4–5
epidemiology 2–3
QoL impact 6
role 1
simultaneous odor percep-
tion enhancing intensity
of 222–223
see also entries under
gustatory
taste agnosia **180**, 180
taste buds (gemmae) 150–151,
152
total number 151
in vivo imaging 174
taste papillae 151–152
circumvallate 151, 152, 154,
172, 191
foliate 151, 152, 154, 168,
172
fungiform 151, 152, 168, 174,
189, 190
innervation 152
taste powders 63–64
taste receptors/receptors
cells 152–153
taste sprays 68
taste strips **69**, *69*, 70, 170
taste tests 53, 68–70, 168–178
expert opinion 215
objective 173–174, 215
psychophysical *see* psychophysical assessment
with qualitative
disorders 191
tasting tablets and wafers 170
temperature dependence,
taste 153

temporal lobe
  contusions 94, 96
  epilepsy 134
thalamus 35, 157–158
  gustation and the 156,
    157–158
    disorders of 183
  nuclei of
    dorsomedial 28
    medioposterior 35
    ventral posteromedial
      (VPM) 156, 157–158
  olfaction and the 28, 35
theophylline, postinfectious
  hyposmia 99
three drops test 68, 169–170
Threshold + Discrimination
  + Identification (TDI)
  score 60–62, 221
  Parkinson's disease 129
  school-age children 121
thyroid drugs see antithyroid
  drugs
tic douloureux 144
tongue (taste areas/function/
  neurons etc.) 150–151, 157
  regional taste function 70
    children 124
topical intranasal drug-induced
  olfactory dysfunction **108**
toxicants 106–107, 144
  diagnosis of disorders caused
    by 55
  gustatory disorders 184
    expert opinion 214
  olfactory disorders 55,
    106–107
    expert opinion 207–208,
      209–210
  see also industrial chemicals;
    occupational disorders
transient receptor potential
  receptors (TRPs) 141
  TRPM5, 19, 46, 141, 153
  vomeronasal organ and 44
trauma, disorders following
  see post-traumatic disorders;
  surgery
tricyclic antidepressants in
  burning mouth syndrome 191
trigeminal nerve/system

(intranasal) 138–148
  assessment/investiga-
    tion 71–72, 141–143
  children 123
  imaging 143, 202–203
  chemical stimulus
    responses 45, 141
  demographic and health
    conditions affecting
    function 143–144
  disorders (neuropathies) 182
    endogenous 144
    exogenous 145–146
  event-related potentials 65,
    72, 142–143, 211
  functional anatomy 138–139
  olfactory system relationship
    with 143, 224–226
  physical stimulus
    responses 141
  somatic and autonomic
    functions 139
trigeminal neuralgia 144
TRP receptors see transient
  receptor potential receptors
tufted (mitral) cells 27, 28, 31,
  32, 35, 36
tumors (neoplasms), 110, **111**,
  111, *112*, 114, 135
  intracranial see intracranial
    tumors
  rhinitis caused by **77**
  trigeminal system 203
  see also antineoplastic
    drug-induced dysfunction
turbo inversion recovery magnitude (TIRM) 197
  gustatory imaging 204–205
  trigeminal imaging 202

U
ultrasound 199
umami substances 150
  gustatory cortex,
    primate 159
  nerve fibers 154–155
  receptors 152, 153
  transduction 153
United States of America,
  expert opinion on olfactory
  disorders 213

University of Pennsylvania
  Smell Identification Test
  (UPSIT) 59, 60, 210–211
USA, expert opinion on
  olfactory disorders 213

V
vagus nerve (VN; Xth cranial
  nerve) 2, 68, 154, 156, 204
  clinical perspectives 223
  stimulation tests 223
  supralaryngeal branch 152,
    154, 155
vasomotor rhinitis 145
ventral posteromedial nucleus
  (VPM) 156, 157–158
ventral striatum 28, 32
viral upper respiratory tract
  infection
  olfactory disorders following
    see postinfectious disorders
  see also common cold
vision and olfaction and
  flavor 223–224
vocal cord dysfunction
  (VCD) 145–146, 146
volatile compounds 106
  inability to detect specific
    ones 2
volumetric assessment of
  olfactory bulb 65–67
vomeronasal receptors 44, 45
vomeronasal system (organ and
  duct) 39–48
  humans 39–48
    damage 46
  non-human animals 39

W
whole-mouth taste tests 68–69,
  169–170
  children 123
wink reflexes 65
work-related disorders see
  occupational disorders
Wrisberg's intermediate nerve
  (IMN) 153–154, 156, 156

Z

zafirlukast, chronic rhinosinusitis with polyps 85–86
zileuton, chronic rhinosinusitis with polyps 85–86

zinc
  in burning mouth syndrome
    deficiency as cause 190
    therapeutic use 191
  in postinfectious
    hyposmia 97
  in taste disorders 185–186
Zürcher Riechtest 59